The Washington Manual™ Pediatrics Survival Guide

Faculty Advisor

Andrew White, M.D.

Assistant Professor of Pediatrics
Department of Pediatrics
Washington University School of Medicine
St. Louis Children's Hospital
St. Louis, Missouri

The Washington Manual™ Pediatrics Survival Guide

Editors

Ana Maria Arbelaez, M.D.

Pediatric Endocrine Fellow
Department of Pediatrics
Washington University School of Medicine
St. Louis Children's Hospital
St. Louis, Missouri

Tami Hutton Garmany, M.D.

Pediatrics Resident
Washington University School of Medicine
St. Louis Children's Hospital
St. Louis, Missouri

Series Editor

Tammy L. Lin, M.D.

Adjunct Assistant Professor of Medicine
Washington University School of Medicine
St. Louis, Missouri

Series Advisor

Daniel M. Goodenberger, M.D.

Professor of Medicine
Chief, Division of Medical Education
Washington University School of Medicine
Director, Internal Medicine Residency Program
Barnes-Jewish Hospital
St. Louis, Missouri

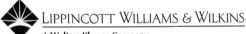

LIPPINCOTT WILLIAMS & WILKINS
A **Wolters Kluwer** Company
Philadelphia · Baltimore · New York · London
Buenos Aires · Hong Kong · Sydney · Tokyo

Acquisitions Editors: Danette Somers and James Ryan
Developmental Editors: Scott Marinaro and Keith Donnellan
Supervising Editor: Mary Ann McLaughlin
Production Editor: Amanda Waltman Yanovitch, Silverchair Science +
Communications
Manufacturing Manager: Colin Warnock
Cover Designer: QT Design
Compositor: Silverchair Science + Communications
Printer: Victor Graphics

Library of Congress Cataloging-in-Publication Data

Arbelaez, Ana Maria.
   The Washington manual pediatrics survival guide / Ana Maria Arbelaez, Tami Hutton Garmany.
       p. ; cm. -- (Washington manual survival guide series)
   Includes bibliographical references and index.
   ISBN 0-7817-4366-4
   1. Pediatrics--Handbooks, manuals, etc. I. Title: Manual pediatrics survival guide. II. Garmany, Tami Hutton. III. Title. IV. Series.
   [DNLM: 1. Pediatrics--Handbooks. WS 39 A664w 2003]
   RJ48.A73 2003
   618.92--dc21

                                                              2003047620

The Washington Manual™ is an intent-to-use mark belonging to Washington University in St. Louis to which international legal protection applies. The mark is used in this publication by LWW under license from Washington University.

Care has been taken to confirm the accuracy of the information presented and to describe generally accepted practices. However, the authors, editors, and publisher are not responsible for errors or omissions or for any consequences from application of the information in this book and make no warranty, expressed or implied, with respect to the currency, completeness, or accuracy of the contents of the publication. Application of this information in a particular situation remains the professional responsibility of the practitioner.

The authors, editors, and publisher have exerted every effort to ensure that drug selection and dosage set forth in this text are in accordance with current recommendations and practice at the time of publication. However, in view of ongoing research, changes in government regulations, and the constant flow of information relating to drug therapy and drug reactions, the reader is urged to check the package insert for each drug for any change in indications and dosage and for added warnings and precautions. This is particularly important when the recommended agent is a new or infrequently employed drug.

Some drugs and medical devices presented in this publication have Food and Drug Administration (FDA) clearance for limited use in restricted research settings. It is the responsibility of health care providers to ascertain the FDA status of each drug or device planned for use in their clinical practice.

10 9 8 7 6 5 4 3 2 1

Contents

CONTENTS

Contributing Authors

Ana Maria Arbelaez, M.D.
Pediatric Endocrine Fellow
Department of Pediatrics
Washington University School of
  Medicine
St. Louis Children's Hospital
St. Louis, Missouri
*Survival in Pediatrics, Admission
  and Event Notes, Admission
  Orders and Writing Prescrip-
  tions, Adolescent Medicine,
  Dermatology, Emergencies,
  Endocrinology, Orthopedics,
  Pulmonary, Rheumatology*

Sangita Basnet, M.D.
Pediatric Critical Care Fellow
Washington University School of
  Medicine
St. Louis Children's Hospital
St. Louis, Missouri
Critical Care

Tami Hutton Garmany, M.D.
Pediatrics Resident
Washington University School of
  Medicine
St. Louis Children's Hospital
St. Louis, Missouri
*How to Calculate IV Fluids and
  Feeds, Calculating Total
  Parenteral Nutrition, Ten Most
  Common Floor Calls, Cardiol-
  ogy, Emergencies, Gastroenterol-
  ogy, Growth and Development,
  Infectious Disease, Newborn
  Medicine, Procedures, Formulary*

**William J. Grossman, M.D.,
  Ph.D.**
Hematology/Oncology Fellow
Department of Pediatrics
St. Louis Children's Hospital
St. Louis, Missouri
Hematology-Oncology

**Christina Ann Gurnett, M.D.,
  Ph.D.**
Pediatric Neurology Fellow
Department of Neurology
Washington University School of
  Medicine
St. Louis Children's Hospital
St. Louis, Missouri
Neurology

Stephanie Hsieh, M.D.
Nephrology Fellow
Department of Nephrology
Children's Hospital and Regional
  Medical Center
Seattle, Washington
Nephrology

Joseph V. Philip, M.D.
Neuroradiology Fellow
Department of Neuroradiology
Massachusetts General Hospital
Boston, Massachusetts
Radiology

Shailaja M. Philip, M.D.
General Pediatric Attending
Department of Pediatric Health
The Children's Hospital
Boston, Massachusetts
Radiology

Shulamit Portnoy, M.D.
Pediatric Neurology Fellow
Department of Pediatric Neurology
Washington University School of
  Medicine
St. Louis Children's Hospital
St. Louis, Missouri
Neurology

Chairman's Note

Medical knowledge is increasing at an exponential rate, and physicians are being bombarded with new facts at a pace that many find overwhelming. The Washington Manual™ Survival Guides were developed in this context for interns, residents, medical students, and other practitioners in need of readily accessible practical clinical information. They therefore meet an important need in an era of information overload.

I would like to acknowledge the authors who have contributed to these books. In particular, Tammy L. Lin, M.D., Series Editor, provided energetic and inspired leadership, and Daniel M. Goodenberger, M.D., Series Advisor, Chief of the Division of Medical Education in the Department of Medicine at Washington University, is a continual source of sage advice. The efforts and outstanding skill of the lead authors are evident in the quality of the final product. I am confident that this series will meet its desired goal of providing practical knowledge that can be directly applied to improving patient care.

Kenneth S. Polonsky, M.D.
Adolphus Busch Professor
Chairman, Department of Medicine
Washington University School of Medicine
St. Louis, Missouri

Series Preface

The Washington Manual™ Survival Guides, a multispecialty series, is designed to provide interns, residents, medical students, or anyone on the front lines of clinical care with quick, practical, essential information in an accessible format. It lets you hit the ground running as you learn the basics of practicing clinical medicine, gain more responsibility, and become a valued team member. Although written individually, they all incorporate series features. Each book takes care to give you an insider's view of how to get things done efficiently and effectively, tips on how to "survive" training, and pearls you will want to pass on in the future. It is similar to receiving a great sign-out from your favorite resident. When faced with an unfamiliar situation, we envision getting timely information and guidance from the survival guide (like you would from your resident) to make appropriate decisions at 3:00 p.m. or 3:00 a.m.

One of the most unique and notable features of this new series is that it was truly a joint effort across subspecialties at Washington University. We were fortunate to have significant departmental support, particularly from Kenneth Polonsky, M.D., whose commitment made this series possible. Every survival guide has the credibility of being written by recent interns, residents, or chief residents in that specialty with input from faculty advisors. We were fortunate to have found outstanding lead authors who were not only highly regarded clinicians and teachers, but who also provided significant leadership and collaborated well together. Their incredible enthusiasm and desire to pass on their hard-earned knowledge, experiences, and wisdom clearly shine through in the series.

Anyone who has been through training will tell you the hours are long, the work is hard, and your energy is limited. With either a print or electronic version of a survival guide by your side, we hope you will work more efficiently, make decisions with more confidence, stay out of trouble, and get that ever-elusive good night's rest.

Tammy L. Lin, M.D., Series Editor
Daniel M. Goodenberger, M.D., Series Advisor

Preface

This book is a conglomeration of the cards, charts, graphs, and cheat sheets we carry around in our pockets. We put them together and added other things that we know are useful to produce a reference that will help get medical students and residents through their next call night or emergency room shift. The information is presented in easy-to-read tables, outlines, and pictures so that you may spend your time taking care of patients, not searching for references. We added chapters on adolescent medicine, rheumatology, and orthopedics that are not often found in pediatric pocket references. An easy-to-use formulary that includes NICU dosing, pain management, and sedation medications can be found in the back of the book. Our goal was to present information as clearly and succinctly as possible so that those taking care of patients will have more time to do just that—take care of patients. Medical science has become so complex that figuring out how to diagnose and treat patients has become ever more challenging, and the proportion of time spent with patients and their families has decreased. The best way to learn pediatrics is to observe children, listen to their stories and the stories of their parents, and examine the children closely and often. This book is meant to be a guide for what to consider in terms of diagnosis and treatment when hearing those stories as well as what to anticipate over the course of a child's illness. Use it in your evaluations of children, in writing their orders, and in considering their diagnostic and therapeutic management. May you have as much fun with your patients and with your role as a pediatrician as we do.

T.H.G.
A.M.A.

"[Y]ou bring me the deepest happiness which a man can experience who believes implicitly that science and peace will triumph over ignorance and war, that people will learn to agree together, not for purposes of destruction but for improvement, and that the future will belong to those who shall have done the most for suffering humanity.

...Young people, young people, confine yourselves to those methods, sure and powerful, of which we as yet know the secrets. And all however noble your career, never permit yourselves to be overcome by scepticism, both unworthy and barren; neither permit hours of sadness which pass over a nation and discourage you. Live in the serene peace of your laboratories and your libraries. First ask yourselves, What have

I done for my education? Then, as you advance in life, What have I done for my country? So that day the supreme happiness may come to you, the consciousness of having contributed in some manner to the progress and welfare of humanity."

—An extract from Louis Pasteur's address
at the celebration of his seventieth birthday

Acknowledgments

The authors thank the following individuals for their assistance in reviewing the manuscript:

Adolescent Medicine: Lynn White, M.D.
Cardiology: Delwin McOmber, M.D., Mark Johnson, M.D.
Critical Care: John McGuire, M.D.
Dermatology: Susan Mallory, M.D.
Emergency Medicine: Mark Hostetler, M.D., Katherine Gnauck, M.D.
Endocrinology: Abby Hollander, M.D.
Gastroenterology: Jack An, M.D.
Hematology-Oncology: David Wilson, M.D., Ph.D.
Infectious Disease: David Hunstad, M.D.
Nephrology: Paul Hmiel, M.D., Ann M. Beck, M.D.
Neurology: Edwin Trevathan, M.D.
Pulmonary: Leonard Bacharier, M.D., St. Louis Children's Hospital AIMES nurses.
Pain Management (Appendix B): Pain Service, St. Louis Children's Hospital.
Radiology: William McAllister, M.D.

The authors extend special thanks to Rick Garmany, M.D., Carlos Bernal, M.D., Kristina Kloos, Pharm.D., Christy Gilcrease, M.S., R.D., Anne Borgemeyer, P.N.P., and Patty Gyr, P.N.P.

Key to Abbreviations

ABC	airway, breathing, and circulation
ABG	arterial blood gas
AIDS	acquired immunodeficiency syndrome
ALT	alanine aminotransferase
ANC	absolute neutrophil count
ASA	acetylsalicylic acid
AST	aspartate aminotransferase
BMP	basic metabolic panel
BP	blood pressure
BUN	blood urea nitrogen
CBC	complete blood count
CF	cystic fibrosis
CNS	central nervous system
CRP	C-reactive protein
CSF	cerebrospinal fluid
CT	computed tomograph
CXR	chest x-ray
ECG	electrocardiogram
ESR	erythrocyte sedimentation rate
FTA-ABS	fluorescein *Treponema* antibody absorption
GI	gastrointestinal
Hct	hematocrit
HEENT	head, ears, eyes, nose, throat
Hgb	hemoglobin
HIV	human immunodeficiency virus
HSP	Henoch-Schönlein purpura
HTN	hypertension
ICP	intracranial pressure
ITP	idiopathic thrombocytopenic purpura
IVC	inferior vena cava
LDH	lactic acid dehydrogenase
LP	lumbar puncture or leukopoor
MAOI	monoamine oxidase inhibitor
MRI	magnetic resonance imaging
NHL	non-Hodgkin's lymphoma
NICU	neonatal intensive care unit
NPO	nothing by mouth
NS	normal saline
NSAID	nonsteroidal antiinflammatory drug
N/V	nausea and vomiting
OFC	occipitofrontal circumference

KEY TO ABBREVIATIONS

PICU	pediatric intensive care unit
PMD	primary medical doctor
PT	prothrombin time
PTT	partial thromboplastin time
RBC	red blood cell
RPR	rapid plasma reagent
SGOT	serum glutamic-oxaloacetic transaminase
SGPT	serum glutamic-pyruvic transaminase
SIDS	sudden infant death syndrome
SSRI	selective serotonin reuptake inhibitor
STD	sexually transmitted disease
TB	tuberculosis
TCA	tricyclic antidepressant
TMP-SMX	trimethoprim-sulfamethoxazole
TPN	total parenteral nutrition
UTI	urinary tract infection
WBC	white blood cell

Keys for Survival

Children are not just little adults.

- First do no harm.
- Make time for meals.
- Sleep whenever possible.
- Call your spouse or significant other when on call.
- It's often easier to look at the patient than try to figure out what is going on over the phone.
- Nurses' kardex and notes contain the true record of what your patients receive and look like during the day and night.
- Your marriage to the admitting diagnosis obscures findings that may point you in other directions.
- You are never alone. *Always* work as a *team* player with all your coworkers (including nurses).

1

Survival in Pediatrics

Planning the day.

HOW TO ORGANIZE YOUR DAY

Preround

- Check with your patient's night shift nurse or the nurse's notes regarding any events that occurred overnight.

- Ask your patient about any new complaints.

- Find out the maximum temperature, vital signs, and inputs/outputs. Examine the heart, lungs, abdomen, and impaired organ system.

Rounds

- Should be concise, but pertinent information should include the following: main problem, positives on physical exam, antibiotics (and day of antibiotic therapy), and plan.

- For initial presentation, include name, age, and comorbidities.

- Write orders during rounds. Write doses in mg, not in mL. Sign all verbal orders carried out the previous night.

- It facilitates patient care if you let the nurse know every time you write a new order.

- NPO orders: *<6 mos old*: 4 hrs for solids and formula, 2 hrs for clears. *>6 mos old*: 6 hrs for solids and formula, 4 hrs for clears.

Post-Rounds

- Make a to-do list.

- Communicating with medical students: Spend 10 mins running through patient plans; encourage early note writing, assign phlebotomy, or schedule tasks.

- Communicating with PMDs: update daily if they are the attending or are very involved; every 2–3 days if not heavily involved or patient status is not changing much.

- Communicating with parents: update daily. If in the NICU or PICU, coordinate updates with the fellow.

- Schedule tests.

- Call consults early in the day whenever possible. Before calling the consult, try to exclude obvious things first.

- Write discharge orders. Nurse's medicine kardex may be helpful. If the patient is going home over the weekend, leave written discharge orders and make follow-up appointments on the preceding Friday.

- Write TPN orders.

Note Writing

- Most of the information for daily notes is from preround information. Admit notes should be inserted in the chart before rounds.

- Remember that patient care is a priority over writing notes.

- Sign students' notes and orders after reading and editing them.

Gather Labs and Test Results

Repeat or treat seriously abnormal labs.

Call the Senior Resident

Give a run down of all your patients, new problems or events, and test results, and discuss plans.

Touch Base with the Attending

Notify the attending any time a patient's condition worsens or a patient needs transfer to the ICU or a surgical intervention.

Sign Out

- Include name, age, weight, allergies, and meds.

- Diagnosis (if known) or chief complaint.

- Attending physician and any consultants involved.

- Issues to expect overnight and to-do list (use highlighter or red pen).

- Identify **sick kids.** State if IV needs to be replaced if access is lost.

Go Home

You've done everything; you will be back too soon.

WHEN ON CALL

- Sign out should take no more than 20–30 mins.

- A "walking signout" is helpful because it gives you the idea of location of the **sick kids.**

- When an admission is called to you and you feel the floor is an inappropriate place for a patient, call the appropriate person for further clarification (e.g., ER attending, chief resident, floor attending).

- If you do not understand a patient's diagnosis and plan: *ask, ask, ask*.

- Never forget to check with the nurses before going to bed.

- If any patient becomes unstable and needs to be transferred to the PICU, remember:

  - ABCs first. Stabilize the patient and remain calm.

  - Use the *entire team*. Delegate tasks.

  - Notify the chief resident, PICU fellow, charge nurse, patient's attending, and the PMD.

  - Notify the parents of the patient's status and the need for a transfer.

  - If called to a code blue, *run*, don't walk. Never assume others will respond before you.

2 Admission and Event Notes

Nothing charted, nothing done.

STUDENTS AND INTERNS

An effective note is concise but contains all of the relevant information. The skill of effective note writing is one that is learned and improved with time. The history of present illness, impression, and plan should be the focus of the note. Always date and time all notes.

- **Chief complaint:** in the words of the patient or caregiver.

- **History of present illness:** Focus on the child's active problem(s). It is helpful to outline events in a chronological manner— e.g., 1 wk before admission, 2 days before admission. Pertinent negatives should follow positive signs and symptoms.

- **Review of systems**

- **Past medical history**

  1. Birth and delivery history.

  2. Past illnesses or surgeries (minor ones can be omitted).

  3. Developmental history (key events only).

  4. Diet history

     - Important in any child with growth problems, abdominal pain, and diarrheal illness.

     - Remember that the Special Supplemental Nutrition Program for Women, Infants, and Children (WIC) provides a monthly voucher for 13-oz. cans of liquid concentrate, each of which is mixed 1:1 with water to yield 26 oz. of formula.

  5. Medications, allergies, and immunizations.

- **Family history:** only pertinent positives and negatives for the current problem.

- **Social history:** Who lives at home? Who has custody? School performance?

- **Physical exam:** Always describe the patient's general appearance and include vital signs. List the weight, length, or height; OFC; and the percentiles every time. Always include a growth chart with your note. Think about your patient's problem when writing your exam; don't just list a lot of normal findings.

- **Lab data:** List only the relevant ones.

- **Impression/Diagnosis** (if known): Do not repeat the patient's history. In complicated patients, it is helpful to approach them through problem lists. Establish your considerations for etiology. In patients with preexisting conditions, it is also helpful to divide them by acute vs established problems or diagnoses—e.g., Acute: pneumonia. Established: static encephalopathy.

- **Plan:** easier to follow when outlined in a list format.

UPPER LEVEL RESIDENTS

- Notes should be short and concise and include only the key points of the patient's history and exam.

- Include a comprehensive list of problems and decision-making processes.

- You should have discussed the findings and plan with the intern and student before writing the orders.

- You do not need to repeat the entire past medical history unless it is relevant for patient care and is not included in the student's or intern's note.

- Your priority is at the patient's bedside; notes can be written later.

- *Never* address yourself as "the cross-covering resident" when you are on call, you are the person responsible for all the patients you cover.

EVENT NOTES

- Describe any change in the patient's status that requires interval assessment and decision making, even if the current treatment plan remains unchanged.

- It is extremely important to date and record the time on these notes.

- These notes can be brief.

- A good event note may serve as a daily note.

3

Admission Orders and Writing Prescriptions

First things first.

ADMISSION ORDERS

There are different mnemonics. Use the one you will remember most easily.

- **Always** write the patient's *weight* at the top of every order sheet.
- Admitting floor and attending.
- Diagnosis.
- Condition.
- Vital signs frequency.
- Allergies.
- Nursing (e.g., daily weights, strict input and output).
- Diet.
- Activities.
- Labs.
- IV fluids.
- Supplemental O_2.
- Medications.

WRITING PRESCRIPTIONS

- Include patient's full name, weight, and allergies.
- Include drug, dose, route, and frequency.
- Describe length of therapy.
- Include the total quantity of medication to be dispensed.
- Do not place zeros after a decimal point. Include a zero before the decimal point when amount is <1.
- Remember that intervals vary: q8h is around the clock, whereas tid is during waking hours only. This is important if a therapeutic response depends on consistent drug levels.
- Print physician's name under the signature.
- Include the U.S. Drug Enforcement Administration (DEA) number on all prescriptions for controlled substances.

4

How to Calculate IV Fluids and Feeds

Grab a calculator; you'll need it.

CALCULATING IV FLUIDS

Composition of Total Body Compartments

- Remember that water represents 60% of total body weight (TBW) (80% in infants).
- Intracellular water corresponds to 40% of TBW.
- Extracellular water corresponds to 20% of TBW of which 4% represents the intravascular space and 16% the interstitial space.

Daily Water Losses

- Insensible (respiration and perspiration): infant, 600 cc/kg; adult, 300–500 cc/kg.
- Fecal: 70–100 cc/kg.
- Urine: 600–1200 cc/kg.
- During fever, losses are 0.2 cc/kg/hr/°C above 37.5°C rectally.

Daily Fluid Requirements

- If <10 kg: 80–100 cc/kg/day = 4 mL/kg/hr
- If >10 kg: 1500–2000 cc/m^2/day

Daily Electrolyte Requirements

- Na: 2–3 mEq/kg/day
- Ca: 0.5–1.5 mEq/kg/day
- Mg: 0.25–0.5 mEq/kg/day
- K: 2–3 mEq/kg/day
- Phosphorus: 1–1.5 mM/Kg/day
- HCO$_3$: approximately 3 mEq/kg/day

Remember:

- Body surface area = m^2 = (weight in kg $\times$ 4 + 7) / (weight in kg + 90) or
- Body surface area = $[\sqrt{(\text{weight in kg} + \text{height in cm})}]/3600$

Suggested Maintenance Solutions

- D_{10} 1/4 NS + 20 mEq/L KCl in premature infants
- D_{10W} in first day of life
- D_5 1/4 NS + 20 mEq/L KCl for infants (most common maintenance solution used)
- D_5 1/2 NS + 20 mEq/L KCl for children and adults

Composition of Commonly Used Parenteral Solutions

See Table 4-1.

HOW TO CALCULATE FEEDS

Neonatal Enteral Feeding Guidelines

- Goals: preterm, 120–130 kcal/kg/day; full term, 110 kcal/kg/day.
- Caloric percentages: carbohydrate 40–50%, protein 10–14%, fat 50–60%.
- Initiation of feeds: Usually on day of life 2–3 in high-risk or premature infants. Table 4-2 gives suggestions. Obviously, careful exams of the infant determine the speed of advancement.
- Postgastric residuals: If the feeds are continuous and the residual is >2 times the rate/hr or if the feeds are bolus and the residual is more than half the bolus amount, examine the infant. If abdominal distension is present, decrease or hold feeds.
- Fortifying enteral feeds: Fortify breast milk or 20 kcal/oz. formula when the infant is tolerating 100 cc/kg/day.
- Polycose increases osmolality and increases CO_2 production if it is >60% of calories.
- Promod increases renal solute load and can contribute to metabolic acidosis.
- Medium-chain triglyceride oil can adhere to tubing and cause ketosis if >60% of calories; also may cause diarrhea.
- All patients that are strictly breast-fed should be supplemented with vitamin D to prevent rickets.

TABLE 4-1.
COMPOSITION OF COMMONLY USED PARENTERAL SOLUTIONS

Solution	Na (mEq/L)	K (mEq/L)	Cl (mEq/L)	HCO$_3$ (mEq/L)	Comments
3% NaCl	513	0	513	0	Used in symptomatic hyponatremia.
0.9% NaCl	154	0	154	0	Isotonic. Used in first phase of fluid resuscitation.
0.45% NaCl	77	0	77	0	$^1/_2$ NS.
0.2% NaCl	40	0	40	0	$^1/_4$ NS.
Lactated Ringer's	130	4	109	28	Calcium: 1.5 mEq/L. Isotonic. Used in first phase of fluid resuscitation.
D$_{5W}$	0	0	0	0	50 g/L dextrose.

TABLE 4-2.
INITIATION OF FEEDS IN THE NEWBORN

Weight (g)	Start	Advance
<750	0.5–1 cc q6h (change to q3h on sixth day of life)	0.5 cc q24h (change to 0.5 cc q12h on sixth day of life)
751–1000	1–2 cc q3h × 24–48 hrs	1 cc q12h
1001–1250	2–3 cc q3h × 24–48 hrs	2 cc q12h
1251–1500	3 cc q3h	1 cc every other feed
1501–2000	3–5 cc q3h	2 cc every other feed
>2000	NG: 5 cc q3h × 24 hrs	5 cc every third feed
	PO: breast milk ad lib; bottle 30 cc q3h	

5

Calculating Total Parenteral Nutrition

If the gut works, use it. If not, use TPN.

CALCULATING HOURLY FLUID INFUSION RATE

cc/kg/day × weight in kg/24 hrs = rate (cc/hr)

FLUID REQUIREMENTS

- Newborns
  - Transition: 80–120 cc/kg/day
  - Maintenance: 150 cc/kg/day
- <10 kg: 100 cc/kg/day
- 10–20 kg: 1000 cc + 50 cc/kg for each kg >10
- >20 kg: 1500 cc + 20 cc/kg for each kg >20

TOTAL PARENTERAL NUTRITION RATE

TPN = Total fluid rate − lipids − drips

CALORIE REQUIREMENTS FOR GROWTH (KCAL/KG/DAY)

Premature Infants

- 120–140 (enteral)
- 90–100 (parenteral)

Term Infants and Children

- 0–1 yr: 80–115
- 1–3 yrs: 100
- 4–6 yrs: 85
- 7–10 yrs: 85
- 11–14 yrs: 50–60
- 15–18 yrs: 40

DEXTROSE

- 3.4 kcal/g.
- Glucose infusion rate (GIR) mg/kg/min = [(% dextrose) × cc/hr] / [(weight in kg) × 6].

- Start at a GIR of 6–8 and monitor blood glucose levels. Adjust up or down as needed.
- Upper limit for GIR: 12–16.
- Increase GIR by 2–3/day in the NICU. Can increase more quickly in other areas of the hospital.
- kcal/kg/day from dextrose = [(% dextrose / 100) × cc/hr × number of hrs/day dextrose is infusing × 3.4 kcal/g] / weight in kg.

PROTEIN

- g/kg/day = [(% protein / 100) × cc/hr × number of hrs/day protein infusing] / weight in kg

  Start:

  - 1 g/kg/day for <1 kg
  - 1.5 g/kg/day for ≥1 kg

  Goal:

  - 2.7–3.5 g/kg/day for preterm infants
  - 2–3 g/kg/day for term infants
  - 1–2.5 g/kg/day for >12 mos

FAT

- 20% intralipid = 2 kcal/cc
- g/kg/day = (0.2 g/cc × cc/hr × number of hrs/day fat is infusing) / weight in kg

  Start:

  - 0.5–1 g/kg/day for <1 kg
  - 1.5 g/kg/day for ≥1 kg

  Goal:

  - 1–2.5 g/kg/day in preterm infants
  - 2–3 g/kg/day in term infants
  - 2–4 g/kg/day for >12 mos

- kcal/kg/day from fat: (cc/hr × number of hrs fat infusing × 2 kcal/cc) / weight in kg

ELECTROLYTES

- mEq/kg/day = (cc/hr × number of hours infusing × mEq/1000 cc) / weight in kg

- Requirements (mEq/kg/day): see Chap. 4, How to Calculate IV Fluids and Feeds

- Ca (mEq/kg/day) 2–4 (preterm infants), 1.5–2 (term infants), 0.5–1.5 (infants/children)

RICKETS PREVENTION IN BABIES <1500 G

- Keep 2.5:1 ratio of Ca (mEq) to phosphorus (mM).

- Start with 20 mEq of Ca and 8 mM of phosphorus, then titrate up.

- Titrate up on Ca/phosphorus q2–3days as amino acids increase.

AMINO ACIDS	CA (MEQ/L)	PHOSPHORUS (MM/L)
0.5–1	20	8
1.1–1.9	30	12
>2	40	16

MONITORING

When beginning or changing total parenteral nutrition, monitor serum electrolytes and blood glucose closely. Remember that abruptly stopping a high GIR can induce hypoglycemia. As TPN becomes stable, you can decrease the frequency of monitoring.

6

Ten Most Common Floor Calls

Just wanted to let you know . . .

INTRODUCTION

- If for any reason a nurse calls you to look at a patient, do so. Do not argue.

- If the nurse has a question about a patient, he or she will ask you the question over the phone. If the nurse is concerned about a patient, he or she will ask you to come look.

- Remember, the nurse has usually been around patients longer than you have and is invaluable in assessing change in a patient he or she has been taking care of.

- Likewise, if the patient you are evaluating is unfamiliar, ask the parent and the nurse how the patient has changed.

- No one knows the child better than the parent. If a parent is worried, you should be, too.

FEVER

The patient has a fever.

- Does this patient have a source for the fever? If not, go examine the patient to look for a source.

- After evaluating the patient, ask yourself which studies might be helpful in identifying the source—i.e., CXR, lumbar puncture (LP), UA, throat, urine, blood, CSF or sputum culture.

- Is this a patient (e.g., neutropenic, sickle cell) in whom you should start empiric antibiotics (after drawing cultures)?

- If the patient has a source and you decide that no new studies are needed, you may give acetaminophen or ibuprofen based on weight. (Obviously, you should first consider whether a patient's medical conditions prohibit either of these medications.) Remember that neutropenic patients should not receive suppositories.

IV LINE

The IV came out.

- Does this patient need the IV replaced? Is the patient receiving any medication that can only be given IV or is he or she at a point clinically that it would be OK to change to a PO or IM medication?

- Does the patient need TPN or fluids through the IV?
- Is the patient unstable and may need an IV acutely (e.g., at risk for arrhythmia, seizure, respiratory distress)?

BREATHING TREATMENTS

Can the patient's breathing treatments be spaced?

- This is an easy one. It just requires some effort on your part. No matter how tired you are, go and listen to the patient's breathing just before the next treatment is due.
- If the patient sounds good and is comfortable, the treatments may be spaced and the patient monitored closely until you and the patient are comfortable with the new schedule.

BLOOD IN STOOL OR EMESIS

The stool or emesis is blood tinged or Gastroccult/Hemoccult positive.

- Think about the patient. Does he or she have a reason for the blood (e.g., was an NG tube just placed, did the patient swallow blood from a recent nosebleed, does the patient have an anal fissure)?
- If the patient is clinically stable and feels well, and the amount of blood in the emesis or stool is small, it is usually safe to watch the patient carefully without immediate intervention.
- Be sure to follow up on this complaint often. If it continues or worsens, it can turn into something serious quickly.

DECREASED URINE OUTPUT

A well-hydrated pediatric patient should make at least 1–2 cc/kg/hr. If you are called about decreased urine output, as always, think about each patient individually.

- Is patient dehydrated and in need of fluid?
- Is patient at risk for renal insufficiency or failure (and if so, think about accompanying problems such as uremia and electrolyte abnormalities)?
- Could the patient have a mechanical obstruction to urine output such as a malfunctioning Foley or recent catheterization making urination painful?
- Go look at the patient. Does the patient have signs of dehydration (tachycardia, dry mouth, sunken fontanel, decreased tear production)? If so, give PO or IV fluids. If not, is patient edematous and in need of diuretics or could there be any of the mechanical problems mentioned above?

- Sometimes, despite your best efforts, you will not be able to tell if patient needs diuretics or fluids. In this case, you may have to make the best decision you can and try it. If it doesn't work, you may have to do the other. Sometimes patients need both things (e.g., a patient with heart failure who is edematous but intravascularly dry).

FEEDING PROBLEMS

The patient is not tolerating feeds (e.g., PO, NG, or GT).

- As always, think about your patient. Is the patient one who has gastroenteritis and needs to be changed to either a rehydration solution or IV fluids? Or could this patient have an obstruction?

- Is this an infant in whom difficulty with feeds is a sign of something else (e.g., bacteremia, meningitis, necrotizing enterocolitis)?

- Based on these considerations, is simply holding feeds and giving IV fluids appropriate or is further evaluation necessary?

- Consider abdominal imaging, electrolytes, CBC, cultures.

- If this could be a surgical issue, get surgery involved early.

- Will the patient benefit from gastric decompression?

- Monitor the patient closely.

CHANGE IN MENTAL STATUS

- Do a bedside Dextrostix and feed or give dextrose if needed.

- Send electrolytes and arterial blood gases stat. Is this a child with an underlying neurological condition (seizure, tumor, shunt, etc.), and if so, could his or her change in mental status be related to the underlying disorder?

- Consider a CT scan and shunt series.

- Call neurosurgery if the patient is a neurosurgery patient.

- Could one of the child's medications be affecting mental status?

- Make sure the airway is protected and provide support if needed.

- If airway is at risk, make patient NPO.

PAIN

- Is this a new pain or an undertreated old pain? If it is a new pain or the pain has changed in character, work up the pain as appropriate. If this is an undertreated old pain, reevaluate the patient's medications.

- Can the patient safely receive more pain medication or more frequent dosing?

- Is anxiety contributing to the pain, and if so, is it being treated?

- If you are at all uncomfortable with changing the patient's pain medications, ask for help (e.g., pain service, pharmacists, attending).

- Remember that the most common side effect of pain medications is respiratory depression. Also, never underestimate the value of non-medical therapies (e.g., change in position, child life).

DIFFICULTY BREATHING
Assess the child.

- Does he or she have decreased air movement or wheezing and need albuterol?

- Does the child have crackles and need either a diuretic to treat pulmonary edema or antibiotics to treat pneumonia?

- Place the patient on pulse oximetry.

- Get a portable CXR and a stat ABG measurement if indicated.

- Provide supplemental O_2.

- Have the appropriate airway equipment in the room and know how to hook it up.

- Remember that, in children, cardiopulmonary arrest is usually due to respiratory arrest, and these children can go downhill quickly.

- If you cannot easily get the child comfortable, consider transfer to the PICU.

PARENTS HAVE QUESTIONS
Parents invariably have questions at night when you are cross-covering, and you may not know that patient's story as well as you know your own patients.

- Ask the nurse if he or she knows what the parent's specific questions are. Then you can be prepared when you enter the room.

- Consult the nurse and the chart to familiarize yourself with the patient.

- Never identify yourself to the parent as the cross-covering resident.

- If you do not know the answer to the parents' question, tell them you will find out and get back to them as soon as possible.

- Update the parents of your primary patients often so that you will not put your colleagues in this position at night.

7

Adolescent Medicine

Sex, drugs, and rock-'n'-roll.

INTRODUCTION

- Adolescence is the time of transition from childhood to adulthood. Typically it begins at 10–14 yrs of age. It is characterized by rapid physical, cognitive, and emotional growth and sexual development (puberty).

- At this age, children start to develop some independence and separation from their parents: They become unwilling to participate in some family activities, they concentrate on peer relationships, and they challenge old behaviors and parental authority.

- They have increased concern about their developing body, peer pressure, independence, and sexual exploration and definition.

TIPS ON CLINICAL INTERVIEW

- Interview the child alone and with the parent. While the patient undresses, you may have a chance to talk to parents alone at that time. Entirely independent visits create suspicion and distrust except in older adolescents.

- Early in the interview and in front of the parents, pledge confidentiality to the child. Be clear to say you will keep complete confidence unless the patient is at risk of hurting himself or others.

- Encourage adolescents to discuss any problems with their parents, and encourage parents to create a daily time away from television or work to share with their child during which the adolescent feels comfortable talking to them.

Clinical History

An adolescent clinical history should include questions about **HEADS:**

- **H**ome dynamics
- **E**ducation: school performance
- **A**ctivities, **a**spirations
- **D**rugs, **d**epression, **d**iet
- **S**ex, **s**uicide

Before the exam give the patient the option of being examined alone or accompanied by a parent. Respect the patient's modesty.

Screening labs at this age include the following:

- Hgb in menstruating girls
- Pap smear, gonococcus, chlamydia yearly in sexually active girls
- Urine dipstick once between 11 and 21 yrs
- Lipid profile (if there are risk factors)

When formulating a plan, it is important to reinforce the strengths and achievements of the child and parent.

Do not forget to give anticipatory guidance on diet, maturation, sex education, injury prevention, good health habits, and good parenting practices.

SEXUALLY TRANSMITTED DISEASES

STDs in adolescents can present as the following:

- Urethritis
- Vulvovaginitis
- Cervicitis
- Genital ulcers or growths
- Pelvic inflammatory disease (PID)
- Epididymitis
- Enteritis or proctitis
- Hepatitis
- Arthritis
- Pharyngitis
- Rash
- Conjunctivitis

All of these entities can be caused by a different variety of organisms.

- **Condoms,** when properly used, can decrease the spread of STDs.
- Long-term sequelae of STDs include infertility, PID, chronic pelvic pain, ectopic pregnancy, cervical dysplasia and cancer, congenital and perinatal infection.
- Adolescents can consent for the evaluation and treatment of STDs without parental consent and notification.
  - Evaluation should include complete history, physical exam (including skin, pharynx, and complete genital exam).
  - In girls, perform a pregnancy test, wet prep, vaginal pH, assay for *Neisseria gonorrhea* and *Chlamydia trachomatis*, Gram's stain of cervical swab and *Trichomonas* culture.

- In boys, send a urethral swab or urine specimen to diagnose infection with *N. gonorrhea* and *C. trachomatis*.

- Consider HIV, RPR, and hepatitis B testing in high-risk populations.

- Detailed information on STDs and their treatment can be found in Table 7-1.

TABLE 7-1.
TREATMENT OF STDS

Disease	Characteristics	Therapy
Gonor-rhea	Caused by *Neisseria gonorrhea*. Patients often are coinfected with chlamydia. Treat sexual partners. Screen for syphilis on all patients. May cause mucopurulent cervicitis.	Uncomplicated urogenital, rectal, or pharyngeal: Ceftriaxone (Rocephin), 125 mg IM single dose **or** Cefixime (Suprax), 400 mg PO single dose **or** Ciprofloxacin (Cipro, Cipro XR),[a] 500 mg PO single dose **plus** Doxycycline (Monodox, Periostat, Vibramycin), 100 mg PO bid × 7 days **or** Azithromycin (Zithromax, Zithromax Z-Pak), 1 g PO single dose Disseminated gonococcal infection: Ceftriaxone, 1g IV or IM qd **or** Cefotaxime (Claforan), 1 g IV q8h 24–48 hrs until symptoms improve, then continue to complete 1 wk of treatment with

(continued)

TABLE 7-1.
CONTINUED

Disease	Characteristics	Therapy
		Cefixime, 400 mg PO bid
		or
		Ciprofloxacin (Cipro),[a] 500 mg PO q12h
		or
		Ofloxacin (Floxin),[a] 400 mg single dose
		Other alternative: Spectino-mycin (Trobicin)
Chlamydia	Caused by *Chlamydia trachomatis*.	Azithromycin: 1 g PO single dose if patient weighs >45 kg
	Asymptomatic infection is very common among men and women.	**or**
		Doxycycline, 100 mg PO bid × 7 days.
	Sexual partners should be treated.	If <45-kg, erythromycin base (E-Mycin, E.E.S., Ery-Tab, Eryc, EryPed, Ilosone), 50 mg/kg/day, divided qid × 10–14 days.
	May cause mucopurulent cervicitis.	
	Sexual abuse must be considered in preadolescent children with chlamydia.	
		Pregnancy: Erythromycin or amoxicillin (Amoxil).
Syphilis	Caused by *Treponema pallidum*.	Primary and secondary syphilis.
	Primary: painless ulcer or chancre. Secondary: rash, mucocutaneous lesions and adenopathy. Early latent syphilis: if within 1 yr preceding the evaluation, patient had seroconversion, or unequivocal symptoms of primary or secondary syphilis or sex partner with primary, secondary, or early latent syphilis. All others should be considered to have late latent syphilis. Tertiary: lesions CNS, cardiac, ophthalmic, auditory, and gummas.	Early latent: Benzathine penicillin G (Bicillin L-A) 50,000 U/kg up to 2.4 million U IM in a single dose (pregnant or not)
Late latent: Benzathine penicillin G 50,000 U/kg up to 2.4 million U IM q wk × 3 wks
Penicillin allergy:
Doxycycline, 100 mg PO bid × 2 wks
or

(*continued*)

**TABLE 7-1.
CONTINUED**

Disease	Characteristics	Therapy
	Diagnosis: VDRL (fourfold change in titers); dark field, FTA-ABS (remain +). All should be tested for HIV. Sexual partners should be treated.	Tetracycline (Achromycin, Panmycin, Sumycin, Tetracap), 500 mg PO qid × 2 wks.
		If duration of infection >1 yr or unknown, patient should receive therapy for 4 wks.
		Tertiary syphilis: Benzathine penicillin G, 2.4 million U IM q wk × 3 wks.
		Neurosyphilis: aqueous crystalline penicillin G, 4 million U IV q4h × 10–14 days.
Bacterial vaginosis	Caused by *Gardnerella vaginalis*. Associated with having multiple sex partners but unclear whether it is an STD. Most prevalent cause of pathologic vaginal discharge. Symptoms include vaginal discharge and odor, vulvar itching and irritation, but 50% are asymptomatic. Partners do not need treatment.	Metronidazole (Flagyl), 500 mg PO bid × 7 days. Other alternatives: clindamycin (Cleocin) cream 2%: (5 g) intravaginally × 7 nights.
Trichomoniasis	Caused by protozoa. 90% of men and 25–50% of female are asymptomatic. Malodorous yellow green discharge and irritation. Diagnosis: wet prep and culture. Treat sexual partners.	Metronidazole vaginal gel, 0.75%, 5-g applicator bid × 5 days or metronidazole 2 g PO single dose **or** Metronidazole, 500 mg PO bid × 7 days if previous treatment fails.
Candidiasis	Symptoms include pruritus, erythema, and white discharge. Partners don't need treatment.	Clotrimazole (Mycelex, Gyne-Lotrimin), 100-mg tab: 2 intravaginal × 3 days or 1 × 7 days. Clotrimazole, 1% cream intravaginally × 7–14 days qhs. Miconazole (Monistat), 200 mg vaginal suppository × 3 days.

(continued)

**TABLE 7-1.
CONTINUED**

Disease	Characteristics	Therapy
		Fluconazole (Diflucan), 150 mg PO × 1.
Epididy-mitis	Usually caused by *Chlamydia* or *Neisseria*.	Ceftriaxone, 250 mg IM × 1 **plus**
	Epydidimal swelling, tenderness, discharge, fever, dysuria.	Doxycycline, 100 mg PO bid × 10 days.
Herpes	Recurrent, incurable viral infection.	Acyclovir (Zovirax), 400 mg PO tid × 7–10 days.
	May manifest as painful genital or oral ulcers, cervicitis, proctitis, or asymptomatic.	Famciclovir (Famvir) or valacyclovir (Valtrex). These therapies may shorten dura-
	Pregnant women who acquire infection near time of delivery have a higher risk of perinatal infection (30–50%). Encourage condom use.	tion of lesions but do not eradicate the virus.
		Daily suppressive therapy: Acyclovir, 400 mg PO bid (decreases frequency of recurrences by 75%).
Chan-croid	Caused by *Haemophilus ducreyi*. ≥1 painful ulcers and tender suppurative regional lymphadenopathy. All patients should be tested for HIV at time of diagnosis and 3 mos after. Partners must be treated.	Azithromycin, 1 g PO single dose **or** Ceftriaxone, 250 mg IM × 1 **or** Ciprofloxacin,[a] 500 mg PO bid × 3 days **or** Erythromycin base, 500 mg PO qid × 7 days.
		If treatment is successful, ulcers improve symptomatically in 3 days, complete healing may require >2 wks.
Genital warts, Condyloma acuminatum	Caused by HPV. There are >20 types. May manifest as visible genital warts, uterine, cervix, anal, vaginal, urethral, laryngeal warts.	External warts. Podofilox 0.5% topical solution bid × 3 days **or**

(continued)

TABLE 7-1.
CONTINUED

Disease	Characteristics	Therapy
	Associated with cervical dysplasia. Condoms reduce but do not eliminate the risk of transmission. Patient might remain infectious even though warts are gone.	Imiquimod 5% cream or cryotherapy or podophyllin resin 10–25% or trichloroacetic acid or surgical or laser removal
		Vaginal, urethral, and anal.
		Cryotherapy or podophyllin resin 10–25%. Trichloroacetic acid or bichloroacetic acid 80–90% can also be used for vaginal and anal warts. Cervical and anal mucosa wart management should be by an expert.
		Treatment may induce wart-free periods but do not eradicate the virus.
Pediculosis pubis	Lice or nits on pubic hair. Patients consult because of pruritus.	Permethrin 1% cream **or** Lindane 1%[b] shampoo. If used for >4 mins, associated with toxicity effects as seizures and aplastic anemia.
Scabies	Produced by *Sarcoptes scabiei*. In adults may be sexually transmitted. Not in children. Pruritus and rash.	Permethrin 5% cream **or** Lindane 1% lotion[b] **or** Sulfur 6% **or** Ivermectin, 200 µg/kg or 0.8% solution.

[a]Do not use in patients <15 yrs due to potential risk of affecting growth plate cartilage.
[b]Do not use in patients <2 yrs or in pregnant or lactating women due to neurotoxicity.

PELVIC INFLAMMATORY DISEASE
Definition

PID is a spectrum of inflammatory disorders of the upper female tract including endometritis, salpingitis, tubo-ovarian abscess, and pelvic peritonitis. It is usually polymicrobial in nature. The most common organisms are *N. gonorrhea* and *C. trachomatis*. Other organisms isolated are *G. vaginalis*, *Haemophilus influenzae*, enteric gram-negative rods, *Streptococcus agalactiae*, and *Bacteroides fragilis*.

Diagnostic Criteria
Minimum Criteria

- Lower abdominal tenderness
- Adnexal tenderness
- Cervical motion tenderness

Additional Criteria

- Oral temp >101°F (38.3°C)
- Abnormal cervical or vaginal discharge
- Elevated ESR or CRP
- Lab documentation of *N. gonorrhea* or *C. trachomatis*

Definitive Criteria

- Histopathologic evidence of endometritis on endometrial biopsy
- Transvaginal U/S or other imaging techniques showing thickened fluid tubes ± free pelvic fluid or tubo-ovarian complex
- Laparoscopic abnormalities consistent with PID

Hospitalization Criteria

- All adolescent patients who are poor follow-up candidates or who are unable to tolerate an outpatient oral regimen.
- All pregnant women.
- All immunocompromised patients.
- If a surgical emergency, such as appendicitis, cannot be excluded.
- If a patient did not respond clinically to oral antimicrobial therapy.
- If the patient has a severe illness, nausea and vomiting, or high fever.
- Patients with a tubo-ovarian abscess.
- Hospitalize the patient for at least 24–48 hrs after substantial clinical improvement.

Parenteral Treatment

- Cefotetan (Cefotan), 2 g IV q12h, **OR** cefoxitin (Mefoxin), 2 g IV q6h **PLUS**

- Doxycycline (Monodox, Periostat, Vibramycin), 100 mg IV or PO q12h × 14 days

    OR

- Clindamycin (Cleocin), 900 mg IV q8h, + gentamicin (Garamycin), 2 mg/kg loading dose followed by 1.5 mg/kg q8h.

- After 24 hours of clinical improvement on IV therapy, discontinue IV therapy and follow with doxycycline, 100 mg PO q12h, to complete a 14-day total course of antibiotics.

- If outpatient therapy is established:

    - Ofloxacin (Floxin), 400 mg PO bid × 14 days, + metronidazole (Flagyl), 500 mg PO bid × 14 days

    OR

    - Cefoxitin, 2 g IM, + probenecid (Benemid, Probalan), 1 g PO as a single dose; or ceftriaxone (Rocephin), 250 mg IM, + doxycycline, 100 mg PO bid × 14 days.

    - Evaluate and treat all sexual partners.

Follow-Up Exam

- Perform within 72 hrs.

- Perform a microbiologic evaluation to rescreen for *N. gonorrhea* or *C. trachomatis* 4–6 wks after completing therapy.

DYSMENORRHEA
Definition

Pain with menstruation. Caused by the release of prostaglandins during menstrual flow.

Primary

When it appears within 1–2 yrs of menarche. Cramping usually starts 1–4 hrs before a period and may last 24 hrs, although some experience these symptoms 2 days before menstruation (may last up to 4 days). Episodes become less severe with increasing age.

Secondary

When painful menstruation appears for the first time or suddenly intensifies in a mature woman, it is nearly always the result of a specific pathologic problem such as endometriosis, chronic PID, benign uterine tumors, intrauterine device (IUD), or anatomic abnormalities.

Treatment

- Mild symptoms: Aspirin or acetaminophen.

- Moderate to severe symptoms: NSAIDs such as ibuprofen, 600 mg PO q6–8h; naproxen, 275–550 mg PO q8–12h; mefenamic acid, 250 mg PO q6h. These are most effective if given before the onset of menses and continued for 2–3 days after.

- Steroidal contraceptives.

CONTRACEPTIVES

See Table 7-2.

TABLE 7-2.
CONTRACEPTIVES

Method	Mechanism of action and characteristics	Failure rate (%)	Adverse effects
None		85	
Rhythm method	Avoidance of coitus during presumed fertile days.	14–20	
	Ovulation occurs 14 days before menses; sperm can survive in the vagina for 3–4 days and oocytes can survive up to 24 hrs after ovulation.		
Barrier/ chemical	Condom: mechanical barrier to sperm.	10–19	Allergic reactions
	Diaphragm (placed intravaginally 1–6 hrs before coitus) or cervical cap (should be used in conjunction with spermicides).	12–40	UTI or vaginal infections
	Sponge and foam or vaginal tablets: inactivate sperm. Allow 10–15 mins for the tablets to dissolve.	21–25	Irritation
IUD	Inhibits sperm transport, and causes direct damage on sperm and ova affecting fertilization and ovum transport. Progesterone release IUD must be replaced every year. Copper-containing IUD must be replaced q10yrs.	2.5–4.5	Dysmenorrhea, PID, uterine perforation copper increases menstrual flow
	Recommended for women who have had at least 1 child and are monogamous.		Ectopic pregnancy if patient becomes pregnant with device in place

(continued)

TABLE 7-2.
CONTINUED

Method	Mechanism of action and characteristics	Failure rate (%)	Adverse effects
Oral contra-ceptives		4–9	
Combined	Suppresses ovulation by inhibiting the gonadotropin cycle and changing the cervical mucus and endometrium.		Estrogen-related risk of thromboembolism, HTN stroke, MI in older smokers
Progestins only	Changes the cervical mucus and endometrium, possible suppression of ovulation.		Irregular bleeding
Medroxy-progesterone	Inhibits ovulation by inhibiting the midcycle rise of LH; it also thickens cervical mucus and causes endometrial thinning. Dose: 150 mg IM q3mos.	<1	Menstrual irregularities, weight gain, headache
Emergency contraception (postcoital)	Ovral, 2 pills; or LoOvral, Triphasil Ovral, Tri-Levlen, Nordette or Levlen, 4 pills after unprotected intercourse (within 72 hrs). Repeat the dose 12 hrs after.		Nausea and vomiting

Contraindications
IUD Insertion
- Pregnancy or suspicion of pregnancy
- Uterine abnormalities
- Multiple sexual partners
- Acute PID or history of PID
- Untreated acute cervicitis
- Postpartum endometritis or infected abortion in <3 mos
- Known or suspected uterine or cervical malignancy
- Wilson's disease (copper IUD)
- History of ectopic pregnancy
- Conditions associated to increased risk of infection

Oral Contraceptive Pills
Absolute Contraindications

- History of thromboembolic disease
- Liver dysfunction
- Undiagnosed uterine bleeding
- Pregnancy
- MI, stroke, pulmonary embolism
- Breast cancer
- Estrogen-dependent neoplasias

Other Strong Contraindications

- Severe HTN
- Cyanotic heart disease
- Sickle cell disease

Relative Contraindications

- Chorea
- Collagen vascular disease
- Diabetes
- Depression
- Lactation
- Hyperlipidemia
- Melasma or other estrogen-related dermatologic disorders
- Gallbladder disease

EATING DISORDERS
Common problem in primary care

Persons at Risk

- Gender: 90–95% female
- Race: >95% white
- Age: >80% adolescent or young adult
- Adolescents with poor self-esteem
- Athletes: gymnasts, ballet dancers, runners (roles in which thinness is related to success)
- Socioeconomic status: predominantly middle to upper class
- Third most common chronic illness in adolescents

Anorexia Nervosa (Pursuit of Thinness)

- Insufficient caloric intake and dietary restriction
- Delusion of being fat
- Does not improve with weight loss
- Obsession of being thinner
- Denial
- Wasting of the body with weight loss or failure to gain weight as expected

Bulimia Nervosa (Avoidance of Obesity)

- Fear of not being able to stop eating
- Recurrent binge eating
- Awareness of abnormal eating pattern
- Depressed mood and poor self-esteem
- Temporary relief via avoidance of weight gain by the following:
  - Fasting
  - Self-inducing vomiting
  - Laxatives or diuretics
  - Exercise

Signs and Symptoms of Eating Disorders

- Low energy level
- Amenorrhea
- Cold hands and feet
- Constipation
- Neutropenia
- Bradycardia
- Loss of muscle mass
- Dry skin/hair loss
- Increased ALT and AST
- Social withdrawal
- Poor concentration
- Fainting/dizziness/orthostasis
- Decreased serum glucose

- Headaches/lethargy
- Irritability/depression
- Decreased ability to make decisions
- QT prolonged
- Binge eating
- Weight gain
- Bloating and fullness
- Guilt/depression/anxiety
- Knuckle calluses
- Lethargy
- Dental enamel erosion
- Enlargement of salivary gland
- Increased CO_2 and decreased K

Complications

- Amenorrhea and infertility: Adequate weight gain should return fertility and menses to normal.
- Birth control pills and other hormonal therapies will result in withdrawal bleeding, not in menses.
- Abnormal heart contractility, prolonged QT, and ventricular dysrhythmias.
- Osteopenia and osteoporosis. Weight gain is the most effective method to increase bone density.

Management

- Take all concerns seriously.
- Focus on overall health, not only on weight.
- Target weight >85% average.
- Team approach: mental health care providers, dietitian, primary care physicians, and/or adolescent medicine specialist.

DEPRESSION

- Prevalence of major depression in adolescents is estimated at 4.7% and dysthymic disorder at 3.3%.
- Often adolescents will not tell or admit that they are depressed, and when confronted they will deny it.

- Patients feel hopeless, worthless, and helpless.
- School problems, social withdrawal, substance abuse, somatic complaints, high-risk behaviors should be red flags that patient may be depressed.
- Patients have problems with **SIG E CAPS:**
  - **S**leep and **s**ex
  - **I**nterest
  - **G**uilt
  - **E**nergy
  - **C**oncentration
  - **A**ppetite
  - **P**sychomotor retardation
  - **S**uicide

Risk Factors

Parental history of affective illness, chronic illness, history of abuse, loss through separation or death, and medications

Definition

Major Depressive Episode

- Depressed mood or loss of interest for ≥2 wks

  AND

- ≥4 of the following:
  - Weight loss/gain
  - Low energy/fatigue
  - Insomnia/hypersomnia
  - Psychomotor retardation/agitation
  - Worthlessness/guilt
  - Poor concentration/indecisiveness
  - Suicidal ideation

Dysthymic Disorder

- Irritable or depressed mood for most of the day, most days, for ≥1 yr, with significant impairment in functioning

  AND

- ≥ 2 of the following:
  - Insomnia/hypersomnia
  - Poor appetite/overeating
  - Low self-esteem
  - Hopelessness
  - Low energy/fatigue
  - Poor concentration/indecisiveness
  - No major depressive episode

Adjustment Disorder with Depressed Mood

- Emotional symptoms within 3 mos of the stressor onset.
- Distress/impairment in social/occupational/academic functioning.
- Once stressor is terminated, symptoms do not persist >6 mos.
- Depressed mood, tearfulness, hopelessness.

Therapy

- Psychotherapy and pharmacotherapy are equally effective in mild to moderate depression.
- Consider pharmacotherapy in those with substantial impairment.
- Major cause of failure is noncompliance. Relapse rate as high as 72% after 5 yrs.
- Treat for at least 6 mos after initial episode or 12 mos if >1 episode.
- TCAs: not recommended since not superior to placebo in children or adolescents.
- MAOIs: only to be prescribed by a psychiatrist. Not to be given with SSRIs.
- SSRIs: fluxetine, sertraline, paroxetine, fluvoxamine, citalopram reveal benefit above placebo.
  - May not see benefits for 4–8 wks.
  - Response to one SSRI does not predict response to different SSRI.
  - Few side effects, most common include
    - GI: Nausea and vomiting, diarrhea, constipation, mouth dryness, appetite change, dyspepsia
    - CNS: Headache, nervousness, tremor, insomnia, confusion, fatigue, dizziness, decreased libido

- Also effective for obsessive disorder.
- Electroconvulsive therapy: no data in adolescents. Of use in refractory major depression in adults.

SUICIDE AMONG ADOLESCENTS

- Is the third most common cause of death in adolescents.
- Rate is 4 times higher in males but attempts are more frequent in females.
- More common in patients with a family history, a psychiatric disorder, or a previous suicide attempt.
- Any patient who talks about suicide should be taken seriously.
- There is always a precipitant factor and a motivation (gain attention, escape, communicate love or anger).
- It is very important to know when evaluating adolescents if they feel depressed. Ask about their family support system. Ask if they have ever thought of hurting themselves, and if so, when, how, if they had a plan, if they would do it again, and if they feel the same way at time of your evaluation.
- When patients are suicidal or you are concerned for their safety, you should
  - Hospitalize
  - Consult psychiatry
  - Involve parents and/or support system
  - Formulate a "no suicide" agreement
  - Consider antidepressant therapy

CONSENT AND CONFIDENTIALITY

- Consent and confidentiality are very important when caring for adolescents.
- Always find out about the specific laws in your state.

Consent

This is an agreement to medical care (exam, testing, treatment, surgical procedures).

- Patients have the right to know about their health and treatment options, and the physician should respect their autonomy, rights, preferences (religious, social, cultural, philosophic), and decisions.

- When obtaining consent it is important to (a) provide relevant information (illness, studies, treatments, risks/benefits, options); (b) assess the patient's understanding; (c) assess the patient's capacity for decision making; and (d) assure the patient's freedom to choose.

- In many states, any patient <18 years of age (minor) must have parental or a legal guardian's permission for any surgical/medical treatment or procedure. In most states, minors who are authorized to consent for their own treatment include

  - Those who have been lawfully married

  - Those who have legal custody of a child

  - Those who are self-supporting and living away from home

  - Those who present requesting treatment for

    - Pregnancy (not abortions or contraception)

    - STDs

    - Drug or substance abuse

    - Emergency care

Confidentiality

This is an agreement between the patient and the health care provider that information will not be shared without explicit permission of the patient.

- When possible, do involve parents in evaluation and treatment.

- The goals of confidentiality are to protect the patient's privacy, assure access to health, and encourage open and honest communication.

- Adolescents like to keep confidentiality because they fear parental retribution, fear damage to their reputation, and are striving for independence and adult status.

- Consider breaching confidentiality when the adolescent poses a severe risk of harm to self or others.

SUGGESTED READING

Centers for Disease Control. Guidelines for treatment of sexually transmitted diseases. *MMWR Morb Mortal Wkly Rep* 1998;47/NoRR-1.

Greydanus DE, et al. Consent and confidentiality in adolescent health care. *Pediatr Ann* 1991;20(2):80–84.

Greydanus DE, et al. Contraception in the adolescent: an update. *Pediatrics* 2001;107(3):562–573.

Kreipe RE. Eating disorders among children and adolescents. *Pediatr Rev* 1995;l6:370–379.

Neinstein, LS. *Adolescent health care: a practical guide*, 3rd ed. Baltimore: Williams & Wilkins, 1996.

8 Cardiology

Oxygen is good.

INTRODUCTION

- Approach to the patient with a possible cardiac lesion: Always remember to take a good history.

- Heart disease in infants and children often manifests as feeding difficulties, growth problems, and exercise intolerance.

- When performing the physical exam, you need to be in a quiet room and wait until the patient is quiet in order to listen to the heart. Then you need to listen in several places until you can really describe what you are hearing.

- Until you are good at listening to hearts, select different components of the exam and listen to them sequentially (i.e., listen to the rhythm first, then listen to S_1, then S_2, then systole, then diastole).

- Think about which studies would be helpful. These often include an ECG, CXR, and echocardiogram. When ordering an echocardiogram, alert the technician to your suspicions so that he or she can give you the most accurate exam (e.g., instead of "murmur," write the indication as "exclude tricuspid regurgitation").

CARDIOLOGY ABBREVIATIONS

AS: aortic stenosis
ASD: atrial septal defect
AV: arteriovenous or atrial-ventricular
BVH: biventricular hypertrophy
IVC: inferior vena cava
JVD: jugular venous distension
LA: left atrium
LAE: left atrial enlargement
LBBB: left bundle branch block
LICS: left intercostal space
LLSB: left lower sternal border
LSB: left sternal border
LUSB: left upper sternal border
LVH: left ventricular hypertrophy
MAP: mean arterial pressure
MPA: main pulmonary artery
MR: mitral regurgitation

MVP: mitral valve prolapse
PAPVR: partial anomalous pulmonary venous return
PDA: patent ductus arteriosus
PS: pulmonic stenosis
RA: right atrium
RAD: right axis deviation
RAE: right atrial enlargement
RBBB: right bundle branch block
RICS: right intercostal space
RUSB: right upper sternal border
RV: right ventricle
RVH: right ventricular hypertrophy
SEM: systolic ejection murmur
SVC: superior vena cava
TAPVR: total anomalous pulmonary venous return
TOF: tetralogy of Fallot
VSD: ventricular septal defect

DEFINITIONS

- Pulse pressure = systolic pressure – diastolic pressure

    - If >40 mm Hg, consider AV fistula, thyrotoxicosis, aortic insufficiency, PDA.

    - If <25 mm Hg, consider AS, pericardial tamponade, pericardial effusion, pericarditis.

- MAP = diastolic pressure + (pulse pressure / 3)

    - A normal MAP in preterm and newborn infants = gestational age + 5.

ACYANOTIC CONGENITAL HEART DISEASE (LEFT-TO-RIGHT SHUNTS)

See Table 8-1.

CYANOTIC CONGENITAL HEART DISEASE (RIGHT-TO-LEFT SHUNTS)

See Table 8-2.

Other cyanotic heart lesions that occur less commonly include pulmonary atresia, Ebstein's anomaly, truncus arteriosus, single ventricle, and double outlet RV.

PALLIATIVE HEART SURGERIES

Atrial Septostomy

- Creates an intraatrial opening to allow mixing.

- *Park*: uses a knife-tipped cardiac catheter.

TABLE 8-1.
ACYANOTIC CONGENITAL HEART DISEASE
(LEFT-TO-RIGHT SHUNTS)

Lesion	Exam	ECG	CXR
VSD	2–5/6 holosystolic murmur at LLSB, loud S_2 if large, ± thrill, ± apical diastolic rumble	Small VSD: normal; medium VSD: LVH ± LAE; large VSD: BVH ± LAE	May have cardiomegaly with increased pulmonary vascular markings
ASD	Wide, fixed split S2; 2-3/6 SEM at LUSB	RAD and mild RVH or RBBB	May have cardiomegaly with increased pulmonary vascular markings
PDA	1–4/6 continuous murmur in infraclavicular area; if large shunt: bounding peripheral pulses with widened pulse pressure	Normal or LVH	May have cardiomegaly with increased pulmonary vascular markings
AV canal	Hyperactive precordium with systolic thrill at LLSB, loud S_2, may have 3–4/6 holosystolic regurgitant murmur along LLSB, may hear MR murmur at apex, may hear middiastolic rumble at LLSB or apex, gallop may be present	RVH and LVH may be present, first-degree AV block, superior QRS axis	Cardiomegaly with increased pulmonary vascular markings
Pulmonic stenosis	Ejection click at LUSB: decreases with inspiration, increases with expiration; S_2 may split widely, SEM ± thrill at LUSB with radiation to back and sides	Mild PS: normal; moderate PS: RAD, RVH; severe PS: RAE, RVH, strain	Normal heart size with normal or decreased pulmonary vascular markings
Aortic stenosis	Systolic thrill at RUSB, suprasternal notch, or over carotids; ejection click which does not vary with respiration; harsh SEM at second RICS or third LICS with radiation to neck and apex, narrow pulse pressure if severe	Mild AS: normal; LVH ± strain as worsens	Normal to increased heart size
Coarctation of the aorta	SEM at LUSB with radiation to interscapular area; BP in lower extremities lower than in upper extremities; weak arterial pulses distal to coarctation; pulse oximetry differs between upper and lower extremities if ductus patent	RVH or RBBB in infancy, LVH in older children	Cardiomegaly and pulmonary venous congestion, rib notching in older children

TABLE 8-2.
CYANOTIC CONGENITAL HEART DISEASE (RIGHT-TO-LEFT SHUNTS)

Lesion	Exam	ECG	CXR
TOF (VSD, overriding aorta, right ventricular outflow obstruction, RVH)	Loud SEM at LUSB, single S_2	RAD, RVH	Boot-shaped heart with normal heart size
Transposition of the great arteries	Extreme cyanosis, single S_2, lower preductal pulse oximetry than postductal	RAD, RVH	"Egg on a string" with cardiomegaly
Tricuspid atresia	Single S_2, murmur of VSD or PDA may be present	Superior QRS axis, RAE, LVH	Normal or slightly enlarged heart, may have boot-shaped heart
TAPVR	Hyperactive RV impulse, gallop, fixed and split S_2, 2–3/6 SEM at LUSB, middi-astolic rumble	RAD, RVH	Cardiomegaly with increased pulmonary vascular markings; "snowman" rarely seen until after 4 mos of age

- *Rashkind*: uses a balloon-tipped cardiac catheter.

Systemic-to-Pulmonary Artery Shunts

- *Classic Blalock-Taussig shunt*: direct end-to-side subclavian artery to pulmonary artery anastomosis on the side opposite of aortic arch.

- *Modified Blalock-Taussig shunt*: Gore-Tex graft placed between the subclavian artery and pulmonary artery.

- *Waterston-Cooley shunt*: ascending aorta to right pulmonary artery anastomosis.

- *Potts shunt*: descending aorta to left pulmonary artery anastomosis.

Cava-to-Pulmonary Artery Shunts

- *Unidirectional Glenn shunt*: SVC to right pulmonary artery anastomosis with ligation of the proximal right pulmonary artery and cardiac end of the SVC.

- *Bidirectional Glenn shunt*: SVC to right pulmonary artery anastomosis.

Transposition Repair Procedures

- Atrial inversion procedures: connects RA to LV (which becomes the pulmonary ventricle) and LA to RV (which becomes the systemic ventricle). *Senning procedure* uses native atrial wall or septum as baffles. *Mustard procedure* uses pericardial or prosthetic intraatrial baffles.

- Arterial switch (*Jatene procedure*): Pulmonary artery and aorta are transected and switched above the valves, and coronary arteries are moved from the old aortic root to the new aorta.

- Transposition with pulmonary artery stenosis (*Rastelli procedure*): VSD is patched such that LV outflow passes through the VSD into the aorta, and a valved conduit is placed between the RV and pulmonary arteries.

SYSTOLIC MURMURS
See Table 8-3.

DIASTOLIC MURMURS
See Table 8-4.

TABLE 8-3.
SYSTOLIC MURMURS

Lesion	Timing and quality	Heard best	Trans-mits to	Miscellaneous
Aortic valve stenosis	Ejection	RUSB	Neck, LUSB, apex	± Thrill, ejection click, possible single S_2
Subaortic stenosis	Ejection	RUSB		No click, may have aortic regurgitant murmur during diastole
Supravalvular aortic stenosis	Ejection	RUSB	Back	± Thrill; associated with Williams syndrome
Pulmonic valve stenosis	Ejection	LUSB	Back	± Thrill, S_2 may be widely split if mild, ± variable ejection click at second LICS
ASD	Ejection	LUSB		Widely split, fixed S_2

(continued)

TABLE 8-3.
CONTINUED

Lesion	Timing and quality	Heard best	Trans-mits to	Miscellaneous
Pulmonary artery stenosis	Ejection	LUSB	Back and both lung fields	P_2 may be loud
Tetralogy of Fallot	Long ejection murmur	Mid-LSB or LUSB		± Thrill, single S_2
Coarctation of the aorta	Ejection	Left inter-scapular area		Pulse disparity
PDA	Continuous	Left infra-clavicu-lar area		± Thrill, bounding pulses
Total anomalous pulmonary venous return	Ejection	LUSB		Widely split and fixed S_2, + S_3 and S_4, diastolic rumble at LLSB
VSD	Regurgitant, harsh, systolic, may be holosystolic	LLSB		May have loud P_2
Complete AV canal	As with VSD	LLSB		Diastolic rumble, may have gallop
Idiopathic, hypertrophic subaortic stenosis	Ejection	LLSB or apex, medium pitch		± Thrill, Valsalva increases murmur, squatting decreases murmur
Tricuspid regurgitation	Regurgitant systolic	LLSB		Triple or quadruple rhythm
Mitral regurgitation	Regurgitant systolic	Mid-precordium	Left axilla	
Mitral valve prolapse	Midsystolic click with late systolic murmur if MR present	Apex		

TABLE 8-4.
DIASTOLIC MURMURS

Lesion	Quality	Heard best	Transmits to
Aortic regurgitation	Decrescendo, high pitched early diastole	Third LICS	Apex
Pulmonary regurgitation	Medium pitched early diastole	Second LICS	Along LSB
Mitral stenosis	Mid- to late diastole	Apex	
Tricuspid stenosis	Mid- to late diastole	LSB	

CONTINUOUS MURMURS

- Begin in systole and continue throughout diastole:

    - Arteriovenous or aortopulmonary connection: PDA, AV fistula

    - Venous hum: turbulent venous flow

    - Turbulent arterial flow: coarctation of the aorta, peripheral pulmonary artery stenosis

BENIGN MURMURS

See Table 8-5.

HEART TONES

See Table 8-6.

ACQUIRED HEART DISEASE

Endocarditis

- **Causes:** Most common cause is streptococcal organisms; staphylococcal organisms are second most common.

- **Symptoms:** malaise, fever.

- **Exam:** new or changed heart murmur, petechiae, splenomegaly, Osler's nodes (tender fingertip nodules), Janeway's lesions (painless macules on palms and soles), splinter hemorrhages, Roth's spots (retinal hemorrhages).

- **Risk factors:** prosthetic heart valves, previous history of endocarditis, complex cyanotic congenital heart disease, systemic-pulmonary shunts, valvular dysfunction, MVP with mitral regurgitation, hypertrophic cardiomyopathy, IV drug abusers.

- **Treatment:** IV antibiotics for 6 wks.

TABLE 8-5.
BENIGN MURMURS

Source	Timing	Heard best	Transmits to	Miscellaneous
Still's vibratory murmur	Grade 2–3/6 systolic ejection murmur, musical, low frequency	LLSB to apex		Louder when supine; usually heard in 3–6 yr olds
Pulmonary ejection murmur	Early to mid-systolic, grade 1–3/6, blowing	LUSB		Usually heard in 8–14 yr olds
Peripheral pulmonic stenosis	High-pitched, blowing, systolic ejection murmur, grade 1–2/6	LUSB	Chest, axillae, back	Heard in newborns
Venous hum	High-frequency, blowing, continuous, grade 1–3/6	Right or left superior infraclavicular area		Disappears when patient is supine and with compression of the neck veins, heard in 3–6 yr olds
Carotid bruit	Systolic, grade 2–3/6	Right supraclavicular area		

TABLE 8-6.
HEART TONES

Sound	Heard best	Represents
S_1	Apex or LLSB	Wide splitting may represent Epstein's anomaly or RBBB.
S_2	LUSB	Physiologic split increases with inspiration; if wide: ASD, PAPVR, MR, PS, RBBB.
		If single S_2: pulmonary HTN, one semilunar valve, severe AS.
		If narrow: pulmonary HTN, aortic stenosis, LBBB.
S_3	Apex or LLSB	Heard in healthy children and adults, can be heard in patients with dilated ventricles.
S_4	Apex	Always pathologic, suggests decreased ventricular compliance.

Myocarditis

- **Causes:** infectious, immune-mediated, collagen vascular disease, toxin-induced
- **Symptoms:** fever, decreased appetite, lethargy, shortness of breath, emesis
- **Exam:** tachycardia, tachypnea, JVD, rales, gallop, hepatomegaly, arrhythmias
- **CXR:** cardiomegaly and pulmonary edema
- **ECG:** low QRS voltages, ST segment, and T-wave changes; QT interval prolongation; arrhythmias
- **Echocardiogram:** atrial and ventricular enlargement, impaired LV function
- **Treatment:** rest, diuretics, inotropics, digoxin, gamma globulin, afterload reduction

Cardiomyopathies

See Table 8-7.

Pericardial Disorders

Pericarditis

- **Etiology:** infectious, uremia, neoplastic disease, collagen vascular disorder, procainamide, hydralazine, postpericardiotomy, post–myocardial infarction
- **Symptoms:** fever, dyspnea, chest pain (classically, radiates to back or shoulder, alleviated by leaning forward, aggravated by lying down)
- **Exam:** pericardial friction rub, tachypnea
- **ECG:** ST segment elevation in most leads, PR segment depression
- **Treatment:** treat underlying condition, rest, analgesia, antiinflammatory agents

Pericardial Effusion

- **Symptoms:** can be asymptomatic, dull ache, or shortness of breath, tachycardia
- **Exam:** if distant heart sounds, be aware of tamponade
- **CXR:** globular, cardiomegaly
- **ECG:** decreased QRS voltage, QRS axis variation with each beat (electrical alternans)

TABLE 8-7.
CARDIOMYOPATHIES

	Dilated	Hypertrophic	Restrictive
Pathophysiology	Myocardial damage leading to atrial and ventricular dilatation	Ventricular hypertrophy with small to normal ventricular size, impaired filling secondary to stiff ventricles	Usually infiltrative or fibrotic disease causes stiff ventricles and thus decreased filling
Contractile function	Decreased	Increased	Normal
Etiology	Infectious, alcohol, doxorubicin, hypothyroidism, muscular dystrophy, collagen vascular disease	Genetic or sporadic	Amyloidosis, sarcoidosis, hemochromatosis, glycogen storage disease, neoplastic infiltration
Symptoms/history	Shortness of breath, fatigue, weakness	Fatigue, shortness of breath, palpitations, chest pain, syncope, family member with sudden death	Shortness of breath, chest pain, weakness, fatigue
Exam	Tachycardia, tachypnea, rales, hepatomegaly, peripheral edema, S_3 gallop, JVD	Often presents in adolescents Exam often with subtle or no findings	Rales, hepatomegaly, tachypnea, JVD, S_3 gallop
CXR	Cardiomegaly and pulmonary congestion	LV enlargement, globular heart	Cardiomegaly, pulmonary congestion
ECG	Rhythm disturbances, tachycardia, possible atrial enlargement	LVH, prominent Q waves, rhythm disturbances, ST segment/T wave changes	Rhythm disturbances
Echocardiogram	Enlarged ventricles, decreased shortening fraction	Hypertrophy, increased contractility	Atrial enlargement with normal ventricular size
Treatment	Digoxin, diuretics, ionotropics	Negative ionotropes (to increase cardiac filling)	Diuretics

- **Echocardiogram:** fluid within the pericardial cavity
- **Treatment:** treat underlying disorder, observation if asymptomatic, pericardiocentesis is symptomatic

Cardiac Tamponade

- **Pathophysiology:** Pericardial fluid causes compression of cardiac chambers, leading to decreased filling, decreased stroke volume and thus, deceased cardiac output.
- **Symptoms:** dyspnea, fatigue.
- **Exam:** JVD, hepatomegaly, peripheral edema, tachypnea, rales, hypotension, tachycardia, muffled heart sounds, decreased capillary refill, pulsus paradoxus (decrease in SBP by >10 mm Hg with inspiration).
- **ECG:** tachycardia, decreased voltage, electrical alternans.
- **Echocardiogram:** RV collapse in early diastole, atrial collapse in late diastole and early systole.
- **Treatment:** pericardiocentesis.

SUGGESTED READING

Behrman RE, Kliegman RM, Jenson HB. *Nelson textbook of pediatrics*. Philadelphia: WB Saunders, 2000.

Critical Care

Run, don't walk, and grab help along the way.

INTRODUCTION

- Critical care is devoted to the understanding of the pathophysiology of life-threatening diseases and to the development of the ability to monitor and treat patients with these diseases.

- Critical care patients require interdisciplinary management.

- Remember that children have tremendous recovery potential and may recover from injuries that adults may not.

- Never underestimate the patient's ability to hear or understand what you verbally or nonverbally say or do when he or she is intubated or sedated.

- Always remember that these children have a family that is anxious and very concerned. Constantly update them and help them cope with their child's disease.

- Remember that there are many different types of ventilators. If you are not familiar with one, always grab the respiratory therapist.

- **Do not panic** if crisis occurs. Always remember the ABCs. *You are not alone*: Call your fellow or attending and use your entire team.

SHOCK

Shock is a clinical syndrome caused by inadequate tissue perfusion that may ultimately lead to deranged homeostatic mechanisms and irreversible cellular damage. It is a clinical diagnosis and should not be judged on the basis of BP alone. Because circulatory function depends on blood volume, vascular tone, and cardiac function, all shock states result from abnormalities in one or more of these factors.

Classification of Shock States

Shock has been classified in many ways, and any classification must allow for overlaps. In other words, any patient in shock, regardless of initial etiology, may have pathophysiologic characteristics of the different types of shock at different periods in the illness. With this preface, shock may be classified according to Table 9-1.

Eventually there is progression to an irreversible stage of shock in which there are abnormalities of multiple organ systems.

TABLE 9-1.
CLASSIFICATION OF SHOCK

| | Types of shock | | | |
	Hypovolemic	Distributive	Cardiogenic	Septic
Etiology	Dehydration Gastroenteritis Deprivation Heat stroke Burns Hemorrhage	Anaphylaxis Neurogenic Drug toxicity Septic	Congenital Ischemic Traumatic Cardiomyopathy Drug toxicity Tamponade	Bacterial Fungal Viral Protozoan
Pathophysiology	Decreased intravascular volume leads to decreased venous return, leading to decreased myocardial preload	Vasomotor tone abnormalities lead to maldistribution of circulatory volume, leading to peripheral pooling and vascular shunting and hypotension	Pump failure Inadequate cardiac output	Invasive organism leads to cytokine release, leading to impaired endothelial, cellular function, leading to circulatory derangements Direct tissue damage
Diagnosis (*history and physical exam* are of utmost importance)	Early compensated Cool extremities Tachycardia Normal BP Increased systemic vascular resistance	Decreased cardiac output Profound hypotension Anaphylaxis leads to other manifestations Spinal shock leads to accompanying bradycardia	Poor perfusion Pulmonary edema Hepatomegaly Cardiomegaly Abnormal heart sounds	Tachypnea Tachycardia, fever, or hypothermia Hyperdynamic circulation followed by hypoperfusion Altered CNS function Oliguria

Decrease in Perfusion Urine Cardiac output Filling pressure (or normal filling pressure)	Increased systemic vascular resistance	Lactic acidemia Impaired organ function Hypoxemia Renal failure Evidence of infection
Uncompensated Hypotension Mental dysfunction Anuria Cardiac and respiratory failure		
Initial treatment	Volume repletion Pressors	Fluid restriction Pressors Diuretics ± after-load reducer	Volume repletion Pressors Antimicrobials

Monitoring

- A high index of suspicion and knowledge of conditions predisposing to shock are important in the early recognition of shock. Once the progression occurs, the likelihood of successful intervention is limited.

- Note assessment of decreased tissue perfusion, changes in body temperature, capillary refill, impaired urine output, tachycardia, tachypnea, decreased pulse pressure and peripheral pulse characteristics, and mental status changes.

- Lab investigations should include serum electrolytes, ionized calcium, CBC, platelet counts, and Hct. ABG analyses and mixed venous O_2 saturation can add further information about the adequacy of tissue perfusion and cardiovascular performance.

- Continuous cardiopulmonary monitoring, pulse oximetry, temperature, and BP measurements are essential. Intraarterial catheters can be used for continuous blood gas and BP monitoring. Consider invasive venous and pulmonary arterial monitoring for determination of cardiac output, volume status, and systemic vascular resistance to guide the management more effectively.

- Urine output of <1 mL/kg/hr suggests renal hypoperfusion.

Treatment

- Management of shock is aimed at optimizing perfusion of critical vascular beds.

- Treatment of the underlying cause is mandatory—e.g., cessation of hemorrhage, antibiotic therapy.

- Fluid resuscitation: 20 mL/kg of isotonic crystalloid (NS, lactated Ringer's) with assessment in between boluses. Colloids and blood products may be necessary. Fluids must be used cautiously if cardiogenic shock is suspected.

- Severe metabolic acidosis may be treated with 1–2 mEq/kg sodium bicarbonate IV. Give sodium bicarbonate cautiously to patients with impaired ventilation because increased intracellular acidosis may occur.

- Use of pressor agents, such as dopamine (Intropin), dobutamine (Dobutrex), epinephrine, and norepinephrine (Levophed), may be used to improve myocardial function and support BP.

- Afterload reduction to improve myocardial performance may be indicated for patients with severe cardiac dysfunction.

- Other abnormalities in the renal, GI, hematologic/coagulation, and CNS systems must be identified and treated, if possible.

MANAGEMENT OF SINGLE VENTRICLES

A variety of congenital heart lesions have the common physiology of complete mixing of the systemic and pulmonary venous returns. These lesions are usually associated with atresia of the atrioventricular or semilunar valves. The result is a single ventricular output that is divided into two parallel circulations, systemic and pulmonary. The relative proportion of flow to these vascular beds is determined by the relative resistances to flow. We can thus divide the single ventricle anatomy into three broad categories (balanced circulation, excessive pulmonary flow, insufficient pulmonary blood flow) that determine the preop management and the surgical treatment.

Balanced Circulation

Balanced circulation occurs when the pulmonary blood flow (Q_p) is equal to the systemic blood flow (Q_s). The aortic saturation will be about 75–85%. Intermediate surgery or medical management may not be needed. See Fig. 9-1A,B.

Excessive Pulmonary Flow

Excessive pulmonary flow occurs when Q_p is greater than Q_s. Arterial saturation is higher, reflecting increased blood flow. If untreated, this may result in congestive heart failure. The primary goal of management is to decrease the pulmonary blood flow.

Medical Management

The goal is to try to decrease systemic vascular resistance so that more blood flows into the systemic circulation. Afterload reduction, such as with nitroprusside (Nipride), may be used. Medications that increase systemic vascular resistance are avoided. Pulmonary vascular resistance may be increased by sedation/muscular relaxation–controlled hypoventilation, mild respiratory acidosis, and decreased inspired O_2. Increased Hct may contribute to increasing pulmonary vascular resistance by increasing blood viscosity.

Surgical Management

Permanent surgical palliation is often necessary after pulmonary vascular resistance decreases after birth, leading to increased pulmonary blood flow. Pulmonary banding is the usual approach. A band is placed around the main pulmonary artery and tightened until O_2 saturation is 75–85% in the aorta or the gradient across the band is 40–60 mm Hg. In hypoplastic left heart syndrome, the pulmonary artery is used in the construction of neoaorta so banding is not performed (Fig. 9-2).

Insufficient Pulmonary Blood Flow

When Q_p is less than Q_s, hypoxemia is present. O_2 saturation may be in the sixties or lower. The goal of management is to increase pulmonary blood flow. See Fig. 9-1C,D.

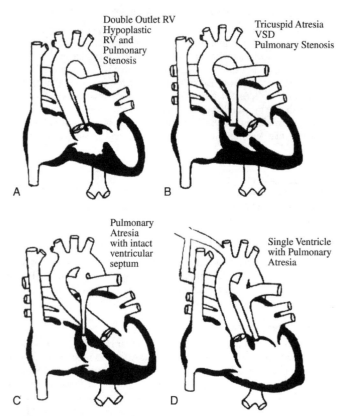

FIG. 9-1.
A,B: Lesions with balanced circulation. **C,D:** Lesions with insufficient
pulmonary blood flow.

Medical Management

The goals are to try to increase systemic vascular resistance and decrease
pulmonary vascular resistance by increasing supplemental O_2, hyperven-
tilating the patient, and inducing a relative alkalosis. Direct pulmonary
vasodilators (e.g., NO and prostacyclin) may be helpful. Systemic vaso-
constrictors (e.g., phenylephrine) may be necessary.

Surgical Management: The Norwood Procedure

Surgical palliation of single ventricles occurs in three steps. The first
includes anastomosis of the proximal main pulmonary artery (MPA) to
the aorta, with aortic arch reconstruction and patch closure of the distal
MPA. A modified Blalock-Taussig shunt is performed to create a sys-

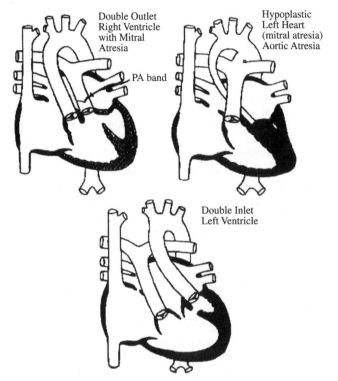

Double Outlet Right Ventricle with Mitral Atresia

PA band

Hypoplastic Left Heart (mitral atresia) Aortic Atresia

Double Inlet Left Ventricle

FIG. 9-2.
Lesions with excessive pulmonary blood flow.

temic to pulmonary shunt. This is followed by the Glenn and Fontan procedures. The ultimate goal is to separate the arterial and venous circulation. This decreases the volume load on the single ventricle that has been pumping blood to both the pulmonary and systemic pulmonary vascular beds. If not corrected, it leads to ventricular failure.

Blalock-Taussig Shunt

A Gore-Tex tube is anastomosed in an end-to-side fashion to both the subclavian artery (innominate artery in hypoplastic left heart syndrome) and the pulmonary artery. This provides adequate pulmonary blood flow. After successful surgery, O_2 saturation is approximately 75–85%, indicative of a balanced circulation.

Glenn Shunt

At about age 4–6 mos, the superior vena cava is anastomosed to the pulmonary artery. At this time, the Blalock-Taussig shunt is taken down. If a pulmonary band was previously done, the surgeon either leaves it alone or transects the main pulmonary artery and oversews the pulmonary valve. These patients will still have cyanosis because the IVC still empties into the heart.

Fontan

- At about age 2–3 yrs, the IVC is anstomosed to the pulmonary artery via either a lateral extracardiac tunnel or a conduit completely excluding the heart. This allows complete separation of the venous and arterial circulations. These patients will have near-normal saturations. The slight reduction in O_2 saturation occurs because the coronary veins, that contain very unsaturated blood, still empty into the heart.

- In many patients undergoing Fontan procedures, a small fenestration is placed between the Fontan circuit and the right atrium, and the atrial septal defect is created or enlarged if necessary. This allows a right-to-left shunt at the atrial level to maintain cardiac output in the event that pulmonary vascular resistance is elevated. BP and cardiac output are maintained while O_2 saturation is decreased. Without this "pop-off" valve, pulmonary blood flow and, subsequently, cardiac output decrease, leading to low O_2 saturation and hypotension with restricted pulmonary flow.

- See Fig. 9-3.

INCREASED INTRACRANIAL PRESSURE

- Elevated ICP is a common sequelae of a variety of CNS insults including trauma, infections, ischemic injury, and metabolic disease.

- ICP results from the interaction of the brain, intracranial blood volume, CSF, and anything else contributing to intracranial volume, such as tumors, hematomas, abscesses, or other mass lesions.

- If the volume of one component of the intracranial vault increases, the volume of the other components, usually blood or CSF, must be reduced to maintain normal ICP. Once the capacity for this mechanism fails, ICP increases. If the pressure is sufficiently high, movement of the brain or brainstem across the tentorium or through the base of the skull can occur. This is defined as *herniation* and can lead to irreversible damage to the brain or brainstem.

Three Types of Cerebral Edema

- **Vasogenic** occurs in tumors, abscesses, intracranial hematomas, and inflammatory conditions such as meningitis and encephalitis. This edema is characterized by increased permeability of brain capillary endothelial cells.

- **Cytotoxic edema** is a result of cellular swelling secondary to cell injury and reflects failure of ATPase-dependent sodium exchange. It

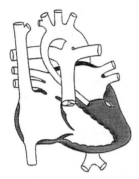

Hypoplastic Left Heart

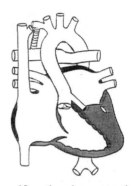

Norwood I: aortic arch reconstruction
with creation of neoaorta from MPA,
Damus-Kaye-Stasel (anastomosis of)
aorta to MPA/neoaorta, atrial
septectomy, BT shunt

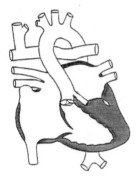

Glenn Shunt (SVC to pulmonary
artery anastomosis)

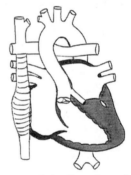

Fontan completion (Lateral tunnel
technique—IVC to pulmonary artery)

FIG. 9-3.
Steps to palliation for hypoplastic left heart syndrome.

may involve all types of cells in the brain and occurs in trauma, diffuse axonal injury, drowning, and hypoxic injury, among others.

- **Interstitial edema** is most often seen in hydrocephalus, where it is the result of increased CSF production.

Cerebral Perfusion Pressure and Cerebral Autoregulation

- The brain depends on a constant blood supply to provide O_2 and metabolic substrates. **Cerebral perfusion pressure (CPP)** must be maintained to keep the integrity of the brain cells.

- **Autoregulation** refers to the brain's ability to maintain cerebral blood flow (CBF) despite fluctuations in mean arterial pressure (MAP). Under normal circumstances, blood flow is well maintained for MAP ranging from 60 to 150 mm Hg. Above and below this range, CBF varies with BP.

- At low BP, the brain blood flow may be inadequate and ischemia occurs.

- In the injured brain, autoregulation may be compromised or completely lost.

- A major factor in autoregulation is the brain's response to changes in arterial O_2 and CO_2 levels. Hypoxia is a potent cerebral vasodilator and hypocapnia is a potent vasoconstrictor. Although other aspects of autoregulation may be lost, these responses are usually preserved in the injured brain.

- CPP is used as a measure of the adequacy of CBF in the injured brain. It is defined by the equation CPP = MAP − ICP.

- Current data suggest that maintaining a CPP >70 mm Hg may be associated with improved neurologic outcome. The optimal CPP in children is unknown, but a goal of keeping CPP >50 mm Hg is probably reasonable.

Increased Intracranial Pressure Monitoring

Maintaining CPP requires monitoring of ICP. This is usually done by a fiberoptic pressure monitor in the brain parenchyma or subdural or epidural space or by an intraventricular catheter (ventriculostomy). The latter offers the advantage of the therapeutic removal of CSF. Monitor-associated complications are rare but include infection, hemorrhage, seizures, and inaccurate readings.

Airway Management for Patients with Elevated Intracranial Pressure

- Stimulation of the oropharynx or larynx produces a vagally mediated reflex increase in ICP; therefore, endotracheal intubation in patients at risk for elevated ICP must include measures to blunt this response.

- This is most commonly done with the use of sedatives and nondepolarizing neuromuscular blocking agents and also administering either sodium thiopental (Pentothal) (1–2 mg/kg IV) or lidocaine (1 mg/kg IV or per ETT), which directly inhibit the ICP response. Avoid drugs, such as ketamine (Ketalar), that increase CBF. Avoid hypoxia: Preoxygenation before intubation is essential.

Treatment of Elevated Intracranial Pressure in Children

The primary goal in caring for patients with elevated ICP is *prevention of secondary brain injury*. This is achieved by maintaining an adequate supply of O_2 and nutrients to the injured brain and avoiding further insults such as ischemia or excessive metabolic demands (e.g., seizures, hyper-thermia). Therapy is directed at maintaining CPP by ensuring that BP (MAP) is adequate and keeping ICP as low as possible. Additional fluid boluses or vasopressor medications may be needed to maintain MAP.

Surgical

Surgical evacuation of mass lesions may occur, but surgical manage-ment is often insufficient as there is often significant residual brain edema leading to elevated ICP.

Medical

Medical management is directed at decreasing ICP by minimizing cerebral metabolism (which increases cerebral blood volume) and con-trolling excessive CBF while maintaining CPP to ensure adequate delivery of O_2 and metabolic substrates to the brain cells.

Temperature Control

Increased metabolic demand from fever can increase CBV and ICP and damage brain cells. A cooling mattress and rectal acetaminophen can be used to maintain normothermia. Shivering can be controlled by muscle paralysis.

Head Position

Head position at 15–30 degrees facilitates venous drainage to help decrease cerebral blood volume.

Seizure Control

Seizures greatly increase cerebral metabolism and blood flow and must be aggressively treated. Consider prophylaxis with phenytoin or phenobar-bital for patients at high risk, including those with penetrating brain injury, intracranial hematomas, and depressed skull fracture. For acute seizure control, lorazepam (Ativan), 0.1–0.2 mg/kg IV repeated at 5 mins; phen-ytoin (Dilantin), 10 mg/kg IV repeated if necessary in 30 mins; and phe-nobarbital (Solfoton), 10 mg/kg IV repeated in 30 mins may be used.

Fluid Management

Overhydration must be avoided. Isotonic fluids like lactated Ringer's or NS must be used. Relative hypotonic solutions such as 0.45% saline may be used in children. Hyponatremia and hypotonic fluids must be avoided. Hyperglycemia should be avoided, and avoidance of glucose-containing IV fluids in the first 24 hrs is recommended. Serum glucose levels must be monitored closely.

Sedation

Decreasing brain metabolism and agitation with sedatives can be very effective in helping control elevated ICP. Benzodiazepines ± opiates are commonly used. A short-acting barbiturate, such as sodium thiopental, may be effective for sedation before noxious procedures such as ETT suctioning or moving the patient. A nondepolarizing neuromuscular blocking agent may be added to prevent coughing or fighting against the ventilator as these are associated with increased ICP.

Cerebrospinal Fluid Removal

CSF removal with intraventricular catheters is often beneficial for ICP control. In patients with severe edema and very small ventricles, CSF removal may be of little benefit.

Osmotic Agents and Diuretics

Mannitol (Osmitrol, Resectisol), given at doses of 0.25–1 g/kg, is the most commonly used osmotic agent to control ICP. It may be given as intermittent doses for acute ICP elevations or scheduled q4–6h, while closely monitoring serum osmolarity, being careful to keep it below 320–325 mOsm/L. Furosemide (Lasix), which directly inhibits CSF production, can be used in addition to mannitol alone for ICP control. Because a brisk diuresis ensues, close monitoring of intravascular volume is important. Hypertonic saline (3%) has also been studied as an osmotic agent with similar efficacy as mannitol.

Hyperventilation

Hyperventilation leads to hypocapnia and cerebral vasoconstriction, leading to decrease in CBV and ICP. $PaCO_2$ levels of 30–35 mm Hg are well tolerated over long periods of time and may produce better overall outcome. Transient aggressive hyperventilation may be used for acute control of increased ICP, but chronic hyperventilation can cause further cerebral ischemia if continued for long periods.

Barbiturate Coma

Barbiturate coma, which decreases CBF by decreasing cerebral metabolism, can be considered for patients with ICP refractory to maximal medical and surgical therapy. A pentobarbital loading dose of 5–10 mg/kg followed by continuous infusions of 1–5 mg/kg/hr with dose titration to clinical effect is an initial starting point. High-dose barbiturate therapy commonly produces hypotension and additional fluid boluses or vasopressor therapy is often necessary.

Steroid Therapy

Steroid therapy is currently only indicated for vasogenic edema.

POSTOP CARE OF CARDIAC SURGERY PATIENTS

Successful postop management of cardiac patients can be achieved by the following:

- Knowledge of preop anatomic diagnosis and pathophysiologic effects of the defect.

- Understanding of operative details and potential complications
- Careful postop ICU management

Preop Details

The ICU team should be familiar with the salient historical details of the patient scheduled for surgery even before the patient is taken to the OR. This includes

- Prenatal course and gestational age, if pertinent
- Age and weight of the patient
- Anatomic details of the lesion
- Pathophysiologic effects before surgery
- General health of the patient
- Noncardiac medical and surgical history
- Results of any diagnostic procedures (echocardiogram, MRI, cardiac catheterization) and radiographic studies

Operative Details

- Note details of the operation, including anesthetics used, the duration of cardiopulmonary bypass, aortic cross-clamp, and circulatory arrest.
- Note details about the surgical approach, ease of coming off bypass, and intraop complications such as dysrhythmias, bleeding, or air embolism.
- A TEE is usually done in the OR to evaluate for residual defects. These and any other problems encountered need to be understood.
- Understanding of the hemodynamics before, during, and after the operation is helpful in the postop care of the patient.

ICU Management

Initial management is directed at stabilizing the patient in the ICU after transport from the OR, including

- Verification of placement of ETT and providing initial ventilator settings if the patient is intubated. Current medications, dosages, and IV fluids must also be verified.
- Physical exam focusing on the cardiovascular and respiratory systems. Heart rate and rhythm, presence of any murmurs and rubs, cardiac impulse, peripheral pulses and perfusion, and presence of hepatomegaly must be noted. Assess adequacy of respiration and breath sounds. Any catheters and pacing wires that the patient might have need to be noted.

- Interpretation of data from bedside monitoring is important—e.g., central venous and left atrial pressures, arterial BP and pulse pressure, wave forms of all transduced catheters, pulse oximeter, mixed venous saturations (if available), urine output, and chest tube drainage/bleeding.

- Chest radiograph for position of the ETT; right and left atrial and central venous catheters and pacing wires, if present, must be checked.

- ECG is performed if the cardiac rhythm is unclear. The requirement for temporary pacing and the underlying rhythm need to be noted.

- Initial lab analysis: arterial blood gas analysis; serum Na, K, Cl; glucose; ionized Ca; Mg levels. Hgb/Hct, WBC, platelets, PT/PTT.

- Document physical exam, lab studies, and evaluate the success of the procedure. Discuss plans for the first postop night with the surgical team.

Maintenance of Cardiac Output

Maintaining adequate cardiac output is a critical determinant of success in managing the recovery of postop cardiac patients. Low cardiac output in the postop patient can result from the following factors:

- Residual or unrecognized structural defects

- Continuation of preop ventricular dysfunction

- Myocardial dysfunction related to intraop procedures, reperfusion injury, effects of bypass, and hypothermia and inadequate myocardial protection

- Type of surgical procedure (e.g., right ventriculotomy)

- Complication of surgery (e.g., compromised coronary artery perfusion)

- Dysrhythmia

- Pulmonary HTN

- Infection

Inadequate cardiac output can be manifested by one or more of the following physical exam features:

- Decreased mental status or irritability.

- Core hypothermia.

- Tachycardia, tachypnea, hypotension, narrow pulse pressure.

- Abnormally increased or decreased cardiac impulse.

- Decreased peripheral perfusion.

- Enlarged liver size.

- Rhythm other than normal sinus rhythm.

- Decreased mixed venous O_2 saturation or increased difference between arterial and venous O_2 saturations (a-v DO_2).

- Metabolic acidosis.

- CXR showing cardiac enlargement and pulmonary edema.

- CVP and LA pressure readings may give insight into the specific causes of low cardiac output. Low readings are seen in hypovolemia. High readings may indicate ventricular dysfunction, poor ventricular compliance, or cardiac tamponade.

One or more factors contributing to cardiac output—heart rate, preload, afterload and contractility—can be manipulated in order to treat a patient with low cardiac output.

Thorough physical exam and interpretation of available data needs to be done. Depending on the reason for low cardiac output, treatment may include

- Judicious use of colloids or crystalloids to increase filling pressure

- Inotropic support for decreased myocardial contractility

- Vasodilators to decrease afterload in patients with increased systemic vascular resistance

- Correction of serum electrolytes, including calcium and magnesium

Echocardiogram and/or cardiac catheterization may be necessary to evaluate for significant residual anatomic lesions and to help determine if reoperation is indicated.

Fluids, Diuretics, and Nutrition

- Patients are kept on routine maintenance fluids, supplemented with boluses as needed.

- Most postop cardiac surgery patients require diuretics after 12–24 hrs.

- Nutrition, either enteral or parenteral, is usually started within 24–72 hrs after operation. If the patient requires prolonged mechanical ventilation, nutrition is given through a NG feeding tube or as TPN, if enteral feeding is not indicated.

MECHANICAL VENTILATION

Mechanical ventilation uses positive pressure to move gas into the lungs. Although modern ventilators offer several different modes, the goal is to select a strategy that maintains oxygenation and ventilation, is comfortable to the patient, and causes minimal trauma to the lung.

Major Indications

- Respiratory failure.

  - Apnea or respiratory arrest

- Inadequate oxygenation, inadequate ventilation (CO_2 removal), or both

- Respiratory pump failure (neuromuscular disease, sedation, anesthesia, or neuromuscular blockade)

- Alveolar disease (pulmonary edema, pneumonia, acute respiratory distress syndrome [ARDS])

- Impaired respiratory drive

- Cardiovascular dysfunction.

- To decrease systemic or myocardial O_2 consumption.

- Clinical condition requiring controlled ventilation (intracranial HTN, surgical, or ICU procedure).

- Upper airway disease requiring intubation.

- A primary objective is avoiding iatrogenic ventilator-induced lung injury or other complications such a pneumothorax, cardiovascular compromise, or respiratory muscle atrophy.

Basic Principles of Mechanical Ventilation

Two basic principles guide ventilator management:

- Lung volume is determined by MAP. MAP is influenced by PEEP, peak airway pressure, and inspiratory time.

- Minute ventilation is determined primarily by the respiratory frequency and the tidal volume.

In all modes of conventional mechanical ventilation, a regulated gas flow generates pressure (airway pressure) that moves a volume (tidal volume) of gas into the lung. The modes differ in which parameter(s)—flow, pressure, or volume—are set by the clinician. The most common modes of ventilation are those in which the clinician sets either the tidal volume (volume control) or the peak airway pressure (pressure control). For most patients, volume control modes are comfortable and provide adequate gas exchange with minimal risk of injury to the lung. For patients with conditions that decrease lung compliance such as severe pneumonia or ARDS, pressure control modes may be safer because they limit the high airway pressures that may be necessary in these conditions. For patients with large leaks around the ETT or tracheostomy tube, pressure control modes can compensate for the volume lost via the leak. Newer ventilators allow setting of both a tidal volume and an airway pressure limit (e.g., pressure-regulated volume control). Most ventilators allow ventilation to be synchronized to respiratory effort in the spontaneously breathing patient to increase patient comfort. Patient effort is sensed either as initiation of inspiratory flow (flow triggering) or as a reduction in the airway pressure (pressure triggering).

In addition to controlling the volume or pressure delivered, the clinician can adjust the timing and pattern of the ventilator delivered breaths. This is described as mandatory, assisted, or supported ventilation.

Mandatory (Controlled) Ventilation

- Volume or pressure controlled.

- The machine provides a set number of breaths with the set tidal volume or pressure limit. Inspiratory time is fixed for mandatory ventilation.

- Useful for patients with limited and/or absent respiratory drive— e.g., patients who are apneic from sedation, anesthesia, CNS injury, drug overdose, and neuromuscular blockade, or for patients whose respiratory drives need to be suppressed.

- **Intermittent mandatory ventilation (IMV)** allows spontaneous breathing between ventilator breaths delivered at a fixed interval.

- **Synchronous IMV** refers to IMV breaths that are synchronized with the patient's breathing effort. If the ventilator does not sense patient effort a mandatory IMV breath is delivered. If the patient makes a respiratory effort between synchronous IMV breaths, spontaneous breathing is allowed.

- See Table 9-2.

Assisted Ventilation

- Volume or pressure controlled.

- For patients with spontaneous respiratory effort assist modes deliver ventilator breaths with a set volume or pressure and with a fixed inspiratory time whenever the ventilator senses patient effort. One drawback is that the inspiratory time is fixed, which may be uncomfortable for the spontaneously breathing patient.

- In **assist control** mode, the machine provides a preset tidal volume or pressure in response to patient-initiated breaths; it also delivers the mechanical tidal volume at a preset frequency if the patient fails to initiate a breath within a preselected time. Patients with weak respiratory effort get complete, maximal support. This allows patient-ventilator synchrony but can lead to hyperventilation and respiratory alkalosis.

Supported Ventilation

- Frequency and inspiratory time of ventilator breaths are regulated by patient effort. Support modes can only be used for patients with adequate respiratory drive.

- **Pressure support ventilation (PSV)** is a commonly used mode of supported ventilation in which the ventilator gives an inspiratory

TABLE 9-2.
MODES OF MANDATORY MECHANICAL VENTILATION

Mode	Volume control	Pressure control
Clinician-set parameter	Tidal volume.	Peak inspiratory pressure.
Variable parameter	Peak inspiratory pressure.	Tidal volume.
Mean airway pressure	Lower for given tidal volume, I-time, and peak airway pressure.	Higher for given tidal volume, I-time, and peak airway pressure.
Other parameters to set	Rate, PEEP, inspiratory time, FIO_2.	Rate, PEEP, inspiratory time, FIO_2.
Flow pattern	Constant inspiratory flow.	Decelerating inspiratory flow.
Advantages	Guaranteed tidal volume and minute ventilation.	Peak airway pressure is limited.
	Changes in respiratory system compliance easily detected (peak inspiratory pressure increases).	Decelerating flow pattern can decrease peak airway pressure and increase mean airway pressure, decreasing risk of further lung injury.
Disadvantages	Peak airway and alveolar pressures may vary excessively. Continuous flow may be low enough to cause patient discomfort, asynchrony, and increased work of breathing.	Tidal volume varies with changes in compliance and may be too high or too low. Changes in respiratory system compliance are not as easily detected.

I-time, inspiratory time.

flow of gas with a decelerating flow pattern whenever the patient triggers a breath, to a preset pressure limit. Patient effort regulates the respiratory cycle. The tidal volume is determined by the patient's effort, preset pressure limit, and respiratory system compliance. PSV may decrease inspiratory work caused by ETT impedance.

• PSV may be combined with synchronous IMV modes of ventilation whereby the spontaneous patient breaths are supplemented with pressure support. These modes may be used in weaning the patient from mechanical ventilation.

Continuous Positive Airway Pressure (CPAP)

• A method of respiratory support whereby a constant level of pressure is maintained in the circuit while the patient breathes spontaneously. *Patients must have an adequate respiratory drive.* CPAP improves gas exchange and decreases respiratory effort by helping maintain end expiratory lung volume. It is used noninvasively for patients with upper airway obstruction or a tendency for airway collapse. CPAP may also be used during weaning from mechanical ventilation before extubation.

Pressure-Regulated Volume Control (PRVC)

- Newer ventilators combine the advantages of a guaranteed tidal volume (like volume control) with a decelerating inspiratory flow pattern to limit airway pressure (like pressure control). This strategy may minimize risks for ventilator-induced lung injury and maximize patient comfort. Mechanical ventilation in these modes can be provided as assist control ventilation with a set inspiratory time and minimum rate or as **"volume support"** ventilation (similar to PSV) with a patient-regulated respiratory cycle and a minute volume guarantee. If patient effort decreases, tidal volume is augmented by increasing gas flow (within preset limits) to maintain minute ventilation. A potential disadvantage is that an unnatural respiratory pattern of slow, large breaths may occur.

- The Servo 300 ventilator combines the pressure-regulated volume control and volume support options with the "auto mode." In this mode, the ventilator provides control ventilation with pressure-regulated volume control until the ventilator senses spontaneous respiratory effort. The machine then switches to "volume support" whereby the patient regulates the respiratory rate and cycle length. If the patient becomes apneic, the ventilator automatically switches to "auto mode off" and returns to the pressure-regulated volume control mode. For some patients, auto mode can be useful as a weaning mode.

Setting Ventilator Parameters

- **Tidal volume:** The average resting tidal volume for a spontaneously breathing nonintubated person is 5–7 mL/kg. To account for volume lost in the ventilator circuit and lack of natural sigh breaths (which expand the lung bases and maintain functional reserve capacity), a larger tidal volume of 10–15 mL/kg is selected. The goal is to achieve a net delivered tidal volume of 8–10 mL/kg. An adequate tidal volume produces an adequate chest rise. For patients with diffuse lung injury, smaller tidal volumes (6–8 mL/kg) may be associated with a decreased risk of further lung injury.

- **Rate:** Physiologic norm for age is selected and then adjusted according to assessment of $PaCO_2$.

- **Inspiratory time:** Physiologic, age-specific I-time resulting in average inspiration to expiration ratio of 1:2 is selected. Reasonable starting points are 0.4–0.5 secs for infants, 0.6–0.8 secs for younger children, and 0.8–1.2 secs for adolescents and adults.

- **FIo$_2$:** Determined by the clinical circumstances. Attempts should be made to keep it below nontoxic levels, usually <60%.

- **PEEP:** 3–5 cm H$_2$O is usually sufficient for most patients. Higher levels may be needed for patients with impaired lung compliance. Increases are made in 1- to 2-cm H$_2$O increments with careful attention to the hemodynamic effects. Excessive PEEP may decrease venous return and cause overdistention of the lung.

- Clinical assessment of aeration and chest wall movement are essential. Evaluation for effective ventilation and oxygenation should be done by ABG analysis or with appropriate noninvasive methods (e.g., pulse oximetry or end-tidal CO$_2$ monitoring).

Discontinuing Mechanical Ventilation

When the reason for beginning mechanical ventilation has resolved, the patient is weaned from the ventilator. While many approaches to weaning are used, the weaning strategy and duration of weaning depend on the clinical condition of the patient. Patients intubated for a short time are often weaned rapidly, whereas after a prolonged illness, weaning may need to be done slowly. A general guideline is to gradually decrease the level of work done by the ventilator to allow increased patient respiratory effort. Depending on the mode of ventilation being used, this is commonly done by decreasing the number of mandatory breaths, or amount of pressure support or tidal volume provided by the ventilator. The patient response to reductions in level of mechanical support is closely monitored to ensure adequate patient comfort, oxygenation, and ventilation. Mechanical ventilation is discontinued when the clinician is confident that the patient can comfortably maintain adequate gas exchange with minimal mechanical support.

SUGGESTED READING

Fuhrman BP, Zimmerman JJ, ed. *Pediatric critical care*. St. Louis: Mosby, 1992.

Nichols DG, et al., eds. *Critical heart disease in infants and children*. St. Louis: Mosby, 1995.

Rogers MC, ed. *Textbook of pediatric intensive care*, 3rd ed. Baltimore: Williams & Wilkins, 1996.

10 Dermatology

If it's wet, make it dry; if it's dry, make it wet.

INTRODUCTION
Skin disorders are one of the most common consults in pediatric practice.

- Never underestimate the parental concerns about rashes. There are many implications: Is it infectious? Is the child sent home from day care due to it? Is it disabling the child? Remember kids with eczema can be irritable, fussy, and hard to take care of.

- Exam of the skin requires observation and palpation of the entire body under good light.

- Description of onset and duration of the primary lesion and its secondary changes should be recorded.

- Clues to the diagnosis may be obtained from the characteristic morphologic arrangement and distribution of the lesions.

- Proximity to a good dermatologic atlas is always helpful.

NEONATAL RASHES
- **Cutis marmorata:** transient mottling when exposed to cold.

- **Erythema toxicum neonatorum:** erythematous macules, papules, or pustules anywhere on the body of unknown etiology. They may range from a few to a confluent eruption. They appear from 3–4 days of life up to 2 wks and last about 2 days. Wright stain shows abundant eosinophils. It is self-limiting.

- **Transient neonatal pustular melanosis:** self-limited vesiculopustular lesions that rupture easily and leave hyperpigmented macules on the neck, chin, forehead, lower back, and shins. The lesions are sterile, and Wright stain shows neutrophils and cellular debris. They fade over several mos.

- **Acne neonatorum:** comedones, pustules, and papules on the face resembling acne vulgaris. May be present at birth and resolve in 6 mos to a year. No treatment required except in severe cases (mild keratolytic agent).

- **Milia:** 1- to 2-mm pearly white papules on nose and cheeks secondary to retention of keratin in the pilosebaceous follicle. Usually disappear spontaneously 3–6 wks of life. The oral counter part are called **Epstein's pearls.**

- **Miliaria:** sweat retention due to keratinous plugging and obstructing sweat glands.

- **Miliaria crystallina:** obstruction at level of stratum corneum. 1- to 2-mm vesicles without erythema on intertriginous areas, neck, and chest.

- **Miliaria rubra:** deeper obstruction in the epidermis. Erythematous papules in same areas. Worsened by heat and humidity.

- **Harlequin color change:** transient erythematous flush on dependent half of the body when patient placed on one side.

BIRTH MARKS

- **Mongolian spots:** blue-black poorly circumscribed macules on lumbosacral areas, or lower extremities. Seen on blacks, Asians, and Hispanics. Present at birth, but they fade some at 1–2 yrs old and disappear when child is 7–13 yrs old.

- **Café au lait spots:** light brown macules anywhere in the body. Six or more >0.5 cm in diameter in prepubertal children, or >1.5 cm in postpubertal, as well as inguinal or axillary freckling are suggestive of neurofibromatosis-1. Association with other disorders: McCune-Albright syndrome, LEOPARD syndrome, Silver-Russell syndrome.

- **Congenital melanocytic nevi:** collection of melanocytes in a macule or papule ± hair, present at birth or first year of life. Up to 8% may transform into melanoma.

- **Port wine stain:** large pink/purple reddish macules. If on face, consider Sturge-Weber syndrome.

- **Telangiectactic nevi/salmon patch ("stork bite"):** flat, pink lesion on scalp or neck. Ones on eyelids usually improve at 3–6 mos and fade out by 3 yrs. Those on back of neck may persist. Treatment: observation, dye laser.

- **Hemangioma:** usually appears within the first month of life and enlarges during the first year, begins to regress after 1 yr of age. Large facial hemangiomas may be associated with posterior fossa malformations. If disfiguring, can be treated.

ACNE VULGARIS

Disorder of the pilosebaceous unit. Etiology is multifactorial: increased sebum secretion, increased propionibacterium acnes (it releases hydrolytic enzymes that damage follicle wall), follicle obstruction, and genetic predisposition.

Clinical Presentation

Primary sites are face, chest, back, and shoulders. There are two types: inflammatory (papules and pustules <5 mm, scarring, and cysts) and non-inflammatory (comedones that are black and open or white and closed).

Treatment

- **Patient education:** Avoid using oil-containing moisturizers, cosmetics, and hair products. Diet plays no role. Premenstrual flare-ups may occur.

- **Medications:**

  - **Topical comedolytics:** (a) benzoyl peroxide: antibacterial effect. Good on inflammatory or mixed acne. Available in 2.5%, 5%, and 10%. Apply once/day and increase strength gradually. Side effects: irritation, dryness, and peeling. (b) Topical retinoids: increased cell turnover normalizing keratinization; reverses comedone formation. Indicated on comedonal acne. Available in tretinoin cream (Retin A) 0.025%, 0.05%, 0.1%; and gel 0.01%, 0.025%, and 0.05%. It should be used qhs, and sunscreen should be recommended.

  - **Topical antibiotics:** kill *Propionibacterium acnes* and decrease inflammation. Useful in mild to moderate inflammatory acne. Are used in conjunction with comedolytics but at different hours. Available: erythromycin solution (Eryderm) 1.5–2%, clindamycin gel (Cleocin) 1%.

  - **Oral antibiotics:** useful in moderate to severe inflammatory acne. Suppress *P. acnes* and decrease free fatty acids, which are the main irritants of sebum. TMP-SMX (Bactrim, Septra), erythromycin or tetracycline (Achromycin, Panmycin, Sumycin, Tetracap) or doxycycline (Monodox, Periostat, Vibramycin) and minocycline (Dynacin, Minocin, Vectrin). Therapy should be continued for 2–3 mos until lesions are improved. Do not use tetracycline, doxycycline, or minocycline in children <8 yrs old.

  - **Oral retinoids:** isotretinoin (Accutane). Ideal therapy for severe nodulocystic scarring acne. Requires close monitoring of lipid profile, SGOT, SGPT, CBC, and strict contraception because it is a teratogenic drug. Dose is 0.5–1 mg/kg/day. Should be administered by dermatologists.

  - **Others:** Oral contraceptives are helpful on severe pustulocystic acne. They suppress the androgenic stimulation of sebum production.

ECZEMA

Atopic Dermatitis

Most common in children. Characterized by pruritic, erythematous, papular, and vesicular lesions with borders merging into the surrounding skin and of unknown etiology that have three clinical phases:

- **Infantile:** onset at 2–3 mos; ends at 18–24 mos old. Patches on cheeks, scalp, trunk, and extensor surfaces of the extremities.

- **Childhood or flexural:** only one-third of patients progress to it. From 2 yrs to adolescence. Patches on antecubital, popliteal fossae, neck, wrists, and feet.

- **Adolescent:** One-third of patients with atopic dermatitis present in the hands only. Atopic dermatitis is most frequent in patients with hypersensitivity, asthma, and hay fever during winter season. Patients can also have other features such as lichenification, keratosis pilaris (cornified plugs of the hair follicles), accentuated palmar creases, and atopic pleats and be hyperactive and restless.

- **Therapy:** bathing without soap, frequent lubrication, low or mid-strength topical corticosteroids, cotton clothing, decreased exposure to smoke and dust mites. Only low-potency steroids should be applied on face and intertriginous areas.

Winter or Asteatotic

Characterized by dry skin with large pruritic, cracked scaly patches with erythematous borders. Frequent in arid climates or in winter. Stratum corneum of skin depends on humidity; when <30%, it loses water and shrinks, predisposing to dermatitis. **Therapy:** humidifiers, petrolatum, and emollients; avoid soap.

Nummular

Numerous coin-shaped plaques of minute scaly pruritic papules and vesicles on an asteatotic skin on the extensor surfaces of the hands, arms, and legs. Etiology is unclear. **Therapy:** frequent lubrication, limited baths, topical corticosteroids (use low potency on face).

Infectious Eczematoid Dermatitis

Second bacterial infection superimposed on lesions of atopic, nummular, or seborrheic dermatitis. Most common organism: *Staphylococcus aureus.* **Therapy:** systemic antibiotics and topical corticosteroid ointment.

PITYRIASIS ALBA

- Discrete hypopigmented patches with well-delineated margins, and fine branny rash on the face, neck, upper trunk, and proximal extremities of unknown etiology. Associated with atopic dermatitis. Lesions usually appear after sun exposure.

- **Therapy:** mild topical corticosteroids, lubrication, and sun exposure.

SEBORRHEIC DERMATITIS

- Oval patches covered by thick, yellow, greasy crusts on scalp (increased sebum production) on face, eyebrows, forehead, nose, diaper area, postauricular area, scalp, intertriginous areas, and perineal areas. Although etiology unknown, it is related to *Malassezia.*

- It appears at 2–10 wks of life and lasts until 8–12 mos and can recur in puberty.
- Called "cradle cap" when confined to scalp of infants.
- Blepharitis is seborrhea on eyelid margins. It is important to differentiate from psoriasis.
- **Therapy:** frequent use of shampoos containing sulfur or salicylic acid, zinc pyrithione, selenium sulfide, ketoconazole, corticosteroids, or tar. Use mild topical corticosteroids. Blepharitis is treated with warm water compresses and baby shampoo.

CONTACT DERMATITIS

- Type IV hypersensitivity (delayed/cell mediated). Occurs within 7–10 days or after months to years of exposure to a sensitizing substance, and within 8–12 hrs of reexposure. Incidence increases with age.
- Acute eczematous lesion characterized by an intense erythema accompanied with edema, papules, and vesiculation mixed with crusting, scaling, and thickening of the skin in the distribution of exposure.
- The major sources are metals (nickel), shoes, preservatives, fragrances, topical medications, and plants (poison ivy).
- **Therapy:** complete avoidance of the offending allergen; topical corticosteroids.

TINEA

Dermatophytoses include the following:

Tinea Capitis

The most common one. A fungal infection of the scalp characterized by round scaling and inflammatory, patchy alopecia in prepubertal children (2–10 yrs old). *Microsporum* and *Trichophyton* species are associated as etiologic agents.

- Kerion: sharply demarcated, painful, inflammatory, boggy tumefaction.
- Diagnosis: clinically and by potassium hydroxide slide preparation. Tiny arthrospores surrounding the hair shaft and within the hair are seen. They can also be grown in Sabouraud agar.
- **Therapy:** griseofulvin microcrystalline (Fulvicin-U/F, Grifulvin V, Grisactin), 10–20 mg/kg/day; ultra-microcrystalline, 5–10 mg/kg/day (maximum, 500 mg PO qd × 4–6 wks. If not well tolerated or ineffective, may try terbinafine (Lamisil) or itraconazole (Sporanox). Topical antifungals are ineffective. Nizoral or selenium sulfide shampoo.

Tinea Corporis

- Asymmetrically distributed superficial fungal infection of the non-hairy skin: face, trunk, limbs. Characterized by one or more annular, sharply circumscribed scaly patches with a clear center and scaly vesicular papular erythematous border.

- Etiology most common in young children: *Microsporum canis, Microsporum audouinii,* and *Trichophyton mentagrophytes.* Transmitted by contact with other individuals, kittens, and puppies.

- **Tinea cruris:** in the groin area.

- **Tinea mannum:** in the hands.

- **Tinea pedis:** in the feet; infrequent in prepubertal age.

- **Tinea barbae:** in the bearded areas.

- **Therapy:** topical application of clotrimazole (Lotrimin), miconazole (Micatin), econazole (Spectazole), terbinafine (Lamisil), or haloprogin (Halotex) applied bid × 3–4 wks or until the affected area is completely clear. Topical antifungals are not helpful for nail or hair infections.

Tinea Unguium and Onychomycosis

- Chronic fungal infection of the nails caused by *Trichophyton rubrum, T. mentagrophytes,* and *Epidermophyton floccosum.* Generally occurs in association with tinea mannum or pedis.

- Infection starts on the lateral edge of the distal tip of the nail as an opaque white-yellow patch that then compromises the nail plate, deforming it and accumulating subungual debris. When caused by *Candida albicans,* it is associated with paronychia.

- **Therapy:** griseofulvin (6 mos for fingernails and 12–18 mos for toenails). Has high incidence of recurrence. Topical therapy is usually ineffective.

WARTS

- Caused by DNA viruses: papillomavirus.

- Verrucae vulgaris: round; discrete; flesh-colored; rough, irregular surface. Commonly in clusters around cuticles and dorsal area of the hands.

- Plantar warts: flat, grapelike appearance with thick keratotic plaques on weight-bearing surfaces of heels, toes, and mid-metatarsal areas.

- Flat warts: slightly tan-colored elevated papules on the face, arms, and legs.

- **Therapy:** There is no single effective treatment for warts; they are resistant to therapy and have a high recurrence rate. Liquid nitrogen, salicylic acid, trichloroacetic acid, cryosurgery, or surgical excision may be tried.

MOLLUSCUM CONTAGIOSUM

- DNA-viral infection of the skin and mucous membranes.

- Characterized by groups of umbilicated pearly papules. A pulpy curdlike core can be extracted from them.

- **Therapy:** removal of the lesion, liquid nitrogen, cantharidin.

ERYTHEMA MULTIFORME

- A hypersensitivity reaction to infection or drugs, characterized by target lesions, which are round with a dusky center as a result of epidermal necrosis. They last >1 wk.

- When there is severe mucous membrane involvement including conjunctiva, oral cavity, and genital mucosa, it is considered **erythema multiforme major** or **Stevens-Johnson syndrome.**

- **Treatment** is symptomatic. Antihistamines, IV fluids, removal of offending drugs, adequate nutrition, treatment of secondary infections, cool compresses, and wet dressings can be useful. The use of intravenous immunoglobulin or steroids is controversial.

PATTERNS OF SKIN DISORDERS

See Fig. 10-1.

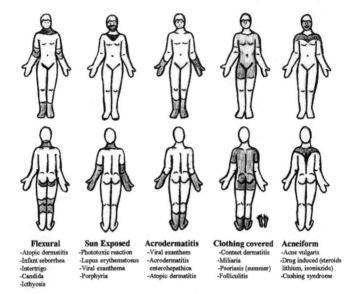

Flexural	Sun Exposed	Acrodermatitis	Clothing covered	Acneiform
-Atopic dermatitis	-Phototoxic reaction	-Viral exanthem	-Contact dermatitis	-Acne vulgaris
-Infant seborrhea	-Lupus erythematosus	-Acrodermatitis	-Miliaria	-Drug induced (steroids
-Intertrigo	-Viral exanthema	enterohepathica	-Psoriasis (summer)	lithium, isoniazide)
-Candida	-Porphyria	-Atopic dermatitis	-Folliculitis	-Cushing syndrome
-Icthyosis				

FIG. 10-1.
Patterns of skin disorders.

SUGGESTED READING

Elewski BE. Tinea capitis: a current perspective. *J Am Acad Dermatol* 2000;42:120.

Hurwitz S. *Clinical pediatric dermatology*, 2nd ed. Philadelphia: WB Saunders, 1993.

Knoell KA, Greer KE. Atopic dermatitis. *Pediatr Rev* 1999;20:46–52.

Mallory S, Leal Khouri S. *An illustrated dictionary of dermatologic syndromes*. New York: Parthenon, 1994.

Roberts LJ. Dermatologic diseases. In: McMillan JA, et al., eds. *Oski's pediatrics: principles and practice*, 3rd ed. Philadelphia. Lippincott Williams & Wilkins, 1999.

Strasburger VC. Acne: what every pediatrician should know about treatment. *Pediatr Clin North Am* 1997;44:1519–1520.

11

Emergencies

Check your own pulse first.

INTRODUCTION

- Remember that ER visits are stressful for parents and children, and if it is a busy day, it can be chaotic; patients and parents can become impatient and restless.

- It is important to prioritize, to be organized and systematic, and to remain calm. *Do not panic!*

- Always think A, A, B, C: anticipation (if possible), airway, breathing, circulation.

- Use your team. Delegate tasks for better patient care.

- If emergent treatment is needed, a brief history relevant to the problem is obtained to institute prompt and appropriate therapy. A more detailed history can be obtained afterward.

- The quiet part of the exam should be done first (lungs, heart, and abdomen); the more threatening parts are examined at the end (ears and throat). If possible, keep the patient on a parent's lap or very close by during physical exam. You may use the parents' help in the exam (e.g., let the parents position the stethoscope on the chest in a scared patient, etc.).

- Keep the parents well informed of the patient's clinical status, management plan, and what to expect.

- Any time you enter a room and find a patient you think is in distress or whom you are uncomfortable dealing with, let your attending or senior resident know immediately.

- Codes: See algorithms in Appendix A.

CARDIOPULMONARY RESUSCITATION

Identification of the cause of cardiopulmonary arrest should be done early because special considerations may affect therapy. Most common causes:

- Traumatic: motor vehicle injury, burns, child abuse, firearm wounds

- Pulmonary: foreign body aspiration, smoke inhalation, near drowning, respiratory failure

- Infectious: sepsis, meningitis

- CNS: head trauma, seizures

- Cardiac: congenital heart disease, myocarditis

- Others: SIDS, poisoning, suicide, dehydration, congenital anomalies

In most patients, hypoxia from respiratory failure causes bradycardia followed by cardiac arrest.

Patients with delayed resuscitation who present in asystole have poor prognosis.

- See algorithms in Appendix A.

Basic Life Support

- The goal is to optimize cardiac output and sustain tissue O_2 delivery (mainly to heart and brain) (Table 11-1).

- See Fig. 11-1 for neonatal resuscitation.

House Officer to House Officer Hints on Airway Management

- Airway management is the first priority in the evaluation of the critically ill or injured pediatric patient.

- Consider all emergency unit patients to have full stomachs.

- Responses to sedation may be difficult to predict.

- Critically ill patients have limited cardiorespiratory reserve.

- Preserve spontaneous ventilation in all potential difficult airways.

- Needle cricothyroidotomy and cricotomy are difficult and have high complication rates. They should not be considered as easy options if intubation fails.

- Always have an escape plan for failed intubation.

- Optimal airway management involves many components, including tracheal intubation, which is a skill that requires a combination of technical expertise, knowledge, and careful clinical judgment to minimize serious complications.

- Do what you do best and keep things simple.

COMA

- **History:** trauma, ingestion, infection, fasting, diabetes, drug use, seizure.

- **Exam:** heart rate, BP, respiratory pattern, temp, pupillary response, rash, abnormal posturing, focal neurologic signs.

- **Management:** airway, breathing, circulation, DextroStick, O_2. If narcotic overdose considered, give naloxone. If infection suspected,

TABLE 11-1.
SUMMARY OF ABC MANEUVERS

Maneuver	Child 1–8 yrs	Infant to 1 yr	Newborn
Airway	Head tilt-chin-lift	Head tilt-chin-lift	Head tilt-chin-lift
	If trauma is present use jaw thrust	If trauma is present use jaw thrust	
Breathing			
Initial	2 breaths at 1–1.5 sec/breath	2 breaths at 1–1.5 sec/breath	2 breaths at 1–1.5 sec/breath
Subsequent	Approx. 20 breaths/min	Approx. 20 breaths/min	Approx. 30–60 breaths/min
Foreign body aspiration	Heimlich maneuver	Back blows and chest thrusts	—
Circulation			
Pulse check	Carotid	Brachial or femoral	Brachial or femoral
Compressions			
Landmark	Lower half of sternum	1 finger width below mammary line	1 finger width below mammary line
Method	Heel of one hand	2 thumbs encircled hands or 2 or 3 fingers	2 thumbs encircled hands or 2 or 3 fingers
Depth	1–1.5 in. or ± one-third to one-half depth of chest	0.5–1 in. or ± one-third to one-half depth of chest	0.5–1 in. or ± one-third depth of chest
Rate	100/min	≥100/min	120/min
Compression/ ventilation ratio	5:1 (pause for ventilation until trachea is intubated)	5:1 (pause for ventilation until trachea is intubated)	3:1 for intubated newborn (two rescuers)

start antibiotics. If diabetic ketoacidosis, consider mannitol. Consider head CT, electroencephalogram.

- **Labs:** CBC, electrolytes, transaminases, ammonia, lactate, toxicology screen, blood gas, blood culture. If infant: plasma amino acids and urine organic acids.

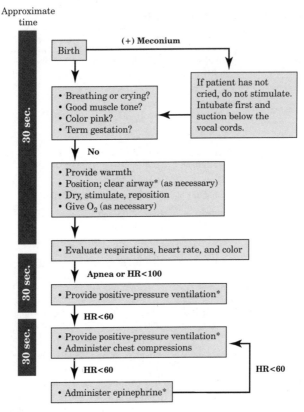

FIG. 11-1.
Neonatal resuscitation. *Endotracheal intubation may be considered at several steps.

TRAUMA

- Most common cause of death during childhood beyond first months of life is injuries.

- Motor vehicle injury is the most common cause of death in all age groups, including children aged <1.

- Drowning ranks second among unintentional trauma deaths with peaks in preschool and late teen years.

Management of the Polytraumatized Patient

Airway, Breathing, and Circulation
Airway

- Immobilize cervical spine.

- Inspect for foreign objects or loose teeth in mouth.

- Intubate if necessary.

Breathing

- Supplemental O_2 if airway patent.

- Consider orogastric tube to decompress stomach.

- Inspect chest for open wounds, pneumothorax.

Circulation

- Direct pressure with sterile gauze to open wounds.

- Heart rate and capillary refill are the best indicator of circulatory status in children (hypotension late).

- IV catheter with two large-bore IVs.

- Intraosseous catheter (if age <8 yrs) or femoral venous line if IV access delayed.

- Rapid infusion of warmed lactated Ringer's or NS at 20 cc/kg for up to three boluses. If patient remains unstable, give colloid and/or blood products and (if not done so already), obtain emergent surgical evaluation.

Secondary Survey

Remove patient's clothing and perform a thorough head-to-toe evaluation.

- **HEENT:** scalp/skull injury, periorbital ecchymosis (? orbital fracture); pinna ecchymosis or hemotympanum (? basal skull fracture); CSF leak from nose or ears; pupil size, corneal reflex, hyphema, cervical spine tenderness or deformity, trachea midline

- **Chest/abdomen/pelvis:** clavicular deformity or tenderness, breath sounds, heart tones, rib tenderness or deformity, chest wall symmetry, SC emphysema, abdominal tenderness or distension, bloody orogastric aspirates, palpate spleen for tenderness, pelvic instability

- **Genitourinary:** rectal tone, blood in stool, blood at urinary meatus

- **Back:** step-off along spinal column, tenderness along spine

- **Extremities:** deformity or pain, neurovascular exam, compartment syndrome
- **Skin:** capillary refill, lacerations, abrasions, contusions
- **Neurologic:** mental status, Glasgow coma scale

Labs

- Hgb/Hct
- Transaminases
- Type and cross
- UA
- Consider toxicology screen

X-Ray Evaluation

- Plain films: cervical spine, chest, pelvis, any extremity with pain or deformity
- CT: low suspicion to obtain head or abdomen CT
- Echocardiogram if indicated

Prevention

- Motor vehicle: <20 lbs: infant seat in rear seat facing backward. >20 lbs: toddler seat in rear seat facing forward. <13 yrs old never in front seat if there is an airbag. Use booster seat and seat belt with shoulder straps.
- Bicycle: Always wear a helmet.

HEAD TRAUMA

- **Concussion:** immediate and transient alteration of consciousness, vision, and equilibrium.
- **Epidural hematoma:** between dura and cranium. Loss of consciousness (LOC) followed by lucid interval. If not treated, results in rapid deterioration. 85% have a skull fracture.
- **Subdural hematoma:** between dura and brain, associated with cerebral contusion and edema. Crescent shape in CT/MRI.
- **Contusion:** associated with skull fractures. Focal symptoms at site of injury or contracoup.

Management

- Minor head trauma with no LOC: (a) thorough history, physical exam, neurologic exam; (b) observe in clinic, office, ER, or home (CT and MRI not recommended).

- Minor head trauma with brief LOC (<1 min): (a) history, physical exam, neurologic exam; and (b) observe or head CT (skull x-rays and MRI not recommended).

- If discharging a patient, it is important that parents understand signs and symptoms for which medical attention should be sought: persistent headache, persistent vomiting 6–8 hrs after injury, drowsiness, weakness, blurry or double vision or ataxia (wake child at 4-hr intervals during night), irritability or change in behavior, neck pain, seizures, fever, watery discharge from nose or ears.

NECK INJURIES

Always rule out a fracture.

Management

- Immobilization of the neck.

- X-ray of the cervical spine (AP, lateral, oblique, and open mouth views).

- If results are normal, obtain flexion extension views to evaluate ligament injury. If the patient is symptomatic, but x-rays are normal, rule out spinal cord hematoma, edema, and stenosis by noncontrast MRI.

- Patients can return to play when they have a full pain-free range of motion, strength, and sensation and normal lordosis of cervical spine.

BURNS

The character of a burn may change over the first few days after the injury. Keep this in mind when deciding whether to admit or not and when discussing prognosis.

General Principles

- Electrical burns often involve tissues in excess of the skin damage.

- High voltage may cause rhabdomyolysis.

- Caution when regarding inhalation when the fire was in an enclosed space, facial burns, singed nares, carbonaceous material in nares or mouth, cough, shortness of breath, and wheezing.

- If there is a chemical burn, clean away remaining chemicals on patient.

Burn Degree

- First: epidermis only; painful and erythematous.

- Second: epidermis and dermis involved, dermal appendages spared. Superficial second-degree burns are blistered and painful. Deep second-degree burns may be white and painless; may require grafting.

- Third: full-thickness burn; leathery and painless. Requires grafting.

Management

- **Airway:** Consider the possibility of airway decline secondary to swelling if inhalational injury. If airway is stable, give humidified 100% O_2. Consider the possibility of CO poisoning if there is a large burn or if the fire occurred in a closed space. In CO poisoning, pulse oximetry may be misleadingly normal. Obtain PaO_2.

- **Breathing:** Monitor closely for signs of distress.

- **Circulation:** 20 cc/kg of lactated Ringer's or NS if body surface area (BSA) >10% in infants or >15% in children. If hypotensive, manage according to trauma principles first. Maintain at least 1 cc/kg/hr.

- **Fluids:**

    - Parkland formula (first 24 hrs): 4 cc/kg × % BSA burned + maintenance fluids, or 5000 mL/m^2 burned area + 2000 mL/m^2 BSA/24 hrs. Give half of this total over the first 8 hrs, then the remaining over the next 16 hrs.

    - Second 24 hrs requirements: usually 50–75% of first day's requirements; calculations should take into consideration urine output, serum electrolytes, weight, and nasogastric losses.

- **Labs:** as indicated by patient status.

- **GI:** Consider NG tube, begin H_2-blocker for stress ulcer prophylaxis.

- **Genitourinary:** Monitor urinary output with Foley.

- **Ophthalmology:** If eye injury suspected, consult ophthalmology.

- **Analgesia:** IV, *not* SC or PO.

- **Burn chart** (see Fig. 11-2).

- **Who to admit?** BSA >10% in infants or >15% in children; electrical or chemical burns; burns involving face, hands, feet, perineum, joints; inhalation injury; children with unsafe environment at home or uncertain if patient will follow up; underlying medical condition.

POISONING
General Approach

- Do not waste time.

- Initial resuscitation and stabilization. ABC, IV access, if comatose bolus of 0.5 g/kg (2 cc/kg D25%) glucose followed by naloxone IV.

- Obtain history, physical exam, and exact information of the substance ingested and its toxicity.

- Obtain ECG and begin lab evaluation to help identify toxic agent or underlying disease.

- Symptomatic treatment if impending death or instability (seizure, arrhythmia, shock).

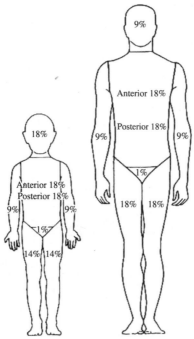

FIG. 11-2.
Rule of nines for child (*left*) and adult (*right*). (Adapted from McMillan JA, et al. *Oski's pediatrics.* 3rd ed. Philadelphia: Lippincott, 1999.)

- Eliminate poison from GI tract, skin, and eyes.

- Discuss case with poison control (1-800-222-1222) or toxicology service.

- Administer antidotes if available.

- Supportive therapy.

Elimination of Ingested Poison

Primary Elimination

- Ideal if <1 hr of ingestion. Not in comatose or obtunded patients.

- Gastric lavage: used to recover pill fragments. Cautiously guard the airway.

- Use normal saline until fluid obtained is clear. Infuse 5–10 mL/kg. May use 0.01 mg/kg of atropine before NG placement.

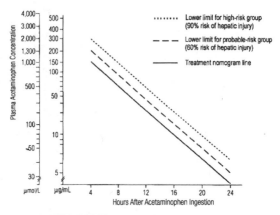

CAUTIONS FOR USE OF THIS CHART:
1. The time coordinates refer to time post ingestion.
2. Serum levels drawn before 4 hours may not represent peak levels.
3. The graph should be used only in relation to a single acute ingestion.

FIG. 11-3.
Nomogram: Plasma or serum acetaminophen concentration vs. time post–acetaminophen ingestion. (From McMillan JA. *Oski's pediatrics: principles and practice*, 3rd ed. Philadelphia: Lippincott Williams & Wilkins, 1999, with permission.)

- Before removal of NG tube, may infuse antidote or activated charcoal.

- Activated charcoal: standard treatment. 0.5–1 g/kg (30–50 g). May repeat 3–4× in first 24 hrs.

- Atropine, barbiturates, chlorpromazine, cocaine, colchicine, digitalis, amphetamines, morphine, phenytoin, salicylates, theophylline, TCAs are known to be absorbed by activated charcoal.

- See Fig. 11-3 for elimination of acetaminophen.

Secondary Elimination

- Cathartics (to increase transit time): magnesium citrate and sorbitol.

- Forced diuresis (caution: some poisons enhance pulmonary edema).

- Alkalinization: for TCA, barbiturates, salicylates, and isoniazide through administering $NaHCO_2$.

- Acidification: for amphetamines, quinine, fenfluramine, and phencyclidine through administering ascorbic acid.

- Hemodialysis, hemofiltration, or peritoneal dialysis: methanol, lithium, ethylene glycol, and salicylates.

- See Table 11-2 for common poisons and antidotes.

TABLE 11-2.
COMMON POISONINGS

Poison	Signs and symptoms	Antidote	Comments
Acetamino-phen	Toxic dose >150 mg/kg N/V, lethargy. >24 hrs: liver damage, jaundice, encephalopathy. >7 days: renal failure See Figure 11-3	N-acetylcysteine 140 mg/kg initial dose, followed by 17 doses of 70 mg/kg q4h. Give activated charcoal if ingestion <4 hrs ago.	If early life-threatening symptoms present, consider multiple drug ingestions. Check level 4 hrs postingestion and repeat q8h if suspect coingestion or if first level is borderline. Check liver enzymes.
Alkaline corrosives	Dysphagia, oral, and esophageal burns	Do not give emetic or do gastric lavage. Controversial use of steroids. If eye or skin contact: rinse with water.	Esophagoscopy 3–5 days afterwards. Esophageal stricture in 15%.
Atropine/antihistamines/anticholinergics	Dry mouth, mydriasis, tachycardia, hyperthermia	Physostigmine 0.02–0.06 mg/kg IV.	Can produce seizures or bradycardia.
Benzodiazepines	Miosis, respiratory depression	Flumazenil (Romazicon), 0.2 mg IV bolus, then 0.2 mg/min up to max 3 mg.	Can precipitate seizures in habituated patients.
Beta blockers	Bradycardia, hypotension	Glucagon, 0.05 mg/kg bolus then 0.07 mg/kg. In adults: 3-mg bolus followed by 5-mg/hr infusion.	—
Barbiturates and anticonvulsants	CNS depression, nystagmus, ataxia, slurred speech	Charcoal, urinary alkalinization.	—
Calcium channel blockers	Hypotension, arrhythmias	Calcium chloride 20 mg/kg.	—

(continued)

TABLE 11-2.
CONTINUED

Poison	Signs and symptoms	Antidote	Comments
Digitalis	Arrhythmia, hyperkalemia	Fab fragments. 80 mg inactivates 1 mg of digoxin.	—
Iron	Nausea, bloody diarrhea, abdominal pain, shock, coma	Deferoxamine (Desferal), 40–90 mg/kg IM q8h or if shock or coma 15 mg/kg/hr × 8 hrs. Hemodialysis if level >180 µmol/L or anuric.	Toxic dose: 20–60 mg/kg iron. High toxic dose: >60 mg/kg. Lethal dose: 200–300 mg/kg.
Narcotics	Miosis, coma, respiratory depression, hypotension	Naloxone (Narcan), 0.1 mg/kg IV.	—
Phenothiazines	As barbiturates and arrhythmia and extrapyramidal reaction	Diphenhydramine (Benadryl, Benylin), 1–2 mg/kg/dose (max 50 mg).	—
Salicylate	Emesis, pyrexia, tinnitus, coma, hyperventilation, seizures, bleeding, metabolic acidosis, and respiratory alkalosis	Gastric emptying if <1 hr. Activated charcoal, urine alkalinization (keep pH 7.5–8), hemodialysis if renal failure, pulmonary edema, salicylate level >100 mg/dL, CNS changes.	Toxic dose >150 mg/kg. Lethal dose >500 mg/kg. Obtain level on admission and 6 hrs postingestion.

BITES

- Contact poison control for advice.

- Tetanus prophylaxis is advisable.

- Antihistamines may help treat minor local symptoms.

Human

- Most common organisms: anaerobes, *Staphylococcus aureus*, and streptococci.

- Management: irrigation and débridement. Leave unsutured.

- Tetanus prophylaxis and antibiotic prophylaxis: (amoxicillin-clavulanic acid [Augmentin] or clindamycin [Cleocin]).

- Joint involvement requires urgent surgical exploration.

Animal

- Most common organisms: anaerobes, *S. aureus*, group A streptococci, *Pasturella multocida*.

- Determine circumstances of attack, animal's state of health. Most animal bites need to be reported; check with your local public health organization.

- Management: high-pressure irrigation and debridement of dead tissue; leave unsutured, especially if in hand or puncture wound. If the wound is on the face, consult a plastic surgeon.

- Tetanus prophylaxis; rabies prophylaxis to be considered.

- Antibiotic prophylaxis: amoxicillin-clavulanic acid or clindamycin.

- Joint involvement requires urgent surgical exploration.

Spiders

- **Brown recluse:** endemic in the southeastern United States; causes local vesicles, redness and swelling in mild cases. Can be painless. In severe cases, local tissue and vascular damage can occur with systemic reactions (hematologic, cardiovascular, and renal): DIC, hemolysis, arthralgias, fever, urticaria, and vomiting. Treatment is supportive; steroid use is controversial. No antivenom available.

- **Black widow:** produces a neurotoxin that causes pain, muscle cramps, and a rigid abdomen rapidly after envenomation. It can also cause ascending motor paralysis, seizures, shock, and fever. Treatment is supportive; diazepam (Valium) and calcium gluconate for muscle spasms; narcotics for pain. Antivenom is available for those not allergic to equine serum.

SEDATION IN CHILDREN

Indications and strategies for procedural sedation should be *individualized* in every patient.

IV Sedations

For IV sedations always remember **AMPLE:**

- Preanesthetic history: **a**llergy, **a**irway history and evaluation, **m**edications, **p**ast medical and anesthetic history (including family history), **l**ast oral intake, recent **e**vents, history, or relevant diagnostic tests.

- NPO time:
  - <6 mos: >4 hrs for solids/formula/breast milk
  - >6 mos: >6 hrs for solids/formula/breast milk
- All age groups can have clear liquids up until 2 hrs before sedation.

Equipment

- Monitoring: pulsoximeter, BP monitor.
- Resuscitation: crash cart, O_2, self-inflating Ambubag with appropriate mask, suction.
- Isotonic IV fluids should be hanging or next to patient.
- Always be ready to manage an emergency airway; remember that the most common side effect of sedatives is *respiratory depression*.

Monitoring

- Heart rate, BP, respiratory rate before sedation, q5–10mins, and until awake. Record this in the patient's sedation record.
- Label all syringes with drug names and dilution concentrations.
- Sedation options: See Table 11-3.
- Sedation medications: See Appendix B, Formulary.

Pain Management

See Appendix B, Formulary.

INTUBATION

Indications

- Facilitate positive pressure ventilation for the treatment of poorly compensated respiratory and cardiac failure.
- Airway protection from aspiration or extrinsic/intrinsic obstruction.
- Tracheobronchial toilet.
- Provide optimal airway control and conditions for diagnostic or therapeutic interventions.

Preparation

- For every intubation prepare the following:
  - Suction
  - O_2

TABLE 11-3.
SEDATION OPTIONS

Type of procedure	Goal	Suggested sedation
Noninvasive		
CT scan, echocardiogram, MRI, electroencephalogram, U/S	Motion control	Comforting alone Age <3 yrs: chloral hydrate Midazolam (Versed) PO, IV, IN; pentobarbital (Nembutal)
Low level of pain and high anxiety		
Dental procedures, IV cannulation, lumbar puncture, foreign body removal, lacerations repair, flexible laryngoscopy, ocular irrigation, and slit lamp exam	Sedation, anxiolysis, motion control	Comforting and topical or local analgesia Nitrous oxide Midazolam PO, IV, IN
High level of pain and high anxiety		
Burn débridement, cardiac catheterization, abscess irrigation and débridement, bone marrow aspiration, endoscopy, fracture reduction, hernia reduction, paracentesis, thoracentesis, chest tube placement, complex laceration repair, sexual assault exam	Sedation, analgesia, anxiolysis, motion control, amnesia	Midazolam and fentanyl (Sublimaze) IV; ketamine (Ketalar) IM, IV

IN, intranasal.
See Sedation/Analgesia section in Appendix B (Formulary) for dosages.

- Airway: face mask, oral airway, ETT (three sizes), stylet, laryngoscope
- Pharmacology: use a minimalist approach with doses and titration
- Monitoring equipment

Never forget complete documentation of summary of patient's relevant clinical status, past medical history, exam, risks and benefits, rapid-sequence intubation algorithm, view of larynx, complications, vital signs, postintubation CXR results, and plan.

These guidelines should be used only within the rubric of the ER airway management polices.

Rapid-Sequence Intubation

Definition

The rapid onset induction of, in sequential fashion, unconsciousness, analgesia, autonomic reflex blockade, and muscle relaxation with two medications: general anesthetic and muscle relaxant combined with cricoid pressure for tracheal intubation. It is indicated in patients considered at risk of pulmonary aspiration of gastric contents.

Contraindications

- Anticipated difficult airway.

- Inexperience or lack of training with advance airway management techniques.

- Relative: cervical spine injury.

- Untreated hypovolemia or other unstable cardiovascular condition.

Techniques

- Classic RSI algorithm: See Fig. 11-4.

- Always have an alternative strategy for securing the airway. See failed intubation escape plan, Fig. 11-5.

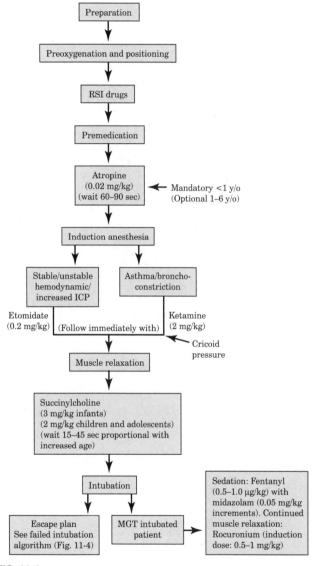

FIG. 11-4.
Classic rapid-sequence intubation algorithm. MGT, management;
RSI, rapid-sequence intubation; y/o, year old. (From McAllister W,
Gnauck K. Rapid sequence intubation of the pediatric patient. *Pediatr
Clin North Am* 1999;46:1249–1284, with permission.)

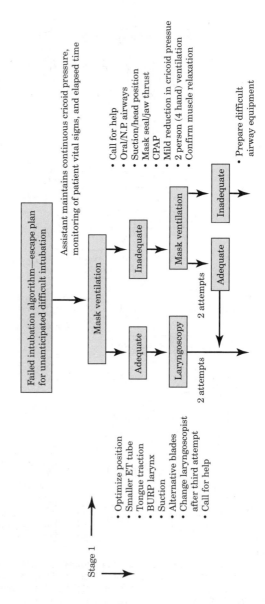

Stage 1 →

- Optimize position
- Smaller ET tube
- Tongue traction
- BURP larynx
- Suction
- Alternative blades
- Change laryngoscopist after third attempt
- Call for help

Failed intubation algorithm—escape plan for unanticipated difficult intubation

Assistant maintains continuous cricoid pressure, monitoring of patient vital signs, and elapsed time

- Call for help
- Oral/N.P. airways
- Suction/head position
- Mask seal/jaw thrust
- CPAP
- Mild reduction in cricoid pressue
- 2 person (4 hand) ventilation
- Confirm muscle relaxation

Mask ventilation

Adequate

Laryngoscopy

2 attempts

Inadequate

Mask ventilation

Adequate

2 attempts

Inadequate

- Prepare difficult airway equipment

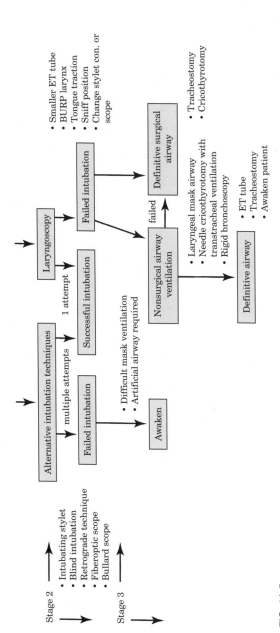

Stage 2
• Intubating stylet
• Blind intubation
• Retrograde technique
• Fiberoptic scope
• Bullard scope

Stage 3

Alternative intubation techniques

multiple attempts ──→ Failed intubation ──→ Awaken
                      • Difficult mask ventilation
                      • Artificial airway required

1 attempt ──→ Successful intubation

Laryngoscopy ──→ Failed intubation

• Smaller ET tube
• BURP larynx
• Tongue traction
• Sniff position
• Change stylet con. or scope

Nonsurgical airway ventilation
• Laryngeal mask airway
• Needle cricothyrotomy with transtracheal ventilation
• Rigid bronchoscopy

failed ──→ Definitive surgical airway
• Tracheostomy
• Cricothyrotomy

Definitive airway
• ET tube
• Tracheostomy
• Awaken patient

FIG. 11-5.
Classic rapid-sequence intubation strategy for failed intubation. BURP, *back up* and *rightward pressure* (on the laryngeal cartilage); CPAP, continuous positive airway pressure; N.P., nasopharyngeal. (From McAllister W, Gnauck K. Rapid sequence intubation of the pediatric patient. *Pediatr Clin North Am* 1999;46:1249–1284, with permission.)

SUGGESTED READING

American Academy of Pediatrics. Guidelines for monitoring and management of pediatric patients during and after sedation for diagnostic and therapeutic procedures. *Pediatrics* 1992;89(6):1110–1115.

American Academy of Pediatrics Committee on Quality Improvement. The management of minor closed head injury in children. *Pediatrics* 1999;104:1415.

American Heart Association Subcommitee on Pediatric Resuscitation. Pediatric basic and advance life support, 1994–1997.

Fleisher GR. The management of bite wounds. *N Engl J Med* 1999;340:138–140.

Guzzetta P, Randolph J. Burns in children. *Pediatr Rev* 1983;4:271.

Krauss B, Green SM. Sedation and analgesia for procedures in children. *N Engl J Med* 342;13:938–945.

McAllister W, Gnauck K. Rapid sequence intubation of the pediatric patient. *Pediatr Clin North Am* 1999;46:1249–1284.

McMillan JA. *Oski's pediatrics, principles and practice*, 3rd ed. Philadelphia: Lippincott Williams & Wilkins, 1999.

Woolf, AD. Poisoning in children and adolescents. *Pediatr Rev* 1993;14:411–422.

12 Endocrinology

A balancing act.

INTRODUCTION

- One of the main functions of the endocrine system is to regulate different enzymatic and metabolic processes to maintain growth, development, reproduction, and homeostasis in the body. That is why a good understanding of the endocrine system is important to differentiate between a disturbance in hormonal action and a normal variation in the time of development.

- Think of each axis as a fun game: Every hormone release is a consequence of a stimuli and its inhibition is a result of a feedback mechanism. Once you know the pathways, it is all very logical.

- Most of the endocrine disorders have a familial component. They can be a challenge to diagnose and manage (especially in adolescents).

- The family and patient's understanding of the condition, cooperation, and interaction are clues to successfully treating these patients. Here is where the "teacher in you" comes out.

- The management of endocrine disorders requires a multidisciplinary approach: social work, psychiatry, nurse educator, home health, and dietitian.

DIABETIC KETOACIDOSIS
Definition

- Acidosis: pH <7.3 or serum bicarbonate <15 mEq/L.
- Hyperglycemia with blood glucose >300 mg/dL.
- Ketonemia in serum >3 mmol/L. Urine ketones positive.

Causes

- In type 1 diabetes mellitus:
  - New onset
  - Failure to take insulin
  - Illness
- In type 2 diabetes mellitus:
  - Severe illness

Clinical Manifestations

- Look for precipitating factors—e.g., infection, stress, noncompliance failure.

- Vomiting.

- Deep-sighing respiration (Kussmaul) with an acetone odor.

- Abdominal pain mimicking pancreatitis or a surgical abdomen without rebound tenderness.

- Somnolence or a loss of consciousness related to the degree of hyperosmolarity.

- In new-onset diabetes: history of polyuria, polydipsia, polyphagia, nocturia, and weight loss.

Lab and Data Evaluation

- Rapid diagnosis: blood glucose (lab, not meter), ketones (urine or blood).

- Testing for glucosuria is not a way of diagnosing diabetes.

- Initial labs:

  - Basic metabolic panel (BMP).

  - Anion gap: $Na - (Cl + HCO_3)$; normal: 8–12.

  - Correction Na level: for each increase in blood glucose of 100 mg/dL above 100 mg/dL; Na decreased by 1.6 mEq/L.

  - Ca^+ and $PO4^-$.

  - Plasma osmolarity if the patient is comatose:

$$2(Na) + \frac{Glucose}{18} + \frac{BUN}{2.8}$$

  - Diabetic ketoacidosis (DKA) patients have a plasma osmolarity >300 mOsm/L.

  - ECG: if potassium is abnormal.

  - Cultures: if febrile or clinical evidence of infection.

Treatment

Mild Diabetic Ketoacidosis

- Ketones large, not vomiting, pH >7.3, HCO_3 >18:

  - Oral hydration

  - Supplemental regular insulin or Humalog SC (0.1–0.2 U/kg q4–6h)

  - Often managed as an outpatient, unless newly diagnosed

Moderate Diabetic Ketoacidosis

- Mild DKA with persistent vomiting or large ketones, pH = 7.2–7.3, HCO_3 = 10–20:

  - Often managed as outpatient or in an ER or short-stay unit.

  - IV hydration is usually necessary.

  - Regular insulin or Humalog, 0.25 U/kg SC q2–6h.

  - Admit to the hospital if not resolving after 3–4 hrs (i.e., HCO_3 not rising and/or unable to take fluids PO), if newly diagnosed, or if the ability of the family caregivers is questionable.

Severe Diabetic Ketoacidosis

- Mild or moderate DKA along with other organ system impairment (altered mental status, impaired renal function, respiratory distress), large ketones, pH <7.2, HCO_3 <10:

  - Admit to hospital for therapy and intensive monitoring (BMP q4h, finger-stick blood glucose level q1h while on insulin drip, neurology status checks q1–2h).

  - PICU admission may be appropriate in many cases (e.g., altered mental status, infant).

IV Hydration

- Hydration is the first and most important step in DKA management. Patients with DKA have volume contraction.

- Simple hydration frequently causes a 180–240 mg/dL drop in glucose.

- *First phase*: NS 20 cc/kg over 30–60 mins continuously until hypovolemia improves.

- *Second phase*: $^1/_2$NS at 3000 mL/m^2/day. Avoid giving >4000 mL/m^2/day. Can decrease amount to 2500 mL/m^2/day if there are concerns for cerebral edema.

- *Third phase*: Once blood glucose is <250, switch to D5$^1/_2$NS at 3000 mL/m^2/day. Maintain blood glucose at 150–250 mg/dL. Continue insulin infusion until anion gap has closed. May increase dextrose in IVFs to 7.5% or 10% if blood glucose drops and patient is still on an insulin drip and acidotic.

Potassium Replacement

- Start if urine flow is established and potassium level is <5.5 mEq/L.

- Potassium level falls with correction of the acidosis, decreased blood glucose, and initiation of insulin.

- Add 30–40 mEq/L of potassium to IVFs as KCl, KPO_4, and/or KAc (acetate) (i.e., second- and third-phase IVFs can be $^1/_2$NS + 20 mEq/L KCl + 20 mEq/L KAc at 3000 mL/m^2/day).

IV Insulin

- IV insulin bolus has a very short half-life. If given, give 0.1 U/kg.

- Once IV access is established, begin insulin drip at 0.1 U/kg/hr. (Remember to give a saline bolus as well.)

- If blood glucose begins falling rapidly and the patient remains acidotic: **Do not stop the insulin drip. Increase the dextrose.**

- Increase insulin infusion rate to 0.15–0.2 U/kg/hr if the blood glucose is not falling over the first 3–4 hrs or the acidosis is not improving.

- Reduce the rate of insulin to 0.05 U/kg/hr when the pH >7.25 or the HCO_3 >15.

- Switch to SC insulin when patient can tolerate oral fluids, the pH >7.25 or HCO_3 >15, and the anion gap has closed.

- Check blood glucose every hour.

Bicarbonate Replacement
Only when absolutely necessary. Use with caution.

- Use with persistent acidosis with pH <7.0 or renal failure after initial volume expansion.

- Never as a bolus, instead add it to the IV fluid (40 mEq/L) and adjust Na in the IV fluid to 75 mEq/L.

- There is some correlation with the use of bicarbonate and cerebral edema.

Complications
Cerebral Edema

- More common in children <10 yrs old, especially <5 yrs old with new-onset diabetes.

- Anticipate cerebral edema in the first 24 hrs after initiation of treatment. Symptoms include change in affect or consciousness, irritability, headache, equally dilated pupils, delirium, incontinence, vomiting, bradycardia, and papilledema.

- Treatment is on a clinical basis, and early intervention is indicated.

  - Mannitol, 0.5–1 g/kg IV push.

  - Decrease IV fluid infusion rate.

  - Consider hyperventilation and dexamethasone (Decadron, Dexamethasone Intensol, Dexone, Hexadrol).

- Brain CT not indicated before treatment or to establish the diagnosis, but consider CT to rule out thrombosis or infarction in addition to the cerebral edema. CT is *not* used to diagnose cerebral edema.

Hints on Diabetes Management

- Diagnostic criteria:
  - 8-hr A.M. fasting glucose ≥126 mg/dL
  - Two random plasma glucose levels ≥200 mg/dL + symptoms
  - Oral glucose tolerance test with 2-hr plasma glucose ≥200 mg/dL
- Hospitalize all new-onset type 1 diabetics for intensive education.
- *Starting* daily dosages for SC insulin: <3 yrs = 0.3–0.4 U/kg/day; 3–6 yrs = 0.5 U/kg/day; 7–10 yrs = 0.6–0.8 U/kg/day; 11–14 yrs = 0.8–1 U/kg/day; >14 yrs = 1–1.5 U/kg/day. After 24 hrs at these doses, adjust doses based on patient's requirements.
- *Total* daily insulin dosages:
  - $^2/_3$ dose in A.M.: $^1/_3$ Humalog, $^2/_3$ NPH
  - $^1/_3$ dose in P.M.: $^1/_2$ Humalog, $^1/_2$ NPH
- Caloric requirements: 1000 Kcal + 100 Kcal/yr up to age 10. After age 10, for females, 45 Kcal/kg/day; for males, 55 Kcal/kg/day.
- Tight diet control is best achieved when patients count carbohydrates. 1 carbohydrate unit = 15 g of carbohydrate.
- Hgb A1c gives an average of blood glucose levels over the 3 mos preceding its measurement.

Hgb A1c (%)	Average blood glucose levels
4–6	Nondiabetic
6	120 (excellent control)
7	150 (very good control)
8	180 (good control)
9	210 (fair control)
10	240 (poor control)

- Time course of action of human insulin preparations: see Table 12-1.

ADRENAL INSUFFICIENCY
Definition

Adrenal insufficiency can be a primary disorder of the adrenal gland (congenital or acquired), or it can be secondary to a deficiency of ACTH or corticotropin-releasing hormone.

TABLE 12-1.
TIME COURSE OF ACTION OF HUMAN
INSULIN PREPARATIONS

Insulin	Onset	Peak	Max (hrs)
Humalog (Lispro)	<15 mins	30–90 mins	4–6
Regular	30 mins	2–3 hrs	6–8
Neutral Protamine Hagedorn (NPH)	2–4 hrs	6–10 hrs	14–18
Ultralente	6–10 hrs	10–16 hrs	20–24
70/30 (70 neutral protamine Hagedorn/30 regular)	30–60 mins	Dual	14–18
Glargine (Lantus)	2 hrs	None	24

Causes

Primary Adrenal Insufficiency (Addison's Disease)

Acute

- Bilateral adrenal hemorrhage
  - With septicemia (Waterhouse-Friderichsen syndrome)
  - Without septicemia
- TB
- Histoplasmosis
- CMV in HIV
- Medications (e.g., ketoconazole)

Chronic

- Autoimmune (e.g., polyglandular autoimmune syndrome)
- Congenital adrenal hyperplasia
- Congenital adrenal hypoplasia
- Adrenal leukodystrophy
- Wolman's disease (lysosomal storage disease that includes calcification of the adrenals)
- Congenital unresponsiveness to ACTH

Secondary Adrenal Insufficiency

- Hypopituitarism
- Congenital
- Acquired

- Tumor (e.g., craniopharyngioma, septo-optic dysplasia)
- Trauma
- Radiation
- Iatrogenic (from chronic steroid therapy)

Clinical Manifestations

A high index of suspicion is crucial, because the presenting symptoms of adrenal insufficiency can be subtle.

Signs

- Weight loss
- Hyperpigmentation
- Hypotension/shock
- Adrenal calcifications (bilateral)
- Vitiligo

Symptoms

- Weakness and fatigue
- Anorexia
- GI symptoms
- Salt craving
- Postural dizziness

Lab Abnormalities

- Hyponatremia (90%)
- Hyperkalemia (60%)
- Hypercalcemia (6%)
- Metabolic acidosis
- Anemia
- Lymphocytosis
- Eosinophilia
- Azotemia

Diagnosis

- Early diagnosis may be life saving.
- A history of steroid use, the presence of another autoimmune endocrine disorder (especially hypoparathyroidism, mucocutaneous candidiasis,

type 1 diabetes mellitus), and a family history of autoimmune endocrinopathies should heighten the suspicion for adrenal insufficiency.

- Random plasma cortisol levels are not very useful except in infants or in shock. They should only be measured when suspecting adrenal insufficiency and before starting treatment. If treatment is not emergent, a fasting 8 A.M. plasma cortisol level is more useful.

- If the patient's condition permits waiting to initiate therapy, do an **ACTH stimulation test** with Cortrosyn, 250 μg/m^2 IV. A plasma cortisol level <18 μg/dL after 60 mins establishes the diagnosis but does not differentiate primary from secondary adrenal insufficiency. Normal ACTH levels rule out primary, but not mild, secondary adrenal insufficiency.

- Secondary adrenal insufficiency can be diagnosed with the help of an endocrinologist using the insulin tolerance test or metyrapone test.

Treatment
Acute Adrenal Insufficiency

- Volume expansion (may use D5NS if there is concomitant hypoglycemia).

- Hydrocortisone: 30–50 mg/m^2/day IV q6h.

- If hypoglycemia persists, increase the amount of dextrose to correct it.

Chronic Adrenal Insufficiency

- The best dose of steroid replacement is the lowest the patient can support without symptomatology.

- Hydrocortisone: 18–30 mg/ m^2/day PO.

- Fludrocortisone: 0.1 mg/day PO in primary adrenal insufficiency. May increase dose as needed.

- Minor illness (nausea, emesis, or fever >100°F): Triple the PO doses or give 30–50 mg/m^2/day of hydrocortisone IV for a short period of time (48 hrs or until symptoms resolve). Can also give dexamethasone equivalent dose IM.

- Major stress (severe illness, general anesthesia, bone fracture): 50–100 mg/m^2/day IV hydrocortisone.

- Patient must wear a medic alert bracelet with diagnoses.

CONGENITAL ADRENAL HYPERPLASIA
Introduction

- Autosomal recessive disorders produced by an enzymatic deficiency in the corticosteroid biosynthesis pathway.

- Characterized by abnormal cortisol and aldosterone synthesis that causes increased ACTH, subsequent adrenal hyperplasia, and over-production of the adrenal steroids that do not require the deficient enzyme activity.

- The excessive adrenal androgen production (androstenedione) by peripheral conversion to testosterone produces virilization, which is the hallmark of this disorder.

21-OH Deficiency

- Is the most common cause of congenital adrenal hyperplasia and is responsible for 90% of the cases.

- The gene is located in the short arm of chromosome 6.

- There are three forms.

Classic Salt-Wasting Form

- Severe mineralocorticoid deficiency as well as glucocorticoid deficiency.

- Females present with virilization and ambiguous genitalia (clitor-omegaly, labial fusion, and rugation).

- Males are phenotypically normal. They present with a salt-losing crisis in the first to second week of life.

- Diagnostic labs: 17-hydroxyprogesterone (17-OHP) (increased, usually >2000 ng/dL after 24 hrs of life); decreased Na, increased K, acidosis, and can have decreased glucose.

- Treatment: glucocorticoid replacement (hydrocortisone, 20–25 mg/m^2/day), mineralocorticoid replacement (fludrocortisone acetate [Florinef], 0.1 mg/day). Infants require NaCl supplements as well.

Classic Simple Virilization Form

- Mild to absent mineralocorticoid deficiency due to partial enzyme deficiency.

- Overproduction of adrenal androgens: Females with ambiguous genitalia are diagnosed in the neonatal period. Diagnosis in males can be missed in early years as they don't have salt-losing crises.

- Males and females have excessive growth and early appearance of pubic hair and pubertal changes.

- Diagnosis: 17-OHP (increased, usually >2000 ng/dL) or significant 17-OHP rise at 60 mins in ACTH stimulation test.

- Treatment: glucocorticoid and mineralocorticoid replacement (see above for dosages).

Nonclassic Form

- Presents later in childhood or in adulthood with premature adrenarche, advanced bone age, severe acne, menstrual irregularities, and hirsutism

- Diagnosis: modestly elevated 17-OHP or excessive rise of 17-OHP after ACTH stimulation test

- Treatment: glucocorticoid replacement

11-Hydroxylase Deficiency

- Accounts for 5% of congenital adrenal hyperplasia.

- The lack of this enzyme results in decreased conversion of 11-deoxycorticosterone and deoxycortisol to cortisol and aldosterone.

- 11-Deoxycorticosterone has some aldosterone-like activity; therefore, salt-wasting syndrome is not present.

- Characterized by HTN and hypokalemia.

- Diagnosis: increased 11-deoxycorticosterone, increased 11-deoxycortisol, increased androstenedione and testosterone.

- Treatment: management of HTN and cortisol replacement.

17-Hydroxylase Deficiency

- Rare cause of congenital adrenal hyperplasia.

- Characterized by decreased cortisol and increased deoxycorticosterone leading to increased Na retention and HTN.

- Males have ambiguous genitalia. Females fail to go through adrenarche and puberty. Both have HTN.

- Treatment: cortisol and sex hormone replacement and HTN management.

DIABETES INSIPIDUS
Etiology

- Central diabetes insipidus (DI): lack of vasopressin: CNS trauma, tumor, surgery

- Nephrogenic DI: kidney unresponsive due to receptor defect response

- Medications, tubular defects, X-linked

- Important to rule out psychogenic polydipsia: primary excess drinking of water

Diagnosis

- Characterized by polyuria and polydipsia.

- Urine osmolality <100 mOsm/kg.

- Urine specific gravity <1.005.

- Serum sodium and osmolality are usually normal or slightly elevated in children with uncomplicated DI and free access to water.

Water Deprivation Test

- See Table 12-2.

- Used to confirm the diagnosis of DI.

- Begin the test in morning after 24 hrs of adequate hydration and after the patient empties his or her bladder.

- Weigh patient and restrict fluid for 7 hrs. Measure weight and urine volume and specific gravity hourly. Check urine and serum osmolality and serum sodium q2h.

- Terminate test if weight loss approaches 3–5%.

Vasopressin Test

- See Table 12-3.

- Used to differentiate between a nephrogenic and central etiology.

- Vasopressin, 0.05–0.1 U/kg SC, is given at the end of water deprivation test after measuring vasopressin level. Urine output, concentration, and water intake are monitored.

Triphasic Diabetes Insipidus

- Occurs after an acute injury to the neurohypophysis (basal skull fracture or status post craniopharyngioma resection with transection of the stalk).

- Initial DI phase is followed by an SIADH phase (up to 5–10 days) and finally a central DI disorder.

Treatment

- Complete central DI: DDAVP (SC, IN, PO).

- Nephrogenic DI: thiazide diuretics, NSAIDs, amiloride (Midamor).

- It is very important to determine that the thirst mechanism is intact in patients and to assure that patients will not become dehydrated and hypernatremic. Monitor sodium daily until a regimen is determined, and follow urine specific gravity.

- Patients with an intact thirst mechanism and free access to water regulate themselves.

TABLE 12-2.
WATER DEPRIVATION TEST

Condition	Urine osmolality (mOsm/L)	Plasma osmolality (mOsm/L)	Specific gravity	Urine:plasma osmolality ratio	Urine volume	Weight loss
Normal/psychogenic polydipsia	500–1400	288–291	1.010	>2	Decreased	No change
Central/nephrogenic diabetes insipidus	<150	>290	<1.005	—	Increased	≥5%

TABLE 12-3.
VASOPRESSIN TEST

Condition	Urine specific gravity	Urine volume	Fluid intake	Vasopressin level
Central diabetes insipidus	>1.010	Decreased	Decreased	Decreased
Nephrogenic diabetes insipidus	<1.005	No change	No change	Increased (10–20 pg/mL)

SIADH
Criteria for Diagnosis

- Hyponatremia and serum hypo-osmolality
- Euvolemia
- Decreased urine output
- High urine osmolality: >200 mOsm/kg of water
- Increase in urine sodium >20 mEq/L
- Normal renal, cardiac, hepatic, adrenal, pituitary, and thyroid function
- No diuretic use
- Progressive weight gain

Etiology

- CNS disorders: meningitis, brain abscess, head trauma, Guillain-Barré, hemorrhage, stroke, acute intermittent porphyrias, brain and spinal surgery, intracranial tumors
- Pulmonary disorders: pneumonia, TB, aspergillosis, respiratory failure, cystic fibrosis (CF), acute respiratory distress syndrome, positive pressure breathing, asthma
- Medications: vasopressin, vincristine, vinblastine, morphine, carbamazepine, haloperidol, cyclophosphamide, tricyclics
- Postop pain and nausea

Management

- Fluid restriction (800 cc/m^2/24 hrs).
- Demeclocycline (takes >24 hrs to start working). Not commonly used in children.
- Avoid raising the serum sodium >2–4 mEq/L per every 4 hrs or >10–20 mEq/L per every 24 hrs due to the risk of central pontine myelinolysis.
- SIADH with severe hyponatremia may cause CNS symptoms (e.g., lethargy, sleepiness, or seizures).
  - When SIADH is symptomatic, correction of hyponatremia with 3% NS (513 mEq/L of sodium) is indicated. There are two ways to calculate the amount of 3% NS to give: 10 cc/kg of 3% NS over 60 mins **OR** amount or 3% NS to give (in cc) = (125 mEq/L – patient's serum Na) × (patient's weight in kg) × (0.66 L/kg).
  - Excessive sodium administration may lead to fluid overload. Concomitant administration of loop diuretics may be necessary.

CONGENITAL HYPOTHYROIDISM

Prevalence 1:4000 births.

Etiology

- Thyroid dysgenesis (75%)

  - Agenesis

  - Hypoplasia

  - Ectopic

- Dyshormogenesis (10%): may resolve; usually an organification defect

- Hypothalamic-pituitary TSH deficiency (5%)

- Transient hypothyroidism (10%)

  - Maternal thyroid disease (antibodies, drugs)

  - Iodine deficiency or excess (premie cleaned with iodine swabs)

Signs and Symptoms

- Most infants completely asymptomatic

- Wide cranial sutures

- Delayed skeletal maturation

- Umbilical hernia

- Prolonged gestation

- Jaundice >7 days

- Hypotonia

- Puffy hands and feet

- Macroglossia

- Hoarse cry

- Goiter (in dysmorphogenesis)

Evaluation

- >15 million infants are screened worldwide yearly by newborn screen.

- If screen is abnormal, obtain T_4 and TSH before starting therapy.

- Presume disease when TSH after 2 days of life is ≥20–25 mU/L (20 µU/mL).

- Sick or very premature infants must be evaluated with free T_4 and TSH when clinical status is stable.

- For low T_4 and normal TSH, consider thyroid-binding globulin deficiency vs hypothalamic/pituitary disturbance (TSH/TRH deficiency).
- If newborn screen normal, consider recheck at 2–6 wks in infants with Down syndrome, family history of dyshormogenesis, or maternal thyroid disorder.

Treatment

- Institute treatment as soon as the diagnosis is confirmed to optimize neurologic development.
- Treat with levothyroxine (Levoxine, Levoxyl, Synthroid). Usual starting dose for a term infant is 37.5 µg/day (can use half of a 75-µg tab).
- For preterm infants, can use 10 µg/kg/day.
- Monitor TSH q1–3mos during first year of treatment or more frequently if dose is adjusted. After 2 yrs, monitoring may be spaced to q6–12mos.
- There is decreased absorption of levothyroxine with soy formulas, iron supplements, calcium supplements.

HYPOGLYCEMIA
Definition

Whipple's triad

- Plasma glucose <50 mg/dL (<45 if whole blood)
- Symptoms consistent with hypoglycemia
- Resolution of symptoms by correction of hypoglycemia

Etiology

High caloric needs, increased or prolonged insulin secretion, disturbances in gluconeogenesis or glycogenolysis.

Neonatal Transient

Inadequate substrate (intrauterine growth rate, premature infants); hyperinsulinism (diabetic mother, erythroblastosis fetalis).

Disorders of Hepatic Glucose Production

- Glycogenolysis: glycogen storage disease, glycogen synthetase deficiency
- Gluconeogenesis: pyruvate carboxylase, fructose 1,6-diphosphatase, phosphoenolpyruvate carboxykinase deficiency
- Ethanol, drugs (e.g., salicylates, beta blockers, valproic acid, cimetidine)
- Galactosemia: hereditary fructose intolerance, ketotic hypoglycemia, prolonged fasting

Abnormal Production of Other Energy Source

- Defects in fatty acid oxidation: carnitine, carnitine palmitoyltransferase, medium chain acyl-CoA dehydrogenase, and long-chain acyl-CoA dehydrogenase deficiency
- Defects in ketogenesis

Hormonal Abnormalities

- Hyperinsulinism: B-cell hyperplasia, dysregulation, B-cell adenoma, Beckwith-Wiedemann syndrome
- Panhypopituitarism, growth hormone deficiency, cortisol deficiency

Miscellaneous Causes

- Propionic acidemia, methylmalonic acidemia, tyrosinosis, maple syrup urine disease
- Severe liver disease (Reye's syndrome, fulminant hepatitis)
- Sepsis in newborns
- Cyanotic heart disease
- Renal failure

Symptoms

Shaky, sweaty, starving, stubborn, sleepy, and seizures.

Labs

See Table 12-4.

Management

- See Fig. 12-1.
- Short term: PO or IV administration of glucose. Glucagon is only useful in hyperinsulinemic patients.
- Long term: treating underlying cause.
  - Ketotic hypoglycemia: feed frequently.
  - Hormonal deficiency: exogenously replace.
  - Enzymatic deficiency: appropriate diet.
  - Hyperinsulinism: octreotide/diazoxide/surgery.

TABLE 12-4.
FEATURES OF CHILDHOOD HYPOGLYCEMIA

Condition	Hypoglycemia	Urine ketones	Reducing substances	Hepatomegaly	Insulin	Beta-hydroxy-butyrate	Lactate	Other
Normal fasting	0	0	0	0	Decreased	Increased	Normal	—
Hyperinsulinemia	Recurrent, severe	0	0	0	Significantly increased	Decreased	Normal	Normal alanine
Ketotic hypoglycemia	Severe with missed meals	Keto-nuria	+++	0	Decreased	—	Normal	—
Hypopituitarism	Moderate with missed meals	Keto-nuria	++	0	Decreased	Significantly increased	Normal	GH and cortisol may be low
Adrenal insufficiency	Severe with missed meals	Keto-nuria	++	0	Decreased	Significantly increased	Normal	Low cortisol
Glycogen storage disease	Varies with disorder	Keto-nuria	++	Yes	Decreased	Increased	Normal or significantly increased	No glucagon response May have increased lactate
Gluconeogenesis defect	Severe with fasting	Keto-nuria	+++	Yes	Decreased	Significantly increased	Significantly increased	—
Fatty acid oxidation	Severe with fasting	Keto-nuria	—	Yes	Decreased	0	Significantly increased	Provoked during intercurrent illnesses
Galactosemia	After milk	0	+	Yes	Decreased	Increased	Normal	Cataracts, *Escherichia coli;* UTIs
Fructose intolerance	After fructose	0	+	Yes	Decreased	Increased	Normal	—

+, mild increase; ++, moderate increase; +++, severe increase; 0, absent.

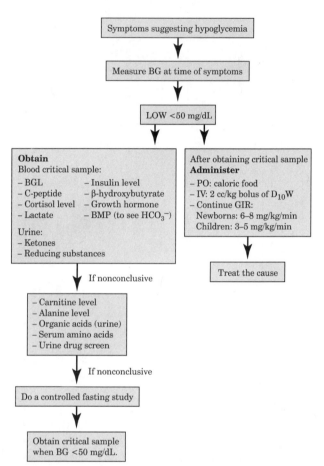

FIG. 12-1.
Management approach to hypoglycemia. BG, blood glucose; BMP, basic metabolic profile; GIR, glucose infusion rate.

SUGGESTED READING

American Diabetes Association. Hyperglycemic crisis in patients with diabetes mellitus. *Diabetes Care* 2001;24(1):154–161.

Fisher DA. Clinical review 19: management of congenital hypothyroidism. *J Clin Endocrinol Metab* 1991;7:523–529.

Levine LS. Congenital adrenal hyperplasia. *Pediatr Rev* 2000;21(5):159–170.

Oelkers W. Adrenal insufficiency. *N Engl J Med* 1996;335(16):1206–1212.

Rudolph AM. *Rudolph's pediatrics*, 20th ed. Stamford, CT: Appleton & Lange, 1996.

13 Gastroenterology

What goes in must come out.

APPROACH TO THE PATIENT WITH GI COMPLAINTS
As always, the most important part of your evaluation is the history. Make sure you ask about diet, vomiting, or nausea; duration and character of any pain; bowel habits; weight loss; occurrence of symptoms at night. An important question to ask yourself is: "Is this a surgical abdomen?"

ABDOMINAL PAIN
Appendicitis

- Symptoms/signs: vomiting, anorexia, vague abdominal pain that then localizes to McBurney's point (one-third the distance from the anterior iliac spine to the umbilicus on a line connecting the two).
- Perforation often follows onset of symptoms in 24–48 hrs.
- Exam: fever, vomiting, irritability, lethargy, right lower quadrant tenderness, and guarding.
- Labs: WBCs may be elevated but are normal in ≥20% of patients.
- Diagnosis: U/S and CT may aid in diagnosis. Surgical consult as necessary.
- Treatment: appendectomy.

Intussusception

- Most common cause of bowel obstruction between the ages of 2 mos and 5 yrs.
- Symptoms/signs: vomiting, colicky abdominal pain with drawing up of the legs, "currant jelly" stools (late in the course of illness), fever, increasing lethargy.
- Exam: abdomen soft and nontender between episodes, sausage-shaped mass in right upper quadrant (RUQ).
- 95% are at the ileocecal junction.
- Diagnosis: In x-rays, the leading outline of intussusception is usually outlined with air. Plain films are often nondiagnostic. Use of contrast enema is diagnostic.
- Treatment: air enema (80–90% success rate) or surgery.

Midgut Volvulus

- Results from improper rotation and fixation of the duodenum and colon (malrotation). Bowel necrosis is due to bowel twisting on itself.

- Most common in the first month of life.
- Symptoms/signs: bilious vomiting followed by abdominal distention and GI bleeding, then peritonitis, hypovolemia, and shock.
- X-ray shows pneumotosis.
- Diagnosis: upper GI with water-soluble, nonionic, iso-osmolar contrast shows a spiral or corkscrew sign.
- Treatment is surgery.
- Often associated with other anomalies (e.g., omphalocele, gastroschisis, diaphragmatic hernia, duodenal atresia).

Gallbladder Disease

- Cholecystitis: usually in adolescent females.
- Symptoms/signs: RUQ pain and tenderness, back pain, or epigastric pain radiating to right subscapular area; bilious vomiting; fever; and RUQ mass.
- Cholelithiasis: associated with hemolytic disease (spherocytosis, sickle cell anemia, thalassemia), obesity, and pregnancy.
- Diagnosis: In the x-ray and U/S, look for gallstones; radioisotope scanning evaluates biliary and gallbladder function.
- Treatment: cholecystectomy and treatment of systemic infection if suspected.

Female Reproductive Tract Pain

- Ectopic pregnancy: abdominal pain, vaginal bleeding, and/or amenorrhea, nausea and vomiting (N/V).
  - Physical exam may reveal abdominal, adnexal, and/or cervical tenderness. 10% present in shock.
  - Diagnose with pregnancy test and U/S.
  - Treat with surgery or methotrexate and close follow-up.
- Ovarian cysts: most common in adolescents. Bleeding into the cyst or cystic rupture causes pain that usually subsides in 12–24 hrs.
  - Physical exam: lower abdominal tenderness; palpable, mobile, cystic adnexal mass on pelvic exam.
  - Diagnose by U/S.
  - Treatment: surgery needed only if bleeding is uncontrolled.
- Adnexal torsion: unilateral, sudden, severe pain; N/V. May have intermittent pain for days. Also, fever and elevated WBCs.
  - Physical exam may reveal muscle rigidity and a fixed mass on pelvic exam.

- Diagnose with U/S.
- Treatment is surgery.
- Pelvic inflammatory disease: See Sexually Transmitted Diseases in Chap. 7, Adolescent Medicine.

Pancreatitis

- Trauma and anatomic obstruction (e.g., gallstone) are the most common causes in children.
- Symptoms/signs: midepigastric abdominal pain, N/V, jaundice.
- Physical exam: epigastric tenderness, abdominal distension, decreased bowel sounds.
- Diagnosis: elevated amylase and lipase.
  - X-ray may show sentinel loop or pancreatic calcifications. U/S shows an enlarged, hypoechoic pancreas. CT shows inflamed pancreas.
- Treatment: NPO, narcotics, IVFs, TPN.

Male Reproductive Tract Pain

- Testicular torsion: Gonad is tender and elevated in the scrotum. *Surgical emergency.*
- Testicular appendix torsion: point tenderness. Treat with bedrest and analgesics.

Other Causes of Abdominal Pain

Think of gastroenteritis, constipation, UTI, basilar pneumonia, hemolytic-uremic syndrome, Henoch-Schönlein purpura (HSP), inflammatory bowel disease (IBD), peptic ulcers, ureteral stones, and mumps.

DIARRHEA
Chronic Nonspecific Diarrhea

- Presents in toddlers between 18 mos and 3 yrs.
- Etiology: excess fluid intake, carbohydrate malabsorption from excessive juice intake, disordered intestinal motility, excessive fecal bile acids, low fat intake.
- Symptoms/signs: frequent large, watery stools (3–6/day) without clinical or lab evidence of malabsorption or infection and without consequences on growth. Stooling does not occur during sleep and there are no associated symptoms.
- Labs (to rule out other etiologies of diarrhea): stool specimen for neutral fat, pH, reducing substances, occult blood, *Giardia* antigen, ova and parasites, culture.
- Spontaneously resolves in 90% of children by 3.5 yrs of age.

Malabsorption

- Causes: CF and celiac disease are the most common. See Cystic Fibrosis in Chap. 21, Pulmonary.

- Symptoms/signs: chronic diarrhea, weight loss, poor appetite, weakness, decreased activity, bloating, flatulence, abdominal pain.

- Diagnosis: acid stool pH, presence of stool-reducing substances, increased fecal fat and PT, decreased serum calcium and vitamin A and E levels.

- Treatment: Treat cause of malabsorption.

CONSTIPATION
In Infants <1 yr

- Causes: Exclude inadequate fluid intake and undernutrition; inspect anus for signs of anal stenosis, renal tubular acidosis, CF, hypothyroidism.

- Hirschsprung's disease: more common in males. 80% develop symptoms in the first month of life.

  - Symptoms/signs include delayed meconium passage and progressive abdominal distension leading to bilious emesis.

  - Physical exam reveals a distended abdomen with palpable fecal masses and an empty anal canal and rectum.

  - Diagnosis: X-ray demonstrates gas and stool in the colon above the rectum. Diagnosis confirmed by biopsy.

  - Treatment consists of surgical resection of the aganglionic bowel.

Older Infants and Children

- Assess fluid and dietary fiber, look for anal fissures, hypotonia, tethered cord.

- Children with stool withholding often have stool incontinence.

- Physical exam to rule out signs of systemic illness. Moveable fecal masses are often felt. Examine lower back for hair tufts or sacral dimples suggesting myelodysplasia. Rectal vault full of hard stool often found in withholding.

Management of Chronic Constipation

- Saline enemas to clear distal impaction.

- Mineral oil (give between meals to minimize the negative effect on fat-soluble vitamin absorption).

- Have the patient sit on the toilet regularly after meals.

GASTROENTERITIS

- Defined as a diarrheal illness with rapid onset and often associated with N/V, fever, or abdominal pain

- Viral gastroenteritis
  - Causes: *rotavirus most common*, then enteric adenovirus, then astrovirus
  - Symptoms/signs: watery diarrhea often accompanied by vomiting and fever
  - Not often associated with blood or leukocytes in the stool
- Bacterial gastroenteritis
  - Causes:
    - Due to toxin production or invasion and inflammation of the mucosa.
    - Secretory diarrheas are caused by enterotoxin, and the patient usually does not have systemic symptoms or WBCs or RBCs in the stool. Symptoms/signs: large volume stools; often associated with N/V.
    - Invasive diarrhea is due to bacterial enteropathogens and is usually accompanied by systemic symptoms such as fever, myalgia, irritability, and anorexia; cramps and abdominal pain common; small amounts of mucousy stool; WBCs and RBCs present in stool.

Evaluation

- Determining the cause of diarrhea is much less important than managing fluid losses, dehydration, and electrolyte abnormalities.
- History should include questions regarding antibiotic use, travel, recent food ingestions, daycare attendance, among others.
  - If fever and abdominal pain (like appendicitis), think *Yersinia*.
  - Bloody stools: Think *Shigella, Salmonella*, enteroinvasive *Escherichia coli*, enterohemorrhagic *E. coli, Camplyobacter, Clostridium, Entamoeba histolytica*.
  - Food poisoning: If <6 hrs, think *Staphylococcus aureus* and *Bacillus cereus*; if >6 hrs, think *Clostridium perfringens*.
  - If there is a history of raw seafood ingestion, think *Vibrio*.
  - If there are risk factors for parasites, think *Giardia, Amoeba, Cryptosporidium, Isospora, Strongyloides*.
  - Lab tests (stool culture) to determine etiology are necessary only if rehydration fails, stools are bloody, systemic signs appear, or diarrhea persists.
  - Evaluation of chronic diarrhea.
    - If bloody, think *E. histolytica, Shigella*, IBD.
    - If malnourished, think inadequate diet, malabsorption.
    - If diet has changed, think milk or protein insensitivity.

Treatment

- For mild to moderate dehydration (5–10%):
  - Oral rehydration with a glucose-electrolyte solution is preferred (i.e., Pedialyte, Rehydralyte [Ross Product Division, Abbott Laboratories, Abbott Park, IL]).
  - For mild dehydratrion, give 50 mL/kg over a 4-hr period. Add to the total for each stool or episode of emesis. For moderate dehydration, use 100 mL/kg.
  - It may be necessary to administer fluid as 1 tsp q2–5mins.
- For severe dehydration (>15%), IV rehydration is required.
  - Begin with an isotonic fluid (lactated Ringer's or NS). Start with 20 cc/kg bolus. Evaluate after bolus. Patients with severe dehydration usually require several boluses.
- Antibiotic therapy
  - *Shigella* can be treated with a third-generation cephalosporin if patient is immunosuppressed or aged <1 mo. Otherwise, no antibiotics are needed.
- Refeeding: Early refeeding of an age-appropriate diet reduces the duration of diarrhea.
  - Early institution of the child's regular formula is recommended. 20% of children develop significant temporary lactase deficiency after an episode of diarrhea and thus require a lactose-free formula temporarily.
- Do not use antidiarrheal compounds to treat acute diarrhea.

GASTROESOPHAGEAL REFLUX

- Normal physiologic event for most infants.
  - 50–65% of all normal infants 2 mos of age vomit ≥3 times/day.
  - Two-thirds of these infants improve by age 18 mos, and almost all improve by age 4 yrs.
- Physiologic reflux occurs in all infants and resolves by 18 mos.
- Pathologic reflux occurs when it causes complications (e.g., bradycardia, apnea, acute life-threatening events, otalgia, recurrent abdominal pain, and Barrett's esophagus).

Diagnosis

- Rule out gastric outlet obstruction; food allergies; malrotation; CNS lesions; metabolic, renal, and infectious disorders.
- If vomiting significant: obtain CBC, electrolytes, BUN, UA, urine culture.
- Esophageal pH monitoring.

- Barium swallow can help exclude structural abnormalities (but does not diagnose reflux).

- If bleeding is present with vomiting, perform upper endoscopy.

Treatment

- Observe the infant being fed: Is the position correct and is the infant being burped correctly?

- Keep baby upright during feed.

- If no response to conservative measures, H_2-blockers and proton pump inhibitors may be used.

- If no response to medication, surgery may be necessary.

INFLAMMATORY BOWEL DISEASE

- Initial evaluation of chronic diarrhea must rule out infectious causes.

- Colonoscopy with biopsy is valuable in the diagnosis of IBD. Ulcerative colitis is associated with an increased risk of colon cancer. Surveillance colonoscopies should begin 8–10 yrs after diagnosis.

- See Table 13-1 for comparison between IBDs.

TABLE 13-1.
INFLAMMATORY BOWEL DISEASES

	Ulcerative colitis	Crohn's disease
GI involvement	Large bowel only	Any portion of the GI tract
Symptoms	Abdominal pain, rectal bleeding, diarrhea, fever, malaise	Abdominal pain, fever, diarrhea, weight loss, fatigue, perirectal fistulas, anal skin tags, anal fissures or ulcerations, perirectal abscesses, growth failure
Sex predominance	Girls > boys	Boys > girls
Endoscopy	Mucosa erythematous, friable, and edematous; superficial erosions and ulcerations; crypt abscesses; pseudopolyps	Transmural involvement, skip lesions, ileal involvement, strictures, cobblestoning, granulomas, fistulas, strictures
Associated symptoms	Peripheral arthritis: migratory, monoarticular, course parallels the colitis; episcleritis, uveitis, iritis, erythema nodosum, pyoderma gangrenosum, aphthous ulcers, hepatic steatosis, sclerosing cholangitis, cholelithiasis, pericholangitis	Same as for ulcerative colitis

- Treatment of mild to moderate IBD: aminosalicylates PO and PR.
- Treatment of severe IBD:
  - Steroids, possibly blood transfusions and rehydration
  - Immunosuppressants (e.g., azathioprine [Imuran] and immuno-modulators)
  - Antibiotics
  - Surgery

PERSISTENT VOMITING
Differential Diagnoses

- Obstruction: malrotation, volvulus, intestinal atresia or stenosis, meconium ileus or plug, Hirschsprung's disease, imperforate anus, incarcerated hernia, pyloric stenosis, foreign bodies, intussusception, Meckel's diverticulum, adhesions
- Infectious/inflammatory GI disorders: necrotizing enterocolitis, gastroesophageal reflux, paralytic ileus, peritonitis, milk allergy, gastroenteritis, pancreatitis, appendicitis, celiac disease, peptic ulcer disease
- Infectious/inflammatory non-GI disorders: sepsis, meningitis, otitis media, pneumonia, pertussis, hepatitis, UTI, pharyngitis
- Neurologic disorders (vomiting often occurs without other GI symptoms): hydrocephalus, kernicterus, subdural hematoma, cerebral edema, intracranial hemorrhage, mass lesion, migraine, motion sickness, hypertensive encephalopathy
- Metabolic and endocrine disorders: inborn errors of metabolism, congenital adrenal hyperplasia, neonatal tetany, adrenal insufficiency, metabolic acidosis, DKA
- Renal disorders: obstructive uropathy, renal insufficiency
- Toxins: digoxin, iron, lead, food poisoning
- Other: pregnancy, anorexia nervosa, bulimia

Bilious Vomiting
Suggests intestinal obstruction at any age.

Necrotizing Enterocolitis
Symptoms/signs include abdominal distention, bilious emesis, vomiting, blood in the stools, lethargy, apnea, temperature instability, and shock.

Inborn Errors of Metabolism
Suggested by early death of sibling, multiple maternal fetal losses, hypotonia, convulsions, lethargy, failure to grow.

Pyloric Stenosis

- 5% have a parent who had pyloric stenosis.
- Occurs more often in boys than girls.
- Symptoms usually begin at 2–3 wks.
- Metabolic alkalosis frequently present.

GI Allergy

- Cow milk allergy is rare in infancy and usually disappears by 2–3 yrs of age.
- Accompanying symptoms may include anaphylaxis, urticaria, angioedema, and wheezing.

Lab Evaluation

- Serum electrolytes
- UA and urine culture
- Plasma amino acids and urine organic acids
- Serum ammonia
- Liver chemistries
- Amylase and lipase

Imaging Studies

- U/S
- Supine and upright plain films
- Upper GI
- Barium enema
- Endoscopy
- Head CT or MRI

Treatment

Treat underlying cause. Maintain adequate hydration.

SUGGESTED READING

Wyllie R, Hyams JS. *Pediatric gastrointestinal disease*. Philadelphia: WB Saunders, 1999.

14 Growth and Development

Pediatric vital signs.

PRIMITIVE REFLEXES

- Palmar grasp: present from birth to 2–4 mos
- Plantar grasp: present from birth to 8 mos
- Moro: present from birth to 4–6 mos
- Tonic neck: present from birth until infant is able to roll over (3–6 mos)
- Galant (ipsilateral trunk curvature with stroking along spine): present from birth to 2–3 mos

GROWTH GOALS IN NEWBORNS

- Infants usually lose weight (5–10% of birth weight) during the first wk of life.
- Preterm infants: weight >15 g/kg/day, length 0.8–1.1 cm/wk, and occipitofrontal circumference 0.5–0.8 cm/wk.
- Full-term infants: weight 20–30 g/day, length 0.66 cm/wk, and occipitofrontal circumference 0.33 cm/wk.

GROWTH

- OFC: should increase 2 cm/mo from 0 to 3 mos, then 1 cm/mo from 3 to 6 mos, then 0.5 cm/mo until 1 yr. From 1 to 2 yrs, 2 cm in diameter should be added.
- Weight: should increase approximately 30 g/day (1 oz/day) for the first 3 mos, then approximately 0.5 kg/mo (1.25 lb/mo) during 3–6 mos of age, then 0.25 kg/mo (0.5 lb/mo) by 1 yr. Birth weight should be doubled by 5 mos and tripled by 1 yr. After 2 yrs, usual gain is 2–3 kg/yr (approximately 5 lb/yr) until puberty.
- Height: length increases by 50% in first year, doubled by 4 yrs. Annual increase in height is 5–7.5 cm/year until adolescent growth spurt.
- The growth pattern may shift significantly in the first 4–18 mos of life. A stable growth percentile should be achieved by 18 mos of age.
- Dentition: central incisors at 6 mos; lateral incisors at 8 mos; first molars at 14 mos; canines at 19 mos; and second molars at 24 mos.

DEVELOPMENT

There are extensive lists regarding normal development. Although it is important during routine, well-child check-ups to evaluate development closely, you will usually be unable to do this on a busy ward rotation. Thus, Table 14-1 is a very brief list of screening developmental questions you can ask during an admission history and physical exam.

TABLE 14-1.
DEVELOPMENTAL SCREENING QUESTIONS

Age	Gross motor	Fine motor	Cognitive and language
1 mo	Head up while prone	Hands fisted	Fixes and follows
2 mos	Chest up in prone	Hands unfisted 50% of the time, grasps rattle placed in hand	Regards speaker, social smile, coos
4 mos	Up on hands in prone, rolls front to back, no head lag	Obtains and retains objects in hand, hand to midline	Reaches for objects, orients to voice, laughs, vocalizes when speaker stops talking
6 mos	Sits with support, rolls back to front	Transfers hand to hand	Discriminates strangers, consonant babbling
7 mos	Sits without support, supports weight while standing, commando crawls	—	Mimics speaker's voice
9 mos	Sits well, pulls to stand, creeps on hands and knees	Brings 2 toys together, finger feeds	Peek-a-boo, uncovers hidden objects, "bye-bye," "dada" and "mama" inappropriately, explores by poking, understands "no," orients to name
12 mos	Cruises, walks with support, may take independent steps	Pincer grasp: objects held between finger-tips	Follows command with gesture, immature jargoning, "dada/mama" appropriately
15 mos	Walks alone, creeps up stairs	Builds tower of 2 cubes, imitates scribble	Follows simple commands, names one object, says "no" meaningfully, points to 1–2 body parts
18 mos	Throws ball while standing, walks up stairs with hand held, sits in chair	Tower of 3–4 cubes, initiates scribbling	Points to 3 body parts and to self, 10–25 words

(continued)

TABLE 14-1.
CONTINUED

Age	Gross motor	Fine motor	Cognitive and language
24 mos	Jumps in place, kicks ball, throws overhand, walks up and down stairs holding rail	Imitates vertical stroke, tower of 6 cubes	Follows 2-step commands, 50+ words, refers to self by name, 2-word phrases, uses pronouns, points to 6 body parts
3 yrs	Pedals a tricycle, alternates feet ascending stairs	Tower of 9 cubes, independent eating, copies circle	Gives full name, knows age and sex, counts to 3, recognizes colors, toilet trained
4 yrs	Alternates feet descending stairs, hops on 1 foot	Tower of 10 cubes, able to cut and paste, copies a cross	Uses "I" correctly, dresses and undresses self with supervision, knows colors
5 yrs	Skips, walks on tiptoes	Copies a triangle	Identifies coins, names 4–5 colors, can tell age and birthday
6 yrs	Tandem walk	Ties shoes, combs hair	Knows left vs right, days of the week, own telephone number
7 yrs	Rides bicycle	Bathes alone	Tells time to the half hour
8 yrs	Reverse tandem walks	—	Tells time within 5 mins, knows the months of the year

- For more reference values, see Vital Signs and Facts (page 368) in Appendix C.

NEWBORN SCREEN

Newborn screening varies by state and changes frequently. For the most up-to-date list, go to http://genes-r-us.uthscsa.edu/resources/newborn/screenstatus.htm.

CHILDHOOD IMMUNIZATION SCHEDULE

Childhood immunization schedule changes yearly. For the most current information, please see the CDC Web site at http://www.cdc.gov/nip/recs/child-schedule.pdf.

TANNER STAGES

See Figs. 14-1, 14-2, and 14-3.

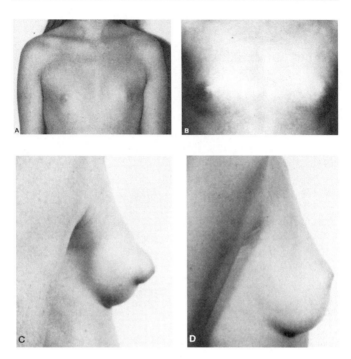

FIG. 14-1.
Stages of breast development. **A–D:** Tanner I–IV, respectively. (From McMillan JA, ed. *Oski's pediatrics*, 3rd ed. Philadelphia: Lippincott Williams & Wilkins, 1999, with permission.)

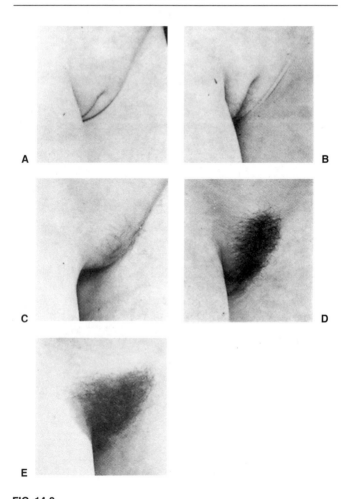

FIG. 14-2.
Development of female anatomy. **A–E:** Tanner I–V, respectively. (From McMillan JA, ed. *Oski's pediatrics*, 3rd ed. Philadelphia: Lippincott Williams & Wilkins, 1999, with permission.)

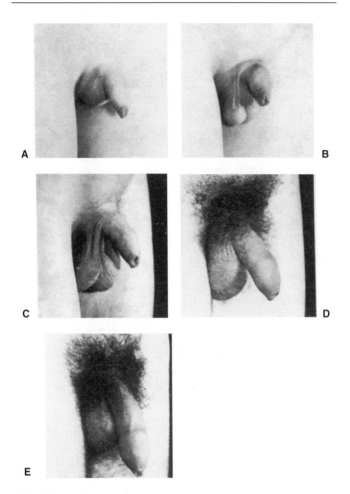

FIG. 14-3.
Development of male anatomy. **A–E:** Tanner I–V, respectively. (From
McMillan JA, ed. *Oski's pediatrics*, 3rd ed. Philadelphia: Lippincott Williams & Wilkins, 1999, with permission.)

15 Hematology-Oncology

Balancing the reds and the whites.

FEVER AND NEUTROPENIA
General Principles

- Risk of infection increases when absolute neutrophil count (ANC) is <1000/mm^3 but rapidly increases when it falls to <500/mm^3.

- Top bugs: *Streptococcus* species, *Pseudomonas aeruginosa*, *Escherichia coli*, *Klebsiella pneumoniae*, *Staphylococcus aureus*, *Staphylococcus epidermidis*, *Enterococcus faecalis*, *Campylobacter jejuni*, *Candida albicans*.

- Time to defervescence in febrile and neutropenic cancer patients: 2–7 days (mean of 5 days); thus, continuation of antibiotic treatment for a minimum of 7 days (and ANC >500 for 72 hrs) is often considered—even in patients with no isolated organism.

Febrile (38.3°C) and Neutropenic Patients

- Obtain blood cultures (from **each** lumen of all indwelling lines; peripheral cultures **not** necessary up front; q24h cultures are usually sufficient); obtain urine culture if patient has symptoms or hematuria (also send urine specimen for BK virus and CMV viral polymerase chain reaction if hematuria is present).

- Discontinue prophylactic antibiotics (e.g., ciprofloxacin [Cipro, Cipro XR], rifampin [Rifadin, Rimactane]). Trimethoprim-sulfamethoxazole (Septra) is usually *continued*.

- Initial treatment: ceftazidime (Fortaz), 50 mg/kg q8h (max. 2 g q8h); alternate lumens if patient has a double lumen Broviac.

- May add vancomycin, 15 mg/kg q8h (renally adjust) after 72 hrs if persistent fever (consider discontinuing if no gram-positive cultures are positive at 72 hrs).

- If febrile >5 days, add fluconazole or amphotericin B (use lipid complex [Abelcet] for all pediatric patients, especially if poor renal function).

- Empiric use of vancomycin: signs of catheter infection, signs of sinus infection (also consider fungal coverage), cutaneous breakdown, prior culture growth of gram-positive organisms (i.e., use your clinical judgment), acute myelogenous leukemia patient on chemotherapy, status post high-dose cytarabine.

- Empiric use of gentamicin or tobramycin: signs of sepsis (e.g., hypotension) and for double coverage of gram-negative infections/ suspected infections until known susceptibilities.

- Patients allergic to penicillin/cephalosporin: Up-front therapy with vancomycin is recommended vs ciprofloxacin (consider age) vs ticarcillin and clavulanate (Timentin) vs imipenem (Primaxin) vs aztreonam (Azactam) and vancomycin.

- *Contine broad coverage until patient no longer febrile and neutropenic or until ANC is rising.*

TRANSFUSION PRINCIPLES
Floor/Bone Marrow Transplant Parameters

- Packed RBCs: Transfuse for Hgb <7g/dL (typically 10–20 cc/kg over 2–4 hrs). (General guidelines: <20 kg receive 0.5 U packed RBCs, and >20 kg receive 1 U.)

- Who requires irradiated cellular components? NICU patients, fetuses, oncology patients, immunodeficient patients (congenital or acquired), solid-organ transplant patients (before and after), BMT patients, patients receiving immunosuppressive chemotherapy or radiation, patients receiving directed donor blood.

- Allo-BMT patients/BMT candidates require single donor (SD)/ CMV negative (for all CMV-negative patients)/irradiated (IR)/leukopoor (LP) blood products.

- Auto-BMT patients can receive CMV-indeterminate RBCs but need SD/IR/LP.

- Solid-organ/auto-BMT patients get LP/IR/CMV indeterminate packed RBCs.

- Hgb SS patients get LP/sickle cell–negative packed RBCs and, if available, minor-antigen compatible.

- CMV-positive transplant patients/candidates need CMV indeterminate/SD/LP/IR RBCs.

Transfusion Reactions

- Allergic (bronchospasm, urticaria, hypotension): **Stop** infusion, treat with antihistamines ± corticosteroids ± epinephrine.

  - Diphenhydramine (Benadryl): treatment of pruritus and hives; no place in treatment of severe reactions; 5 mg/kg/day PO or IV divided q6h

  - Epinephrine: for severe reactions (e.g., bronchospasm, hypotension, shock): 0.1 mg/kg/dose up to maximum of 0.4 mg SC/IV

  - Fluids: for hypotension

  - Narcotics (for rigors): 0.1 mg/kg IV morphine or 0.5–1 mg/kg of meperidine (Demerol)

- Acetaminophen (Tylenol): to treat fever, 10–15 mg/kg/dose PO q4–6h
- Steroids: for moderate to severe reactions (severe urticaria, reactions with fever, chills, diaphoresis, and pallor); 1–2 mg/kg of methylprednisolone (Medrol) (or equivalent dexamethasone [Decadron] or hydrocortisone [Cortef, Hydrocortone])

- Febrile nonhemolytic (fever, chills, diaphoresis) patients: **Stop** infusion; send sample of blood from patient for Coombs' testing; treat with Tylenol, antihistamines, narcotics (for rigors), ± corticosteroids.

- Acute hemolytic reaction (primarily from ABO incompatibility; fever, chills, diaphoresis, abdominal pain, hypotension, hemoglobinuria): **Stop** infusion; send sample to blood bank to ensure correct type; IV fluids for hypotension/ensure adequate urinary output (may need mannitol, 0.25–0.5 g/kg/dose IV q4–6h).

- Delayed transfusion reaction (occurs 3–10 days after transfusion; unexplained anemia, hyperbilirubinemia, abdominal pain): Confirm with positive Coombs' test.

Platelets

- Transfuse for platelets ≤10,000 (in the setting of decreased bone marrow production—i.e., not necessary for ITP).
- Typical dose is 10–20 cc/kg.
- No time constraint—can infuse very fast if needed.
- General guidelines: 0.5 unit SD platelets to patients <20 kg; full unit SD platelets to patients >20 kg; dosing decreases the amount of wasted platelets.
- Allo-BMT patients/BMT candidates require SD/CMV negative (unless known positive)/LP.
- Solid-organ/auto-BMT patients get LP/IR/CMV indeterminate platelets.
- Causes for poor response: fever, sepsis, amphotericin administration, hepatosplenomegaly, alloantibody, autoantibody, blood loss, hemolytic-uremic syndrome, thrombotic thrombocytopenic purpura, necrotizing enterocolitis.
  - To determine effectiveness of transfusion, obtain platelet count at 1 hr and 24 hrs posttransfusion.

Fresh Frozen Plasma

- May need for patients in disseminated intravascular coagulation (DIC) (e.g., contains clotting factors, Ig, albumin).
- Typical dose is 10–20 cc/kg (may also require parental vitamin K); does not need to be screened for CMV.

Cryoprecipitate

- May need for patients in DIC (enriched in fibrinogen, von Willebrand factor, large molecules).

- 1 U is 10–15 cc.

- Dose is approx. 1 bag/5 kg.

ONCOLOGIC EMERGENCIES
Superior Vena Cava Syndrome/Superior Mediastinal Syndrome (SMS)

- Rule out infection, malignancy, iatrogenic causes.

- Symptoms of SMS: cough, hoarseness, dyspnea, orthopnea, chest pain.

- Signs of SMS: swelling, plethora, and cyanosis of the face, neck and upper extremities; diaphoresis, wheezing, and stridor.

- Due to risks of anesthesia, obtain diagnosis with least invasive means possible.

- Associated with giant cell tumors and lymphomas. Check alpha-fetoprotein and human chorionic gonadotropin to differentiate.

- Treatment

  - High-risk: empiric therapy (steroid—prednisone [Deltasone, Orasone, Sterapred], 40 mg/m^2/day divided qid; radiation therapy [XRT]: 100–200 cGy bid): as soon as possible after stabilization of patient. Then biopsy lesion (if not diagnosed, treat for clinical diagnosis).

  - Low-risk: biopsy then treat.

Pleural/Pericardial Effusions

- Evaluation

  - Thoracentesis or pericardiocentesis: send for protein content, specific gravity, cell count, lactic acid dehydrogenase (LDH), cytology, culture, and other biologic/immunologic assays

  - If tamponade, CXR shows waterbag cardiac shadow and ECG shows low-voltage QRS complexes

Massive Hemoptysis

- Most common cause is invasive pulmonary aspergillosis (incidence with hemoptysis is 2–26%).

- Evaluation: CXR, chest CT.

- Treatment: Lay patient on side with hemorrhage to prevent collection in normal lung, correct low platelets, transfuse packed RBCs to maintain normal Hgb.

Gastric/Duodenal Ulcers (Stress, Cushing's Ulcers)

- Children taking high-dose corticosteroids should always be on H_2/H^+ blockers.
- Correct low platelets/coagulation abnormalities for bleeding risk.

GI/Intestinal

- Agranulocytic necrosis seen with typhilitis.
  - Typhilitis: right lower quadrant pain (vs appendicitis) in setting of severe neutropenia, often with fever
    - Usually follows cytotoxic chemotherapy; CT and U/S more sensitive than plain films
    - High mortality: 20–100%
    - Treatment: broad-spectrum antibiotics to cover gram-negative pathogens and clindamycin to treat GI anaerobes ± surgical intervention (persistent bleeding, clinical deterioration, surgical abdomen)
    - *Clostridium septicum* is most common bacterial species; others: gram-negative (*Pseudomonas*); often add oral metronidazole or oral vancomycin to cover *Clostridium difficile*

Hemorrhagic Cystitis

- Diagnosis by UA, U/S (boggy, edematous bladder), direct exam
- Treatment: stop XRT/chemotherapy; hydration, transfusion, correction of low platelets and coagulopathy; removal of clots by catheter/cytoscope
- Prevention: acidification of urine with ascorbic acid before infusing chemotherapy, vigorous hydration during/after treatment, IV and/or PO 2-mercaptoethane sulfonate sodium (mesna) (often mixed in same bag as chemotherapy)

Altered Consciousness

- Etiologies (most common to least): metastatic disease, sepsis/DIC, primary CNS fungal/bacterial infection, metabolic abnormality, viral encephalitis, leukoencephalopathy, intracranial hemorrhage, cerebrovascular accident, oversedation, hepatic failure (e.g., hyperammonemia), chemotherapy induced (ifosfamide: acute somnolence, neurologic deterioration, coma—worse in poor renal clearance that leads to buildup of toxic metabolite chloracetoaldehyde; others: carmustine, cisplatin, thiotepa, high-dose cytarabine, amphotericin, interleukin-2, all-*trans*-retinoic acid)
- Treatment of increased ICP: hyperventilation (to CO_2 of 20–25 mm Hg), IV dexamethasone (1–2 mg/kg), mannitol (Osmitrol, Resectisol) (20% solution at 1.25–2 g/kg)

Cerebrovascular Accident

- Etiologies: cerebral arterial/venous thrombosis, intracranial hemorrhage, chemotherapy-related (L-asparginine–related CNS DIC), sepsis/DIC (intracranial DIC least recognized cause—not always seen in lab values), XRT-induced vascular occlusions.

- Stabilize, then evaluate with CT or MRI (study may need to be repeated in 7–10 days to evaluate full extent).

- Treatment: corticosteroids, mannitol, FFP (± antithrombin III concentrate in patients with L-asparginine cerebrovascular accident), platelets, (?)low-dose heparin.

Seizures

- Etiologies: metastatic disease, cerebrovascular accident, infections, chemotherapy (vincristine, intrathecal methotrexate, cisplatin, cytarabine), SIADH/hyponatremia.

- Evaluation: CT with and without contrast ± MRI; CSF analysis after imaging.

- Treatment: Treat underlying problem (e.g., infection).

- Anticonvulsants (use first three for their rapid onset in secs-mins):

  - Lorazepam (Ativan): 0.05–0.1 mg/kg IV over 2 mins; watch for respiratory depression/hypotension

  - Diazepam (Valium): 0.1–0.3 mg/kg (max. 10 mg) at 1 mg/min (max. 3 doses); rectal preparations available; short duration; watch for respiratory depression/hypotension

  - Fosphenytoin (Cerebyx): loading dose of 15–20 mg/kg of phenytoin equivalent at 100–150 mg/min; watch for cardiac depression; maintenance is approximately 6–8 mg/kg/day q12h (therapeutic level required: 10–20 mg/L)

  - Phenobarbital: 20 mg/kg IV or IM (max. 150 mg or 40 mg/kg); watch for respiratory depression—long half-life/delayed effect (consider pentobarbital); maintenance is approx. 5 mg/kg/day (therapeutic level required: 15–40 mg/L)

Spinal Cord Compression

- Symptoms: back pain in 80% (local or radicular); any patient with cancer and back pain should be considered to have spinal cord compression until proved otherwise; local tenderness in 80–90%.

- Evaluation: spine radiographs (not very sensitive), bone scan, MRI (with and without gadolinium), if not ambulatory should undergo emergent MRI (or myelography).

- Treatment: dexamethasone bolus dose of 1–2 mg/kg immediately, followed by MRI.

Hyperleukocytosis (Count >100,000)

- Complications: early death, CNS hemorrhage, thrombosis, pulmonary leukostasis, metabolic derangements (hyperkalemia, hypocalcemia/hyperphosphatemia), renal failure, GI hemorrhage.

- Evaluation: Examine for signs of hypoxia, dyspnea, blurred vision, agitation, confusion, stupor, cyanosis.

- Treatment: hydration, alkalinization, allopurinol or urate oxidase, platelet transfusion if platelets <20,000, packed RBCs with extreme caution (keep Hgb <10 to minimize viscosity); leukopheresis.

Tumor Lysis Syndrome

- Triad: *hyperuricemia*, *hyperkalemia*, and *hyperphosphatemia* (resulting in secondary renal failure and symptomatic hypocalcemia). Tumor lysis syndrome also may trigger DIC, especially in patients with high tumor burden.

- Risk factors: bulky abdominal tumors (e.g., Burkitt's), increased uric acid and LDH levels, poor urinary output.

- Lab evaluation: CBC, BMP, calcium, phosphorus, uric acid, UA, LDH, PT/PTT (consider fibrinogen/fibrinogen degradation product).

- Other evaluation: ECG if K^+ >7, U/S to rule out kidney infiltrations or ureteral obstruction.

- Treatment

  - Hydration: D5¼NS at 2–4× maintenance + $NaHCO_3$, 20–40 mEq/L (as much as 50–100 mEq/L may be required)

  - Allopurinol (Zyloprim): 10 mg/kg/day or 300 mg/m²/day (divided tid), or urate oxidase 0.2 mg/kg/dose IV qd (as often as bid)

  - Monitor metabolites: BMP, phosphorus, calcium, uric acid, UA

  - If K^+ >6, uric acid >10 mg/dL, creatinine >10× normal, phosphate >10 mg/dL, or symptomatic hypocalcemia, proceed to dialysis, chemotherapy

  - If uric acid <7 mg/dL, specific gravity <1.010, and urine pH 7–7.5, proceed to chemotherapy, then discontinue $NaHCO_3$, monitor metabolites q4–6h

  - Hyperkalemia treatment: stop all K^+ infusion, Kayexalate (1 g/kg PO with 50% sorbitol), calcium gluconate (100–200 mg/kg/dose; for cardioprotection only), insulin (0.1 U/kg + 2 cc/kg of $D_{25}W$)

Hypercalcemia

- Effects: anorexia, nausea and vomiting, polyuria, diarrhea leading to dehydration leading to GI/renal impairment leading to rise in calcium; others: lethargy, depression, hypotonia, stupor, coma, bradycardia, nocturia.

- Treatment: Levels >14 mg/dL require correction (<14 may respond to loops diuretics alone).
  - Pamidronate (considered first-line therapy).
    - Levels <12: 30 mg.
    - Levels >12: 40 mg over 4 hrs.
    - Levels >18, give 90 mg over 24 hrs (wait 7 days for second treatment; repeat q2–8wks).
    - Monitor for hypocalcemia. Infusion may cause fever.
  - Hydration with NS (3× maintenance) and loop diuretics (2–3 mg/kg as often as q2h).
- Glucocorticoids: 1.5–2 mg/kg/day of prednisone; requires 2–3 days to work.

SPECIFIC BONE MARROW TRANSPLANTATION ISSUES
Veno-Occlusive Disease of the Liver

- Most common life-threatening complication related to BMT.
- Syndrome
  - Usually occurs in first 30 days post-BMT
  - Clinical presentation
    - Hepatomegaly or right upper quadrant pain
    - Jaundice (usually hyperbilirubinemia without any other liver function abnormalities until end stage)
    - Ascites/weight gain
    - Platelet consumption
- Risk factors include preexisting hepatitis, antibiotic usage before treatment (vancomycin, acyclovir), age >15 yrs, positive CMV status, female sex, pretreatment radiation to abdomen, intensive conditioning (single-dose total body irradiation, total body irradiation, use of busulfan), second BMTs.
- Treatment: mainly supportive.

Fluid Management

All BMT patients are fluid restricted starting 12–24 hrs posttreatment to 1500/m^2/day, which is continued until engraftment occurs.

Vaccinations

- Given to BMT patients >1 yr posttreatment.
- Patients should avoid family members who have received a live virus vaccine for one month post vaccination.
- For immunization information, please see the CDC Web site at http://www.cdc.gov/nip/recs/child-schedule.pdf.

Graft-Versus-Host Disease

Acute

- Usually 20–100 days posttransplant
- Symptoms: dermatitis (rash on palms, soles, face/neck/upper torso), hepatitis, colitis (diarrhea)
- Treatment: steroids, cyclosporin A (Neoral, Sandimmune) (target range of 250–350), antithymocyte globulin (Atgam), tacrolimus

Chronic

- Usually 150 days posttransplant
- Sicca syndrome: thickened skin, lichen planus, papules, cholestatic jaundice, scleroderma-like skin, eye and GI lesions
- Treatment: steroids, cyclosporin A, azathioprine (Imuran), thalidomide (Thalomid) (although most treatment is discouraging), psoralens + UV light of A wave length (skin), hydroxychloroquine (Plaquenil)

NON-HODGKIN'S LYMPHOMA

- Non-Hodgkin's lymphoma (NHL) encompasses >12 neoplasms.
- It is the most frequent malignancy in children with AIDS; thus, perform HIV screening in all children with NHL.
- See Table 15-1 for lineage categorization and median survival time.

Classification

Low Grade

Clinical presentation: painless, diffuse peripheral lymphadenopathy in older adults.

Intermediate Grade

Clinical presentation: painless peripheral lymphadenopathy, but localized extranodal disease is also common (e.g., GI and bone). Median age is 55 yrs but is also common in children and young adults.

High Grade

Clinical presentation:

- Lymphoblastic lymphoma: disease of children and young adults. Approx. two-thirds are boys, and most (50–75%) have mediastinal involvement at presentation (manifesting as shortness of breath, dyspnea, wheezing, stridor, dysphagia, and head/neck swelling).
- Small noncleaved cell (Burkitt's/non-Burkitt's): usually a childhood disease, but a second peak occurs after 50 yrs. Burkitt's commonly presents in the abdomen and GI tract (approx. 80%) vs non-Burkitt's presents in the bone marrow and with peripheral lymphadenopathy. Presentation in right lower quadrant is common and can be confused with appendicitis.

TABLE 15-1.
LINEAGE CATEGORY (% OF CHILDHOOD NHL)

Lineages (immunophenotype/genotype)	Median survival (yrs)
B lineage (nodal)	
Low grade	
Small lymphocytic	5.5–6
Lymphoplasmocytic/lymphoplasmacytoid	4
Follicular small cleaved cell	6.5–7
Follicular mixed small cleaved/large cell	4.5–5
Intermediate grade	
Follicular large cell	2.5–3
Diffuse small cleaved/mixed small and large	3–4
Intermediate lymphocytic/mantle cell	3–5
High grade	
Diffuse large cell lymphoma	1–2
Immunoblastic	0.5–1.5
Small noncleaved cell	0.5–1
T lineage	
Lymphoblastic	0.5–2
Peripheral T-cell lymphoma	1–2
Primary extranodal lymphoma (classified by site; most are B-cell and MALT lineages)	

Staging Studies

- Essential workup: physical exam, CBC, complete metabolic panel, LDH, uric acid, CXR, chest CT (if CXR is abnormal), abdominal CT (or abdominal U/S), bilateral bone marrow aspirate/biopsy, CSF analysis, gallium scan

- Suggested: bone scan, MRI for bone marrow involvement, PET scan

Treatment

Treatment of NHL depends on pathologic subtype and stage.

HODGKIN'S DISEASE
Definition

- Lymphoma with pleomorphic lymphocytic infiltrate; Reed-Sternberg cells are multinucleated giant cells and are considered to be the malignant cells of Hodgkin's disease.

- Distribution: bimodal, with early peak in mid- to late 20s and second peak after 50 yrs.

Epidemiology

Most cases outside of United States are associated with EBV in Reed-Sternberg cells vs approx. one-third in United States.

Clinical Presentation

- Usually painless adenopathy (common in the supraclavicular/cervical areas; usually firm; usually spreads contiguously).

- Many patients have some degree of mediastinal involvement (approximately two-thirds), some have systemic symptoms (e.g., B symptoms—see below), cough (need to fully assess airway before procedures), generalized pruritus.

- Primary subdiaphragmatic disease is rare (approx. 3%), as is ethanol-induced pain in the lymph nodes (pathognomonic).

- B symptoms: presence of fever >38°C for 3 consecutive days, night sweats, or unexplained weight loss of ≥10% in the past 6 mos preceding admission (denote presence of B symptoms by "B" after stage, or "A" for asymptomatic).

Evaluation

Workup: physical exam and determination of history for B symptoms, measurement of lymph nodes, CBC (idiopathic thrombocytopenic purpura [ITP] is commonly associated), LDH, ESR, and UA (more commonly elevated in NHL), renal and hepatic function tests, neck/chest/abdomen/pelvic CT, gallium scan, bone scan (for those with bone pain or elevated alkaline phosphatase), PET scan (more commonly used), bilateral bone marrow aspirate and biopsy (not just aspirate; performed usually just in patients with stage III–IV or with B symptoms, or at relapse).

Treatment

Treatment of Hodgkin's disease depends on stage.

WILMS' TUMOR AND RENAL TUMORS
Clinical Presentation

Primary presentation is abdominal mass, usually not crossing midline (vs neuroblastoma, which often crosses midline).

Clinical Syndromes Associated with Wilms' Tumors

As many as 10% of Wilms' tumors are associated with malformation syndromes.

- Beckwith-Wiedemann syndrome (approx. 5% incidence): macroglossia, organomegaly, umbilical hernia, gigantism, neonatal hypoglycemia. Approx. one-fifth present with bilateral Wilms' tumors and are also at increased risk for metachronous recurrence.

- WAGR syndrome (>30%): **W**ilms' tumor, **a**niridia, **g**enitourinary anomalies, mental **r**etardation.

- Sporadic aniridia (33%): absence of the iris.

- Denys-Drash syndrome (>90%): intersex disorders, nephropathy.

- Hemihypertrophy (approx. 5%): asymmetric overgrowth syndrome.

Workup

Abdominal CT, CXR.

NEUROBLASTOMA
Clinical Presentation

75% of cases present before 5 yrs and 97% are diagnosed before 10 yrs (peak is 2–4 yrs).

- Palpable abdominal mass, bone pain from metastases, and mass effects from the tumor or metastases (e.g., proptosis and periorbital ecchymosis from retrobulbar metastases, HTN). Other symptoms: fever, anemia, diarrhea, Horner's syndrome, cerebellar ataxia, opsoclonus/myoclonus.

- Metastatic disease: Approx. 70% have metastatic disease at presentation (majority are N-myc amplified).

Workup

- Investigations needed before treatment: bilateral bone marrow aspiration/BMB, bone scan, abdominal CT, CXR, urine vanillylmandelic acid and homovanillic acid, LDH, histologic exam of palpable lymph nodes

- Considerations: chest CT if positive CXR or bone scan, pelvic CT if notable extension, CT/MRI of other metastatic sites, skeletal survey

OSTEOSARCOMA
Natural History

Occurs primarily in adolescents and young adults, with approximately 50% occurring in the bones around the knee. Approximately 80% of patients with apparently localized tumors have disease recurrence if treated only with surgical excision, indicating that the majority of patients have disseminated disease at presentation.

- Peak incidence: occurs in second decade of life during adolescent growth spurt

Clinical Presentation

Most present with pain over involved area (usually for many mos). 15–20% of patients have detectable metastatic disease at presentation (poor prognosis), of which ≥85% are pulmonary metastases.

Radiologic Workup

- Highly variable with no pathognomonic radiologic features

- Common presentations (plain films): periosteal new bone formation (lifting of cortex, forming of Codman's triangle), soft tissue masses, invariable involvement of the metaphyseal portion (<10% involve the diaphysis), ossification in the soft tissue in a radial or "sunburst" pattern, osteosclerotic (approx. 45%), osteolytic (approx. 30%), and mixed sclerotic/osteolytic (approx. 25%)

  - MRI is invaluable to assess intraosseous extent of the tumor and distinction of muscle groups/fat, joints, and neurovascular structures.

  - Bone scan is important to examine extent of primary tumor and detect metastases.

  - CXR/chest CT is important because the lung is the first metastatic site in approx. 90% of cases.

Treatment

- Surgery: Primary management is surgical excision with wide margins because of the unresponsiveness to radiation. Refer to an orthopedic surgeon.

- Adjuvant chemotherapy: usually given pre- and postsurgery.

Follow-Up

Needed for at least 5 yrs after therapy.

- Perform CXR monthly × 2 yrs, with decreased frequency after.

- Perform chest CT q4–6mos for the first 2 yrs.

- Evaluate the primary site at intervals determined by the orthopedic surgeon.

RHABDOMYOSARCOMA
Definition

Soft tissue malignancy of skeletal muscle origin.

Presentation

Primary sites include the head and neck (e.g., parameningeal, orbit, pharyngeal), genitourinary tract, and extremities. Other sites include trunk, intrathoracic, GI tract (liver, biliary, and perianal/anal).

Workup

CT of the area under suspicion, bone scan, CXR, chest CT, bone marrow aspirate, and biopsy.

Treatment

- Surgery: Basic principle is for complete resection with negative margins.

- Chemotherapy options: All patients receive chemotherapy (extent/ duration depends on risk factor analysis).

- XRT: effective for microscopic and gross residual disease after initial surgical resection or chemotherapy.

EWING'S SARCOMAS/PERIPHERAL NEUROECTODERMAL TUMOR
Definition

Ewing's sarcoma refers to tumors of either bone (Ewing's tumor of bone) or soft tissue (extraosseous Ewing's; "classic Ewing's") origin, and are derived from primitive pluripotent cells from neural crest origin (postganglionic parasympathetic autonomic nervous system). Peripheral primitive neuroectodermal tumor is considered to be a more differentiated form of this entity and can occur as a primary tumor of bone or soft tissue.

Presentation/Clinical Symptoms

Pain, palpable mass, pathologic fracture, and fever (often for many mos).

Evaluation

- Imaging: x-ray of bone (usually destructive lesion of the diaphysis with cortex erosion and multilaminar periosteal reaction—i.e., "onion peel"), MRI of primary (better than CT), bone scan, chest CT, CXR
- Labs: LDH, urine catecholamines (to distinguish from neuroblastoma), bilateral bone marrow aspiration/bone marrow biopsy

Treatment

Requires combination chemotherapy in addition to XRT and possible surgery.

MULTIPLE ENDOCRINE NEOPLASIA (MEN) SYNDROMES
See Table 15-2.

RETINOBLASTOMA
Variants
Hereditary

Positive family history (found in 6–10% of retinoblastoma patients); however, 30–40% of "sporadic" may be hereditary. Mean age of 14–15 mos at diagnosis, usually bilateral/multifocal, high risk of developing nonocular tumor.

Nonhereditary

Negative family history. Mean age of 7–23 mos at diagnosis, always unilateral/unifocal (note: 15% of patients with unilateral tumors may have hereditary disease), no increased risk of nonocular tumors.

Presentation/Clinical Symptoms

Leukocoria, proptosis, strabismus.

TABLE 15-2.
MULTIPLE ENDOCRINE NEOPLASIA (MEN) SYNDROMES

Site of origin	MEN I (Werner's)	MEN IIa (Sipple's)	MEN IIb
Pituitary	Prolactinoma, soma-totropinoma, corti-cotropinoma	—	—
Thyroid	—	C-cell hyperplasia, medullary carcinoma	Medullary carcinoma
Parathyroid	Parathyroid hyperpla-sia and adenoma	Parathyroid hyper-plasia and adenoma	—
Adrenal cortex	Adrenal adenoma and hyperplasia	—	—
Adrenal medulla/gas-troentero-pancreatic	Gastrinoma, insuli-noma, vasoactive intes-tinal polypeptide tumor, glucagonoma	Pheochromocytoma	Pheochro-mocytoma
Other	Lipomas, carcinoids	—	Mucosal neu-romas, gan-glioneuromas

Evaluation

- Consult pediatric ophthalmology for direct and indirect ophthal-moscopy, exam under anesthesia.
- CBC, head MRI.
- If tumor extension outside of globe, LP and bone marrow.

Treatment

Radiation therapy, cryotherapy, photocoagulation, enucleation, chemo-therapy.

SICKLE CELL DISEASE
Outpatient Management of Febrile Illness (Temp >38.5°C) in Child with HbSS
History and Physical Exam

Vital signs (with O_2 saturation), pallor, evidence of infection, cardio-pulmonary status (e.g., signs and symptoms of acute chest syndrome), spleen size (vs normal baseline), neurologic exam.

Evaluation

CBC with differential, reticulocyte count (to exclude aplastic crisis due to parvovirus B19), blood culture, UA and urine culture (if indicated), CXR (especially if symptoms of cough, chest pain, history of acute chest syndrome, toxic appearing, <95% saturation or 4% less than baseline, fever), CSF analysis (if indicated), extra purple top for type and cross-match if pallor/acute spleen/respiratory or neurologic symptoms.

Treatment

- IV ceftriaxone (50–75 mg/kg, 2 g max.) after obtaining blood culture; observe 1 hr after chemotherapy administration with repeat vital signs and assessment; may substitute clindamycin (Cleocin) (10 mg/kg, max dose: 600 mg) for those with cephalosporin allergy.

- The presence of a focus of infection (e.g., otitis media) does *not* alter urgency of administration of parenteral antibiotics.

- Acetaminophen (Tylenol), 15 mg/kg (if not given in last 4 hrs). Avoid ibuprofen if contraindicated (e.g., gastritis, renal impairment, coagulopathy, ulcers).

- Admission considerations

  - Most infants aged <3 yrs with HbSS or S-beta thalassemia

  - Most infants with previous episodes of bacteremia/sepsis

  - Most infants with temp >40°C, WBC >30,000 or <5000, and/or platelets <100,000 (except in patients with HbSC and long-standing splenomegaly and thrombocytopenia)

  - Evidence of: severe pain, aplastic crisis (reticulocyte count <5% in HbSS or <2% in HbSC), splenic sequestration, acute chest syndrome, stroke, priapism

  - No hematology visit within last 12 mos regardless of age (indication of poor compliance)

  - O_2 saturation <92% on room air or 5% difference from baseline

  - Hgb <5g/dL or ≥2g/dL below baseline (particularly HbSC disease)

Inpatient Management of Febrile Illness in Child with HbSS
History and Physical Exam

See Outpatient Management (page 142).

Evaluation

- CBC with differential and reticulocyte count (both daily until improving), CXR, blood culture, UA, urine culture, consider lumbar puncture

- Consider LFTs and DIC screen (especially with signs of encephalopathy)

- Consider abdominal U/S, amylase/lipase for upper quadrant/severe abdominal pain (rule out cholelithiasis, cholecystitis, pancreatitis)

- Type and crossmatch if Hgb is 1–2 g/dL below baseline or if evidence of acute chest syndrome (positive CXR infiltrate and fever)—remember to request, if available, minor antigen–matched blood (e.g., "Charles Drew" units if available, or Kell/C/e negative units)

- Consider orthopedic consult to rule out osteomyelitis or septic arthritis.

Monitoring

- Vital signs q4h
- Consider cardiorespiratory (CR) monitor/ICU for signs of cardiovascular instability
- Daily input and output and weight
- Pulse oximetry for severe illness or respiratory symptoms/O_2 saturations <92% on room air or 4% less than baseline

Fluids

D5 $\frac{1}{4}$NS or D5$\frac{1}{2}$NS at 1500 cc/m^2/day (avoid excess fluids).

Treatment

- Antibiotics: ceftriaxone, 50 mg/kg IV q12h; **OR** cefotaxime, 50 mg/kg IV q8h (substitute clindamycin, 10 mg/kg IV q6h for patients with known or suspected cephalosporin allergy). Add azithromycin (Zithromax, Zithromax Z-Pak) (despite age), 10 mg/kg × 1 day, followed by 5 mg/kg × 4 days if patient has CXR infiltrate with fever, or fever with respiratory symptoms. Consider vancomycin, 15 mg/kg IV q8h, for severe illness or suspected CNS infection.

- Discontinue prophylactic antibiotics while patient is receiving broad-spectrum antibiotics.

- Pain: acetaminophen, 15 mg/kg q4h; may add ibuprofen, 10 mg/kg q6h if no contraindication (e.g., gastritis, renal impairment, coagulopathy, ulcer).

- O_2 to keep saturation ≥92% **OR** patient's baseline value (O_2 saturation measured using pulse oximetry often is not correlative to partial pressure of O_2 and central arterial O_2 saturation). Investigate etiologies (e.g., repeat CXR) for any new or increasing O_2 requirement. Avoid excess O_2 (exacerbates anemia and suppress reticulocytosis).

Current Management of Acute Chest Syndrome

Definition

Appearance or new infiltrate on CXR in a patient with sickle cell disease.

Evaluation

- *Watch carefully!* Acute chest syndrome is the primary cause of death with a mortality rate of 1–4%.
- Monitoring: vital signs with BPs q2–4h, continuous pulse oximetry, input and output.
- Labs:
  - Type and screen patients with new CXR infiltrate in anticipation of probable simple transfusion and/or exchange; consider

type and crossmatch for severe illness or Hgb >1 g/dL below baseline (request minor antigen–matched if available, sickle negative, LP).

- Daily CBC with differential and reticulocyte counts (may require more frequent CBCs with reticulocyte counts to monitor Hgb level), blood gas for severe illness, complete metabolic panel and fractionated bili for severe illness (rule out multiorgan failure syndrome).

Treatment

- IV fluids: maintenance (1500 cc/m^2/day) or maintain euvolemia.
- Begin on double antibiotic coverage (cefotaxime/ceftriaxone + azithromycin/erythromycin; substitute clindamycin for ceftriaxone/cefotaxime in cephalosporin-allergic patients).
- Begin incentive spirometry (10×/hr while awake)—write this as an order.
- Steroids at 2 mg/kg/day is controversial.
- Adequate pain control with bowel regimen.
- Consider scheduled albuterol—especially if patient has history of asthma/reactive airway disease or wheezing on exam (a trial is often indicated).
- Supplemental O$_2$ to keep saturation ≥92% or patient's baseline (watch carefully for increased O$_2$ requirement, as that is a signal of poor O$_2$ delivery and the need for probable transfusion)—*call fellow/attending immediately!*

Acute Splenic Sequestration
Definition
Acute illness with Hgb of ≥2 g/dL below patient's baseline with acutely enlarging spleen. Mild to moderate thrombocytopenia is often present. Usually with reticulocytosis (consider aplastic crisis if decreased).

Evaluation

- Consider ICU admission for observation/requirement for partial exchange. Type and crossmatch STAT (consider minor antigen–matched if time permits).
- Monitoring: daily CBC with differential and reticulocyte count, serial abdominal/cardiovascular exams q2–4h, pulse oximetry, CR monitor, vital signs with BPs q2h.

Treatment

- Fluids: D5^1/$_4$NS or D5^1/$_2$NS at 1500/m^2/day (more if dehydrated, fever). Incentive spirometry.

- Medications
  - Packed RBC transfusion of 10 cc/kg for Hgb <4–5 and/or signs of cardiovascular compromise. In severe cases, urgent initiation of transfusion before inpatient admission may be life saving.
  - Antibiotics if febrile (see above). O_2 to keep saturation ≥92% or patient's baseline.
  - Treatment of pain with analgesics.

Aplastic Crisis

Definition

Acute illness associated with Hgb below patient's baseline with substantially decreased reticulocyte count (often <1%)—most are due to parvo B19 virus.

Evaluation

- Place patient on contact/respiratory isolation if suspected.
- Daily CBC with differential and reticulocyte count; parvo B19 PCR or titers; consider blood culture, UA, urine culture if febrile (also CSF).
- Type and crossmatch (consider minor antigen–matched blood, and sickle-negative/LP).

Treatment

Packed RBC transfusions for symptomatic anemia or Hgb <5 with no evidence of erythroid recovery. Repeated transfusions may be required. Transfusion may need to be repeated. Avoid transfusion of Hgb >10.

Acute Stroke or Neurologic Event

- Occurs in 7–11% of patients with HbSS.
- Consult neurology.

Evaluation

- Consider ICU and/or CR monitoring until stable or first 24 hrs; neurologic checks q2h.
- Labs: CBC with differential, reticulocyte count, RBC minor antigen–phenotype, consider coagulation workup, blood and urine cultures if febrile, type and screen, daily BMPs, consider lumbar puncture/CSF analysis.
- Studies: MRI and MRA; if not immediately available, CT **without** contrast to exclude intracranial hemorrhage.

Treatment

- Fluids: $D5^1/_4NS$ or $D5^1/_2NS$ at 1500 cc/m^2/day (caution with fluid overload)

- Medications
  - Seizure treatment if needed.
  - Steroids if signs of increased ICP.
  - Erythrocytapheresis/partial exchange to Hgb of 10 should be considered for patients with Hgb <6–7 (do not transfuse if Hgb >10).
  - Simple transfusion with packed RBCs to Hgb of 10 may be considered as an alternative to partial exchange for stable patients with Hgb <6–7 (do not transfuse Hgb >10).
  - Antibiotics: if febrile or suspected CNS infection.

Immunizations and Prophylactic Meds for Sickle Cell Disease

- Penicillin prophylaxis: 125 mg penicillin VK PO bid for <3 yrs; 250 mg PO bid for 3–5 yr olds
- Folic acid: 400 μg–1 mg PO qd for children with significant hemolysis (e.g., HbSS, S-beta thalassemia; these patients have 5–6× normal bone marrow RBC turnover)

Pain Management in Sickle Cell Disease

Physical Exam

Always consider etiologies other than sickling for pain (e.g., cholecystitis, appendicitis, trauma); compare to prior vascular occlusive crisis pain episodes; exam for hydration/evidence of infection/pallor/spleen size/priapism/neurologic.

Labs

See Inpatient Management of Febrile Illness in Child with HbSS and Current Management of Acute Chest Syndrome above.

IV Fluids

Start with 10 cc/kg bolus over 1 hr, then at 1500 cc/m^2/day (higher if dehydrated).

Mild to Moderate Pain

- Acetaminophen (Tylenol #3 [codeine at 1 mg/kg]) PO, then q4h; if inadequate relief in 30 mins, use morphine or alternatives below.
- Consider ibuprofen/NSAIDs if no contraindication exists.

Moderate to Severe Pain

Start morphine or other alternative analgesics below (e.g., hydromorphone [Dilaudid], ketorolac [Toradol], fentanyl [Duragesic]). Consider pain team consultation.

Morphine

- Discuss with pediatric hematologist or PMD.

- Start at 0.05–0.15 mg/kg q2h and titrate (many patients require *a lot more*)—ensure continuous pulse oximetry and consider CR monitoring; reassess pain q15–30mins.
- In most cases, prn analgesic orders are **not** appropriate.
- If pain relief with 1 or 2 doses of morphine, consider T#3 (1 mg/kg based on codeine) or other PO narcotics in planning outpatient therapy.

Fentanyl Drips

Bolus with 1 mg/kg, then start at 0.75–1 mg/kg/h and titrate up (may need to adjust titration frequently in the first few hrs).

Others

Consider hydromorphone (Dilaudid), 0.015–0.02 mg/kg IV q3–4h; ketorolac (Toradol), 0.5 mg/kg (30 mg max.) IV q6–8h in addition to opioid (do not use with ibuprofen).

ANEMIAS

See Fig. 15-1 for diagnostic algorithm.

History

- Past medical history
- Dietary history (including mother and newborn; iron-deficiency anemia in term infants never is the etiology before 6 mos—rare in preemies)
- Gender (consider X-linked: G6PD, pyruvate kinase deficiency)
- Race (Hgb S–, C–, beta-thalassemia, in blacks/Mediterraneans; alpha-thalassemia in blacks/Asians)
- Neonatal (history of hyperbilirubinemia suggests congenital hemolytic anemia such as hereditary spherocytosis, hereditary elliptocytosis, G6PD)
- Trauma/blood loss
- History of transfusions
- Medications
- Illnesses (e.g., infections such as hepatitis-induced aplastic anemia)
- Family history (anemia, jaundice, gallstones, splenomegaly, surgeries, and transfusions)

Evaluation

- CBC, reticulocyte count, evaluation of smear, Coombs', creatinine.
- Others after initial evaluation:
  - Hgb electrophoresis
  - Infectious workup
  - Osmotic fragility

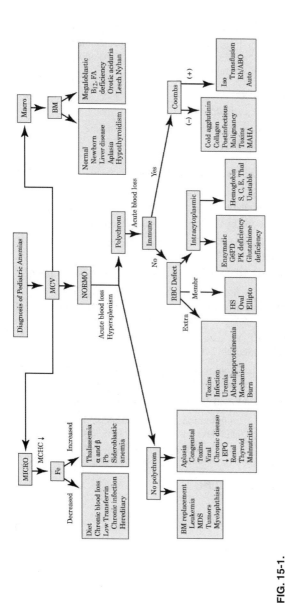

FIG. 15-1.

Diagnosis of pediatric anemias. BM, bone marrow; Ellipto, elliptocytosis; EPO, erythropoietin; FA, folic acid; HS, hereditary spherocytosis; macro, macrocytic; MAHA, microangiopathic hemolytic anemia; MCHC, mean corpuscular hemoglobin concentration; MCV, mean corpuscular volume; MDS, myelodysplastic syndrome; micro, microcytic; normo, normocytic; Oval, ovalocytosis; PK, pyruvate kinase; polychrom, polychromasia; Thal, thalassemia.

- G6PD test
- Bone marrow aspirate/biopsy
- Hgb stability
- Others: bilirubin panel, LDH, haptoglobin, serum B_{12}, RBC folate, ferritin, iron, total iron-binding capacity, circulating transferrin receptor, serum Pb, RBC zinc protoporphyrin, RBC enzyme panel, membrane protein studies

LEAD POISONING
Treatment for Asymptomatic Children
- See also American Academy of Pediatrics guidelines.
- See Table 15-3.

Treatment for the Symptomatic Child
- Patients with clinical symptoms suggesting encephalopathy require inpatient chelation therapy.
- Lead encephalopathy is a life-threatening emergency.
- **Treatment** includes monitoring of increased ICP and hemodynamic stability.
  - Control convulsions with diazepam, 0.15 mg/kg, repeat prn q20–30mins).
  - Maintain diuresis with D10W or D5^1/4NS to keep urinary output at 350–500 cc/m^2/day.
  - Chelation therapy should be administered as per the guidelines for blood lead levels ≥70 mg/dL.
  - Parenteral chelation should be continued with both BAL and $CaNa_2$ EDTA until the patient is clinically stable.
- Ensure follow-up for all children receiving chelation therapy.
  - A period of reequilibration of 10–14 days should occur, then another blood lead level should be drawn. Further treatment should be based on this level and should proceed according to the recommendations for the new blood lead level.

WORKUP FOR BLEEDING
Screening Tests
CBC (platelet count), PT, aPTT, fibrinogen level, fibrinogen degradation product.

- If abnormal platelet number: ITP, bone marrow suppression/replacement (rule out drug role), bone marrow hypoplasia, von Willebrand's disease IIb.

TABLE 15-3.
LEAD POISONING TREATMENT

Blood level (mg/dL)	Action	Treatment
0–9	No immediate concern	None.
10–14	Environmental survey	None.
15–19	Educational intervention, monitor periodically	None.
≥30	Education, removal of lead source	None.
29–45	Medical attention, removal of lead source	Begin iron replacement if iron deficient.
45–69	Medical attention, removal of lead source	PO: succimer (DMSA) 10 mg/kg/dose q8h × 5 days. Then 10 mg/kg/dose q12h × 14 more days. **OR** IM: $CaNa_2$ EDTA. Begin multivitamin. $CaNa_2$ EDTA at 25 mg/kg/day × 5 days.
≥70	Emergency hospitalization	Initiate therapy with IM BAL at 25 mg/kg/day divided into 6 doses. The second dose of BAL is given 4 hrs after the first dose and is followed immediately by IV $CaNa_2$ EDTA at 50 mg/kg/day as a continuous infusion. Therapy must be continued for ≥72 hrs. After 72 hrs, two options exist: continue therapy with both drugs for a total of 5 days **OR** continue therapy with $CaNa_2$ EDTA alone for a total of 5 days. If BAL and $CaNa_2$ EDTA are both used for the full 5 days, a minimum of 2 days with no treatment should elapse before further treatment is considered.

BAL, British antilewisite; EDTA, ethylenediaminetetraacetic acid.

- If normal platelet number: Is there a deficient coagulation factor or platelet dysfunction (acquired, congenital—e.g., gray platelet syndrome)?
- If abnormal morphology ± abnormal number: check PT/aPTT.
- If abnormal platelets, PT, aPTT, thrombin time: consider DIC, liver disease, dysfibrinogenemia.
- If normal platelets, PT, aPTT: consider factor XIII, $alpha_2$-antiplasmin.

DISSEMINATED INTRAVASCULAR COAGULATION

Definition

- Generalized dysregulation with activation of coagulation and fibrin as well as fibrinolysis; thus, may experience bleeding, thrombosis, both or none
- Triggered by exposure of tissue factor on tissue (subendothelium, brain, placenta, activated endothelial cells)

Labs

PT/PTT are prolonged, fibrinogen <100 mg/dL, platelet count is low, D dimer >2 mg/cc (commonly positive in infants without DIC), factor II/factor V/factor VIII/antithrombin III/protein C are usually low, microangiopathic hemolytic anemia on peripheral smear.

Treatment

- Fresh frozen plasma, cryoprecipitate, platelet transfusions (heparin treatment has shown no benefit)
- General guidelines: platelets: keep >50,000; fibrinogen: keep >100 mg/dL; PT: keep within normal range for age

HEMOPHILIA

Factor VIII Deficiency (Hemophilia A)

Labs

- Bleeding time: normal.
- PT: normal.
- PTT: prolonged.
- PTT corrects with 50:50.
- An infant with factor VIII deficiency must be evaluated for von Willebrand's disease (because neonates have higher vWF levels, and only severely affected patients might show bleeding problems).

Treatment

Each U/kg raises blood level approx. 2%.

- Limited oral bleeding: aminocaproic acid (Amicar), 100 mg/kg PO q6h (antifibrinolytic agent: epsilon-aminocaproic acid)
- Mild to moderate bleeding: factor VIII, 20–25 U/kg IV; and/or DDAVP, 0.3 μg/kg/dose IV or DDAVP nasal spray (<50 kg: 150 μg in one nostril; >50 kg: 150 μg in each nostril), in those who respond
- Severe to life-threatening bleeding: factor VIII, 50 U/kg IV followed by repeated infusions of 20–25 units/kg IV q12h
- Surgical patients: 50 U/kg IV; usually require repeat administration q6–12h for a total of 10–14 days or until healed

Factor IX Deficiency (Hemophilia B; Christmas Disease)
Labs
- Bleeding time: normal.
- PT: normal.
- PTT: prolonged.
- Thrombin time: normal.
- PTT corrects with 50:50.

Treatment
Each U/kg raises blood level approx. 1%.
- Limited oral bleeding: aminocaproic acid (Amicar), 100 mg/kg PO q6h
- Mild to moderate bleeding: factor IX, 30 U/kg IV
- Severe to life threatening: factor IX, 80 U/kg, followed by 40 U/kg q24h (note: longer half-life)

Factor XI Deficiency (Hemophilia C)
- Rare autosomal recessive disorder (Ashkenazi Jews, Noonan syndrome)
- Treatment: FFP

Factor XIII Deficiency
- Often presents with umbilical cord bleeding (80% with homozygous deficiency): one-third with intracranial hemorrhage; autosomal dominant inheritance
- Diagnosis: with 5M urea exam of clot stability
- Treatment: cryoprecipitate

THROMBOCYTOPENIAS
Etiologies in Newborns
- Decreased production
- Immune mediated: maternal ITP, maternal SLE, maternal hyperthyroidism, maternal drugs, maternal preeclampsia, neonatal alloimmune thrombocytopenia
- Nonimmune (probably related to DIC): asphyxia, aspiration, necrotizing enterocolitis, hemangiomas, thrombosis, respiratory distress syndrome, Kasabach-Merritt syndrome, hemolytic uremic syndrome, heart disease (congenital/acquired)
- Unknown: hyperbilirubinemia, phototherapy, polycythemia, Rh disease, congenital thrombotic thrombocytopenia, total parenteral nutrition, inborn errors
- Hypersplenism

- Fatty acid–induced thrombocytopenia
- Decreased production

Idiopathic (Immune) Thrombocytopenic Purpura

- Peak age of diagnosis of acute ITP is 2–4 yrs (although any child can develop ITP; those aged <1 yr or >10 yrs are more likely to develop chronic ITP, possibly in conjunction with other immune disorders—e.g., SLE, angiolymphoproliferative syndrome, or *Helicobacter pylori*).
- Acute ITP: occurs in approximately 90% and is self-limited disease, resolving in 6 mos—whether or not therapy is given.
- If treatment is given, there are several options. Fresh blood or platelet concentrates may be given but are of transient benefit. IVIG (1 g/kg/day for 1–2 days) increases the platelet count. Corticosteroids (prednisone, 1–2 mg/kg/day) reduce the severity and shorten the initial phase of the disease. Steroids are given until the platelet count is normal or until 3 wks of treatment have elapsed, whichever occurs first.

CAUSES OF LYMPHADENOPATHY

- Infection:
  - Bacterial: streptococcus, staphylococcus, mycobacteriosis, brucellosis, tularemia, bartonella, syphilis
  - Viral: EBV, CMV, HIV, rubella
  - Fungal: histoplasmosis, coccidioidomycosis
  - Protozoan: toxoplasmosis, malaria
- Autoimmune disease: rheumatoid arthritis, SLE, serum sickness, autoimmune hemolytic anemia.
- Storage disease: Niemann-Pick and Gaucher's diseases
- Drug reactions (e.g., phenytoin).
- Malignancy: lymphoma, leukemia, metastatic (rhabdomyosarcoma, neuroblastoma, thyroid, carcinomas), histiocytosis (Langerhans' cell histiocytoma, malignant histiocytosis).
- Others: sarcoidosis, Kawasaki's disease, cat-scratch disease.
- Evaluation: Based on history and examination, perform lab tests to look for above causes. Lymph node biopsy may be necessary.
- Management: Treat etiology.

SUGGESTED READING

Pizzo PA, Poplack DG. *Principles and practice of pediatric oncology*, 3rd ed. Philadelphia: Lippincott–Raven, 1997.

16 Infectious Disease

Remember to wash your hands.

INTRODUCTION

When evaluating the patient with a presumed infectious condition, always get a detailed exposure history, including travel, animals, day care attendance, food intake (and how the food was prepared), and sick contacts. Always think about current outbreaks in the community. Also, remember to isolate the child sooner rather than later.

EPSTEIN-BARR VIRUS (INFECTIOUS MONONUCLEOSIS)
Signs and Symptoms

Fever, exudative pharyngitis, lymphadenopathy, malaise, hepatosplenomegaly.

Labs

- Monospot may be falsely negative, especially if age <5 yrs. Need IgG and IgM.
- Consider CMV if patient seronegative for Epstein-Barr virus (EBV).

Treatment

Supportive; avoid contact sports if splenomegaly, corticosteroids if severe pharyngeal swelling.

SEPTIC ARTHRITIS
Signs and Symptoms

Painful joint, fever, decreased range of motion, swelling/warmth/tenderness/erythema at joint.

Diagnosis

Joint aspiration with elevated WBCs, positive Gram's stain.

Serum Labs

Elevated ESR, C-reactive protein, and WBCs.

Imaging

Plain films may show widened joint space; U/S may show increased fluid in joint space.

Treatment

Analgesia and IV antibiotics

- Neonate: Antibiotics effective against *Staphylococcus aureus*, group B streptococci, *Escherichia coli*.

- Age <5 yrs: Antibiotics effective against *S. aureus*, *Streptococcus pyogenes*, pneumococcus, *Haemophilus influenzae*.

- Age >5 yrs: Antibiotics effective against *S. aureus, S. pyogenes*, *Streptococcus pneumoniae*, *Neisseria meningitidis*.

- Adolescent: Also consider *Neisseria gonorrhoeae*.

- Sickle cell disease: Also consider *Salmonella*.

- Consult orthopedic surgery early.

TUBERCULOSIS
Definition of Positive Mantoux Skin Test

See Table 16-1.

Drug Therapy

Prophylaxis if positive tuberculin test but no evidence of disease, or recent contact with TB infected person even if tuberculin test negative. See Table 16-2.

TABLE 16-1.
DEFINITION OF POSITIVE MANTOUX SKIN TEST

≥5 mm	≥10 mm	≥15 mm
Children in close contact with people who have known or suspected TB	Children at increased risk of dissemination (age <4 yrs, Hodgkin's lymphoma, diabetes, CRF, malnutrition)	Children >4 yrs without any risk factors
Children suspected to have TB based on CXR or other clinical evidence of TB Children with immunosuppressive conditions	Children with increased environmental exposure (born or having parents who were born in areas with increased TB rates, those who travel to high-prevalence regions, those frequently exposed to adults who are HIV infected, homeless, street drug users, medically indigent, residents of nursing homes, incarcerated, institutionalized, or migrant farmers)	

TABLE 16-2.
THERAPEUTIC REGIMENS FOR TB

Category	Regimen	Remarks
Asymptomatic	6–9 mos (12 mos if HIV infected): isoniazid qd or rifampin if isoniazid resistant qd	If daily therapy is impossible, therapy 2×/wk may be used. Repeat tuberculin skin test 12 wks after contact with TB is broken; if negative, may discontinue prophylaxis; if positive, complete regimen.
Pulmonary	6 mos: 2 mos of isoniazid (Laniazid, Nydrazid), rifampin (Rifadin, Rimactane), and pyrazinamide (pms-Pyrazinamide, Tebrazid) qd followed by 4 mos of isoniazid and rifampin qd	If possible drug resistance, add ethambutol (Myambutol) or streptomycin to original 3-drug regimen until drug susceptibilities known.
	9 mos (if hilar adenopathy only): 9 mos of isoniazid and rifampin qd or 1 mo of isonaizid and rifampin qd followed by 8 mos of isoniazid and rifampin 2×/wk	—
Extrapulmonary	2 mos of isoniazid, rifampin, pyrazinamide, and streptomycin qd followed by 10 mos of isoniazid and rifampin qd	—

HEPATITIS B SEROLOGIES

- HBsAg indicates acute or chronic infection.
- HBeAg indicates active HBV infection, indicates high infectivity.
- HBV-DNA indicates HBV replication.
- Anti-HBc indicates active HBV infection.
- Anti-HBe indicates resolution of hepatitis.
- Anti-HBs indicates clinical recovery or immunization.

COMMON PEDIATRIC INFECTIOUS DISEASES AND THEIR CAUSES

See Table 16-3.

TABLE 16-3.
COMMON INFECTIOUS DISEASES IN CHILDREN

Infection	Common etiologies	Remarks
Bacteremia (well-appearing child)	*S. pneumoniae, H. influenzae, N. meningitidis, E. coli, Salmonella*	—
Human bite	Streptococci, *S. aureus, Staphylococcus epidermidis,* anaerobes, *Eikenella corrodens*	—
Dog/cat bite	Human bite etiologies, *Pasteurella multocida*	15–20% of dog bites become infected, 30–40% of cat bites become infected
		Clean wound
		Do not primarily close wounds >24 hrs old, infected wounds, or hand wounds
		Consider need for rabies and tetanus prophylaxis
Cellulitis	Group A streptococci, *S. aureus*	—
Conjunctivitis (neonatal)	Chemical irritation	—
	Chlamydia trachomatis, N. gonorrhoeae, HSV	—
Conjunctivitis (suppurative)	*S. pneumoniae, H. influenzae, S. aureus, Moraxella catarrhalis,* adenovirus	Bacterial more common in the preschooler and more likely to be bilateral
Gastroenteritis (community acquired)	Viruses, *E. coli, Salmonella, Shigella, Yersinia, Camplyobacter*	—
Gastroenteritis (nosocomial)	*Clostridium difficile*	—
Meningitis <1 mo	Group B streptococci, *E. coli, Listeria monocytogenes*	—
Meningitis 1–3 mos	Group B streptococci, *S. pneumoniae, H. influenzae, N. meningitidis,* Enterobacteriaceae, HSV	—
Meningitis >3 mos	*S. pneumoniae, N. meningitidis, H. influenzae,* enteroviruses	—
Orbital cellulitis	*S. pneumoniae, H. influenzae, M. catarrhalis, S. aureus,* GAS, anaerobes	Proptosis, ophthalmoplegia, pain with eye movement
		Obtain ophthalmological consult

(continued)

TABLE 16-3.
CONTINUED

Infection	Common etiologies	Remarks
Osteomyelitis	*S. aureus*, group A streptococci	—
Osteomyelitis age <5 yrs	Add *H. influenzae* type B	—
Osteomyelitis foot puncture	Add *Pseudomonas*	—
Osteomyelitis sickle cell disease	Add *Salmonella*	—
Otitis media	*S. pneumoniae, H. influenzae* (nontypeable), *M. catarrhalis*	Most common 6 mos–3 yrs
Otitis externa	*Pseudomonas, S. aureus,* Enterobacteriaceae, *Proteus*	—
Periorbital cellulitis	*S. aureus*, group A streptococci, *H. influenzae, S. pneumoniae*	Most common <2 yrs, eyelid swelling, fever
Pharyngitis	Adenovirus, enteroviruses, EBV, RSV, parainfluenza viruses, influenza viruses, group A streptococci, *Chlamydia pneumoniae, Mycoplasma pneumoniae*	—
Pneumonia (neonatal)	*E. coli*, group B streptococci, *S. aureus, L. monocytogenes*	—
Pneumonia (3 wks–4 mos)	*C. trachomatis*	—
Pneumonia (6 wks–4 yrs)		
Lobar	*S. pneumoniae*	—
Atypical	*Bordetella pertussis*, RSV, adenovirus, parainfluenza, *M. pneumoniae*	—
Pneumonia (>4 yrs)		
Lobar	*S. pneumoniae*	—
Atypical	*M. pneumoniae* or *C. pneumoniae*	—
Septic arthritis	*S. aureus*, group B streptococci (also consider *N. gonorrhoeae* in adolescents)	—
Sinusitis	*S. pneumoniae, H. influenzae, M. catarrhalis* (anaerobes if chronic)	—

MENINGITIS
Etiology
See Table 16-3.

Signs and Symptoms
- In newborns: hyper- or hypothermia, lethargy, listlessness, irritability, vomiting, respiratory distress, often lack meningismus.
- Older infants and children: fever (usually >38.3), vomiting, lethargy, headache, altered sensorium, meningismus. Kernig's and Brudzinski's positive in 50%.

Diagnosis
- Lumbar puncture (CT first if elevated ICP suspected).
- See Table 16-4 for CSF analysis.
- Associated workup: CBC, serum electrolytes (as baseline and to exclude SIADH), blood cultures.

Treatment
- Age <1 mo: ampicillin (Principen, Totacillin) and cefotaxime (Claforan) or gentamicin (Garamycin); age 1–3 mos: ampicillin and cefotaxime; age >3 mos: cefotaxime or ceftriaxone (Rocephin). See Appendix B, Formulary, for dosing information.
- Complications: cerebral edema, subdural empyema (usually in infants with severe gram-negative meningitis), ventriculitis (common complication of gram-negative and group B streptococcus meningitis in neonates).

RETROPHARYNGEAL ABSCESS
Definition
Infection of the space between the posterior pharyngeal wall and the prevertebral fascia.

Etiology
Staphylococcus and *Streptococcus*.

Signs and Symptoms
History of pharyngitis, high fever, dysphagia, sore throat, stridor, drooling. A bulging posterior pharynx wall is usually visualized.

Diagnosis
History, physical exam, inspiratory neck films.

TABLE 16-4.
CEREBROSPINAL FLUID ANALYSIS

Condition	Color	WBCs/mm^3	Glucose (mg/dL)	Protein (mg/dL)	Gram's stain	Culture
Normal infant	Clear	<10	>40	90	Negative	Negative
Normal child or adult	Clear	0	>40	<40	Negative	Negative
Bacterial meningitis	Cloudy	200–10,000	<40	100–500	Usually positive	Positive
Viral meningitis	Clear	25–1000 (<50% polymorphonu-clear neutrophils)	>40	50–100	Negative	Negative
Cryptococcal meningitis	Clear	50–1000 (<50% polymorphonu-clear neutrophils)	<40	50–300	Negative	Negative

Treatment

IV nafcillin (Nafcil, Nallpen, Unipen) or clindamycin (Cleocin), incision, and drainage. See Appendix B, Formulary, for dosing information.

PHARYNGITIS
Viral or Bacterial?

Associated symptoms of rhinitis, conjunctivitis, and cough are indicative of viral infection and antibiotics can appropriately be withheld. Streptococcal infection is more common if the pharyngitis was of sudden onset and is associated with fever, headache, N/V, abdominal pain, tonsillar exudate, tender anterior cervical lymph nodes, scarlet fever. A rapid strep test can aid in diagnosis. Send throat culture as appropriate.

Treatment

To speed recovery and prevent rheumatic fever: if streptococcal infection is present, treat with penicillin or erythromycin.

URINARY TRACT INFECTIONS
Etiology

E. coli most common. Also, *Klebsiella*, *Enterococcus*, *Staphylococcus saprophyticus*.

Signs and Symptoms

- In the newborn: late-onset jaundice, hypothermia, sepsis, failure to thrive, vomiting, and fever
- In older children: frequency, dysuria, urgency, enuresis, vomiting, diarrhea

Physical Exam

Should include

- BP (chronic renal failure due to UTIs may cause HTN)
- Abdominal exam (a mass may indicate an enlarged bladder or obstructed urinary tract)
- Genitalia (for signs of vaginitis, labial adhesions, local irritation, sexual abuse, a tight phimosis)
- Rectal tone (to evaluate for a possible neurogenic bladder)

Lab Evaluation

Significant pyuria if any bacteria on suprapubic aspiration, >10,000 CFU/mL on catheterization or >10^5 CFU/mL on clean catch. Check BUN and/or creatinine in hospitalized patients.

Treatment

If severe symptoms, treat with IV antibiotics. If mild symptoms, treat with PO antibiotics. Begin with empiric treatment based on most common etiologies (e.g., IV ceftriaxone or cefotaxime or PO TMP-SMX or amoxicillin/clavulanate) and change if necessary when culture sensitivities return.

Follow-Up

Imaging studies are recommended in males, infants, patients with pyelonephritis, and patients with recurrent UTIs. Renal U/S and voiding cystourethrogram evaluate for hydronephrosis and reflux.

Prevention of Recurrent UTIs

- Increase fluid intake and frequent voiding.

- Treat constipation. (See Constipation in Chap. 13, Gastroenterology.)

- If grade 1 reflux or frequent recurrences, nitrofurantoin (Macrodantin), 2 mg/kg qd.

HIV

- See Table 16-5 for CDC guidelines in the diagnosis of HIV in children.

- Lab testing: HIV DNA polymerase chain reaction (PCR) is the preferred test to diagnose HIV infection in infants and children aged <18 mos. It is highly sensitive by 2 wks of age. HIV RNA PCR is not recommended in infants and children because a negative test cannot be used to exclude infection.

Protocol for HIV-Exposed Newborns

- Start the newborn on zidovudine (Retrovir) as soon as possible after birth and continue q6h.

  - Term infant dose: 2 mg/kg PO or 1.5 mg/kg IV q6h × 6 wks.

  - Preterm infant dose: 1.5 mg/kg PO or IV q12h (0–2 wks of life), then 2 mg/kg q8h after 2 wks of age. At an estimated gestational age of 37 wks, dose 2 mg/kg q6h.

- Labs: CBC with differential, rapid plasma reagent, HIV DNA PCR, urine CMV culture.

Intrapartum/Postpartum

- Mother should receive zidovudine, 2 mg/kg IV load for 1 hr, then 1 mg/kg/hr intrapartum until baby is born.

- Avoid invasive procedures (fetal scalp electrode, artificial rupture of membranes, episiotomy) if possible.

- No breast-feeding.

TABLE 16-5.
DIAGNOSIS OF HIV IN CHILDREN

This revised definition of HIV infection is intended for public health surveillance only.

I. In adults, adolescents, or children aged ≥18 mos,[a] a reportable case of HIV infection must meet at least one of the following criteria:

Lab criteria:

Positive result on a screening test for HIV antibody (e.g., repeatedly reactive enzyme immunoassay), followed by a positive result on a confirmatory (sensitive and more specific) test for HIV antibody (e.g., Western blot or immunofluorescence antibody), **or**

A detectable quantity of HIV nucleic acid (DNA or RNA)[b]

Clinical or other criteria (if the above lab criteria are not met)

Diagnosis of HIV infection, based on the lab criteria above, that is documented in a medical record by a physician, **or**

Conditions that meet criteria included in the case definition for AIDS

II. In a child aged <18 mos, a reportable case of HIV infection must meet at least one of the following criteria:

Lab criteria:

Definitive

Positive results on 2 separate specimens (excluding cord blood) of HIV nucleic acid (DNA or RNA detection)

Presumptive

A child who does not meet the criteria for definitive HIV infection but who has

Positive results on only 1 specimen (excluding cord blood) using the above HIV virologic test and no subsequent negative HIV virologic or negative HIV antibody tests, OR

Clinical or other criteria (if the above definitive or presumptive lab criteria are not met)

Diagnosis of HIV infection, based on the lab criteria above, that is documented in a medical record by a physician, **or**

Conditions that meet criteria included in the 1987 pediatric surveillance case definition for AIDS

III. A child aged <18 mos born to an HIV-infected mother is categorized for surveillance purposes as "not infected with HIV" if the child does not meet the criteria for HIV infection but meets the following criteria:

Lab criteria:

Definitive

At least two negative HIV antibody tests from separate specimens obtained at ≥6 mos of age, **or**

(continued)

TABLE 16-5.
CONTINUED

At least two negative HIV virologic tests[c] from separate specimens, both of which were performed at ≥1 mo of age and one of which was performed at ≥4 mos of age, **and**

No other lab or clinical evidence of HIV infection (i.e., has not had any positive virologic tests, if performed, and has not had an AIDS-defining condition) **or**

Presumptive

A child who does not meet the above criteria for definitive "not infected" status but who has

One negative enzyme-linked immunoassay HIV antibody test performed at ≥6 mos of age and **no** positive HIV virologic tests, if performed, **or**

One negative HIV virologic test[c] performed at ≥4 mos of age and **no** positive HIV virologic tests, if performed, **or**

One positive HIV virologic test with at least two subsequent negative virologic tests,[c] at least one of which is at ≥4 mos of age; or negative HIV antibody test results, at least one of which is at ≥6 mos of age, **and**

No other lab or clinical evidence of HIV infection (i.e., has not had any positive virologic tests, if performed, and has not had an AIDS-defining condition), **or**

Clinical or other criteria (if the above definitive or presumptive lab criteria are not met)

Determined by a physician to be "not infected," and a physician has noted the results of the preceding HIV diagnostic tests in the medical record, **and**

No other lab or clinical evidence of HIV infection (i.e., has not had any positive virologic tests, if performed, and has not had an AIDS-defining condition)

IV. A child aged <18 mos born to an HIV-infected mother is categorized as having perinatal exposure to HIV infection if the child does not meet the criteria for HIV infection (II) or the criteria for "not infected with HIV" (III).

[a]Children aged ≥18 mos but <13 yrs are categorized as "not infected with HIV" if they meet the criteria in III.
[b]In adults, adolescents, and children infected by other than perinatal exposure, plasma viral RNA nucleic acid tests should **not** be used in lieu of licensed HIV screening tests (e.g., repeatedly reactive enzyme immunoassay). In addition, a negative (i.e., undetectable) plasma HIV-1 RNA test result does not rule out the diagnosis of HIV infection.
[c]HIV nucleic acid (DNA or RNA) detection tests are the virologic methods of choice to exclude infection in children aged <18 mos. Although HIV culture can be used for this purpose, it is more complex and expensive to perform and is less well standardized than are nucleic acid detection tests. The use of p24 antigen testing to exclude infection in children aged <18 mos is not recommended because of its lack of sensitivity.
Source: CDC guidelines for national human immunodeficiency virus case surveillance, including monitoring for human immunodeficiency virus infection and acquired immunodeficiency syndrome. *MMWR Morb Mortal Wkly Rep* 1999;48(RR-13):29–31, with permission.

TABLE 16-6.
PEDIATRIC HIV CLASSIFICATION FOR CHILDREN AGED <13 YRS

Clinical classifications[a]					Immunologic categories					
					Age-specific CD4 lymphocyte count and percentage of total lymphocytes[b]					
					<12 mos		1–5 yrs		6–12 yrs	
Immunologic definitions	N: Number of signs and symptoms	A: Mild signs and symptoms	B: Moderate signs and symptoms	C: Severe signs and symptoms	μL	%	μL	%	μL	%
1. No evidence of suppression	N1	A1	B1	C1	≥1500	≥25	≥1000	≥25	≥500	≥25
2. Evidence of moderate suppression	N2	A2	B2	C2	750–1499	15–24	500–999	15–24	200–499	15–24
3. Severe suppression	N3	A3	B3	C3	<750	<15	<500	<15	<200	<15

[a]Children whose HIV infection status is not confirmed are classified by using this grid with a letter E (for perinatally exposed) placed before the appropriate classification code (e.g., EN2).
[b]To convert values in microliters to Système International units (×10⁹/L), multiply by 0.001.

Source: Modified from CDC. 1994 revised classification system for human immunodeficiency virus infection in children less than 13 years of age official authorized addenda: human immunodeficiency virus infection codes and official guidelines for coding and reporting ICD-9-CM. *MMWR Morb Mortal Wkly Rep* 1994;43(RR-12):1–19.

Pediatric HIV Classification

See Table 16-6 for children aged <13 yrs.

NATIONALLY NOTIFIABLE INFECTIOUS DISEASES

These change yearly. For the most recent list, go to http://www.cdc.gov/epo/dphsi/phs/infdis.htm.

SUGGESTED READING

Feigin RD, Cherry RD, eds. *Textbook of pediatric infectious diseases*, 4th ed. Philadelphia: WB Saunders, 1998.
Pickering LK, ed. *2000 Red book: report of the Committee on Infectious Diseases*, 25th ed. Elk Grove Village, IL: American Academy of Pediatrics, 2000.

17

Newborn Medicine

Welcome to the world.

INTRODUCTION

When assessing the newborn, first get a prenatal and delivery history. Then inspect the infant from head to toe, noting any abnormalities. Remember, the newborn is in a transition period, so his or her exam can change quickly. Be sure to examine the newborn frequently.

NORMAL NEWBORN FINDINGS

- **Many caused by the trauma of delivery.**

- Caput succedaneum: SC edema (crosses suture lines) on head. Usually resolves in 2–3 days.

- Cephalohematoma: subperiosteal swelling (does not cross suture line) on head. Usually appears on second day of life, may progress for several days, and usually resolves by 2–3 mos. May cause jaundice if large.

- Molding: overlapping sutures. Usually resolves in a few days.

- Fontanelles: Anterior usually closes by 9–18 mos, posterior usually closes by 4 mos. Delayed closure/large fontanelles seen in Down syndrome and hypothyroidism.

- Subconjunctival hemorrhage: scleral hemorrhage, resolves over 2–3 wks.

- Edematous eyelids: usually resolves in a few days.

- Blocked tear duct (dacryostenosis): watery eye without other symptoms. Treat with daily eye duct massage. If resistant to massage therapy, may need surgery.

- Eye color: permanent eye color usually not attained until age 6 mos.

- Ebstein's pearls: small white cysts or ulcers on gums or hard palate. Resolve in 1–2 mos.

- Neonatal teeth: extra teeth without roots or prematurely erupted teeth. Remove to prevent aspiration.

- Sucking blister: usually disappears as diet advances to cup feeding.

- Lanugo: more often in preemies; usually disappears at 2–4 wks.

- Scalp hair: can shed at about age 1 mo. Permanent hair may be a different color.

- Gynecomastia: due to maternal hormones; may produce milk; resolves in 4–6 mos.

- Phimosis: tight foreskin. Do not force foreskin retraction. Most are retractable by age 3 yrs.

- Swollen labia: due to maternal hormones; often resolve by 1 mo.

- Vaginal discharge: due to maternal hormones (clear or whitish) or their withdrawal (bloody).

- Cutis marmorata: transient mottling when exposed to cold.

- Telangiectatic nevi/salmon patches ("stork bite"): flat, pink on scalp or neck; those on eyelids usually disappear by age 1–2 yrs; those on back of neck may persist.

- Hemangioma: usually appears within the first month of life and enlarges during the first year; begins to regress after age 1 yr. Large facial hemangiomas may be associated with posterior fossa malformations. If disfiguring, can be treated.

APGAR SCORES

- The Apgar score is a tool that can be used to define the state of an infant at given times, usually at 1 and 5 mins of life. It should not be used to determine resuscitation, which should begin as soon as there is evidence that the infant cannot ventilate sufficiently to maintain an adequate heart rate.

- A 10-min Apgar score should be assigned if the 5-min score is <7.

- A *persistently* low Apgar score is associated with higher mortality and morbidity.

SCORE	0	1	2
Heart rate	Absent	<100 bpm	>100 bpm
Respiratory effort	Absent, irregular	Slow, crying	Good
Muscle tone	Limp	Some flexion	Active motion
Reflex irritability (nose suction)	No response	Grimace	Cough or sneeze
Color	Blue, pale	Acrocyanosis	Completely pink

Devised by Virginia Apgar, M.D.

TRANSIENT TACHYPNEA OF THE NEWBORN

- Pathophysiology: delayed absorption of fetal lung fluid.

- Risk factors: caesarean delivery.

- Symptoms: tachypnea, retractions, nasal flaring, grunting, cyanosis.

- Labs: ABG reveals respiratory acidosis and mild hypoxemia.

- Chest x-ray: perihilar streaking; fluid in the interlobar fissures.

- Clinical course: marked improvement in 12–24 hrs. CXR normal within 2–3 days. Symptoms rarely last >72 hrs.

- Treatment: Symptomatic: O_2 therapy, continuous positive airway pressure, intubation.

RESPIRATORY DISTRESS SYNDROME

- Pathophysiology: surfactant deficiency. Surfactant is produced by type 2 alveolar cells in increasing quantities after 32 wks' gestation and serves to decrease surface tension in the alveoli, thus preventing collapse.

- Risk factors: prematurity, male sex, white, maternal diabetes, c-section without labor, perinatal asphyxia, previous infant with respiratory distress syndrome, second twin.

- Symptoms: tachypnea, nasal flaring, retractions, grunting.

- Labs: ABG reveals hypoxia and hypercarbia.

- Chest x-ray: ground-glass pattern.

- Clinical course: Respiratory distress syndrome worsens during first few hours of life, then progresses for up to 3 days before improving.

- Treatment: surfactant administration; support ventilation and oxygenation.

- Prevention: administration of steroids to mother antenatally >24 hrs and <7 days before delivery.

PERSISTENT PULMONARY HYPERTENSION OF THE NEWBORN

- Pathophysiology: increased pulmonary vascular resistance.

- Risk factors: history of fetal distress, hypoxemia, acidosis, sepsis, meconium aspiration, polycythemia, pulmonary hypoplasia.

- Clinical course: usually presents within 12–24 hrs of birth.

- Diagnosis: severe hypoxemia (PaO_2 <35–45 mm Hg in 100% O_2) disproportionate to x-ray findings, structurally normal heart with right-to-left shunt at foramen ovale or ductus arteriosus, decreased postductal saturations compared to preductal saturations.

- Therapy: Minimal stimulation and procedures, sedate and paralyze if necessary, maintain systemic BP, optimize O_2-carrying capacity, broad-spectrum antibiotics, maintain slightly alkalotic blood gases, nitrous oxide for pulmonary vasodilation, consider extracorporeal membrane oxygenation.

TABLE 17-1.
MANAGEMENT OF HYPERBILIRUBINEMIA
IN THE TERM NEWBORN

Age (hrs)	Serum bilirubin level (mg/dL)			
	Consider phototherapy	Phototherapy	Exchange transfusion if phototherapy fails	Exchange transfusion and phototherapy
25–48	≥12	≥15	≥20	≥25
49–72	≥15	≥18	≥25	≥30
>72	≥17	≥20	≥25	≥30

UNCONJUGATED HYPERBILIRUBINEMIA

- Physiologic: During the first 3–4 days of life, an infant's serum bilirubin increases to 6.5 ± 2.5 mg/dL, then decreases to normal by 10–14 days. Asian and Native American infants often have a more exaggerated and prolonged physiologic jaundice.

- Breastfeeding jaundice: abnormal condition occurring within the first week of life thought to be due to poor caloric intake.

- Breast milk jaundice: normal extension (up to 1–2 mos) of physiologic jaundice occurring in the breast-fed infant. Thought to be due to a factor in breast milk that enhances the absorption of unconjugated bilirubin.

- Pathologic: appears within the first 24 hrs, rapidly rising serum bilirubin (>5 mg/dL/day), prolonged (>7–10 days in a full-term infant).

- Risk factors: Asian ancestry, prematurity, breast-fed infants

- Evaluation: blood typing for mother and baby, maternal screen for serum isoimmune antibodies; infant blood smear, direct Coombs' test, consider G6PD assay if hemolysis and anemia are otherwise unexplained.

- Treatment: Intensive phototherapy should produce a decline in total bilirubin of at least 1–2 mg/dL within 4–6 hrs. The bilirubin level should continue to fall and if it does not, this is considered a failure of phototherapy. See Tables 17-1 and 17-2.

TABLE 17-2.
MANAGEMENT IN THE PRETERM NEWBORN

Weight (g)	Serum bilirubin level (mg/dL)	
	Phototherapy	Exchange transfusion
<1500	5–8	13–16
1500–1999	8–12	16–18
2000–2499	11–14	18–20

SEPSIS

- Etiology: Group B streptococcus and *Escherichia coli* account for the majority of neonatal sepsis.

- Maternal risk factors: premature rupture of membranes >24 hrs or >18 hrs if mother is group B streptococci positive, chorioamnionitis, maternal temp >100.4°F, foul-smelling amniotic fluid or placenta, multiple gestation, group B streptococci colonization, fetal tachycardia, previous infant with group B streptococcus disease, maternal UTI.

- Infant risk factors: prematurity <37 wks, any of the above symptoms.

- Signs and symptoms: feeding intolerance, temperature instability, respiratory distress, tachycardia, lethargy, hypoglycemia, jaundice, petechiae, poor perfusion, cyanotic spells.

  - If a subtle sign is present, do CBC q12h × 2 or careful observation.

  - If more than one subtle sign or risk factor, blood culture ± IV antibiotics. If antibiotics started, strongly consider lumbar puncture.

  - Concerning CBC: if WBC >33,000–35,000 or <5000–10,000, or if bands/bands + segmented neutrophils (I:T ratio) >0.2, or neutropenia.

- Management: Perform a complete workup if the CBC is concerning: blood culture, lumbar puncture, and treat with IV antibiotics (ampicillin **PLUS** gentamicin or cefotaxime).

NECROTIZING ENTEROCOLITIS

- Definition: intestinal inflammation and injury

- Risk factors: prematurity, asphyxia, hypotension, polycythemia, umbilical vessel catheterization, exchange transfusion, infection, patent ductus arteriosus, respiratory distress syndrome, CHF

- Signs and symptoms: temperature instability, apnea, bradycardia, metabolic acidosis, thrombocytopenia, hypotension, neutropenia, large pregastric residuals, abdominal distension, blood in stool, abdominal tenderness, absent bowel sounds

- Abdominal x-ray: ileus, intestinal pneumatosis, ascites, pneumoperitoneum

- Treatment: NPO, antibiotics (i.e., ampicillin, gentamicin, clindamycin; see Appendix B, Formulary, for dosages), gastric decompression, surgery

INTRAVENTRICULAR HEMORRHAGE

- More common the lower the birth weight. Most occur within the first 72 hrs of life; <1% occur after 1 wk of life.

- Routine screening (with U/S) recommended if <32 wks' gestational age.

- Signs and symptoms: hypotonia, hyperreflexia, irritability, seizures, hyperpyrexia; often is asymptomatic.

Classification

- Grade I: hemorrhage in germinal matrix only
- Grade II: intraventricular hemorrhage (IVH) without ventricular dilatation
- Grade III: IVH with ventricular dilatation
- Grade IV: IVH with periventricular hemorrhagic infarct

Management

- Identical to that of any sick, premature infant. Maintain adequate perfusion pressure and ventilation.
- There is no treatment.
- If IVH is present, weekly ultrasounds are indicated to measure ventricular size. If ventricular size is increasing, intervention is necessary.
- Complications of IVH include posthemorrhagic hydrocephalus, learning disabilities, and neuromotor disabilities.

RETINOPATHY OF PREMATURITY

- Definition: interruption of the normal progression of retinal vascularization.
- Who should be screened?
  - All infants <35 wks' gestation or weighing <1800 g at birth who received O_2 therapy >6 hrs and all infants <30 wks' gestation or weighing <1300 g at birth regardless of O_2 therapy.

SPECIAL NEWBORN CIRCUMSTANCES

- If no prenatal care: Infant should receive CBC q12h $\times$ 2 ± blood culture. Also, give hepatitis B vaccine while waiting for maternal serologies.
- If mother has chorioamnionitis: CBC q12h $\times$ 2, blood culture, IV antibiotics, ± lumbar puncture.
- If rupture of membranes >18 hrs: CBC q12h $\times$ 2, blood culture.

SUGGESTED READING

American Academy of Pediatrics Practice Guidelines, Vol. 94, No. 4, Oct 1994.

Avery GB, Fletcher MA, MacDonald MG, eds. *Neonatology pathophysiology and management of the newborn*, 5th ed. Philadelphia: Lippincott Williams & Wilkins, 1999.

Gomella TL, Cunningham MD, Eyal FG, Zenk, KE, eds. *Neonatology: management, procedures, on-call problems, diseases, and drugs*, 4th ed. New York: McGraw-Hill, 1999.

Zitelli BJ, Davis HW, eds. *Atlas of pediatric physical diagnosis*, 3rd ed. St. Louis: Mosby, 1997.

18

Nephrology

It's all about the beans.

EVALUATING RENAL FUNCTION AND URINE ANALYSIS

Three Essential Attributes to Renal Function

- Glomerular ultrafiltration
- Tubular absorption of filtered solutes and water
- Tubular secretion of organic/nonorganic ions

Evaluating Urine

Abnormalities of Appearance

- Hematuria (confirm with urine analysis and microscopic exam as brown color could result from Hgb, myoglobin, porphyria, beet root, certain food colorings)
- Cloudy, offensive odor
- Stone or gravel (in the United States, most stones due to calcium)

Abnormalities of Urine Volume

- Oliguria and anuria
  - Oliguria: insufficient urine for homeostasis (usually <500 cc/24 hrs for adults or 1 cc/kg/hr in infants)
  - Anuria: complete cessation of urine
- Polyuria: increased fluid intake, failure of antidiuretic hormone (ADH) release, resistance to ADH, osmotic diuresis

Abnormalities of Urination

- Incontinence/enuresis
- Poor urinary stream
- Frequency/dysuria

History

- Often asymptomatic
- General: malaise, growth failure

- GI: feeding difficulties, vomiting, anorexia
- Neonatal history
  - Antenatal diagnosis: Most common prenatal diagnosis is hydronephrosis.
  - Edematous/hypertrophied placenta (>25% of birth weight) suggests congenital nephrotic syndrome.
  - Maternal infection.
  - Perinatal asphyxia with macroscopic hematuria in neonatal period might suggest renal venous thrombosis in the same child with hematuria when older.
- Family history
- Past medical history
- Dietary history

Physical Exam

- Growth and nutritional status.
- Hydration status (edema or dehydration).
- Circulation: including four extremity pulses, precordium, lungs (pulmonary edema), abdominal palpation.
- Careful physical exam.
- In newborns: Concentrate on palpating abdomen, as many renal diseases are associated with other congenital defects (e.g., GI: imperforate anus, single umbilical artery).

Lab Evaluation of Renal Function

- **Glomerular function:** BUN, serum creatinine, creatinine and inulin clearance.
- **Tubular function:** water metabolism (urine specific gravity, urine osmolality, maximal urine-concentrating ability), acid-base metabolism (urine pH, urine titratable acid excretion, urine ammonium excretion, urine-blood PCO_2, fractional excretion of bicarbonate at normal serum bicarbonate level).
- **Hormonal function:** erythropoietin (Hct, reticulocyte), vitamin D, serum 1,25-$(OH)_2D_3$ concentration, serum calcium concentration.
- Urine analysis with spun urinary sediment.
- Calculating creatinine clearance.

- Schwartz formula: glomerular filtration rate (GFR) = $(k)(L)/P_{(Cr)}$, where L = length in cm; k = constant of proportionality; $P_{(Cr)}$ = plasma creatinine.

- k values:

  - Full-term newborn through first yr: 0.45

  - Children <13 yrs: 0.55

  - Adolescent boys (13–21 yrs): 0.7

  - Adolescent girls (13–21 yrs): 0.57

- GFR = U × V/P

  - To standardize for growth:

  - $C_{(Cr)}$ (mL/min/1.73 m^2) = $[U_{(Cr)}$ (mg/dL) × V (mL) × 1.73]/[$P_{(Cr)}$ (mg/dL) × 1440 × BSA (m^2)]

    - $U_{(Cr)}$ = urinary concentration of creatinine; V = urine volume in 24 hrs; $P_{(Cr)}$ = plasma concentration of creatinine; BSA = body surface area.

  - If a child aged >3 yrs has <15 mg/kg/day of creatinine in a 24-hr urine collection, it probably means the collection was not for 24 hrs or not all the urine was collected.

- BUN: not as accurate as a predictor of renal function.

  - Factors that *increase* serum BUN: GI hemorrhage, dehydration, increased protein intake, increased protein catabolism (systemic infection, burns, glucocorticoid therapy, early phase of starvation)

  - Factors that *decrease* serum BUN: decreased protein intake, advanced starvation, liver disease

- Normal values of GFR: See Table 18-1.

Urinalysis

- **Blood:** tests for heme moiety (Hgb and myoglobin). If positive, must confirm RBC by microscopic exam.

- **Protein:** Standard Clinistix detects albumin; works less well with free light-chain proteins (Bence-Jones) or low-molecular-weight "tubular" proteins.

- **Glucose:** Standard Clinistix detects glucose alone. To test for other sugars, need a Clinitest.

- **Nitrite:** 90% of common urinary pathogens are nitrite-forming bacteria.

- **Urinary concentration:** tested by specific gravity, but osmolality is more accurate with large molecules such as glucose.

TABLE 18-1.
NORMAL VALUES FOR GLOMERULAR FILTRATION RATE

Age	GFR (mL/min/1.73 m^2)
Birth	20.8
1 wk	46.6
3–5 wks	60.1
6–9 wks	67.5
3–6 mos	73.8
6 mos–1 yr	93.7
1–2 yrs	99.1
2–5 yrs	126.5
5–15 yrs	116.7

- **Urine bilirubin:** elevated in any disease that causes increased conjugated bilirubin in the bloodstream (negative in hemolytic disease).

- **Urine urobilinogen:** increased in conditions that increase the production of bilirubin or decrease the liver's ability to remove reabsorbed urobilinogen from the portal circulation (positive in both liver disease and hemolytic disease).

Microscopic Exam

- In healthy children: 1–2 RBC/high-power field or 1–2 WBC/high-power field is normal.

- Casts: precipitation of debris in renal tubules.

  - Hyaline casts: fever, after exercise, dehydration, diuretic use, congestive heart failure, nephrotic syndrome.

  - Waxy casts: many chronic renal diseases and nondiagnostic.

  - Red cell casts: Hematuria of glomerular origin suggests glomerulonephritis.

  - Fatty casts (Maltese cross structures): commonly seen in nephrotic syndrome.

- Crystals

  - Calcium oxalate: hypercalciuria

  - Uric acid crystals: hyperuricosuria

  - Hexagonal (benzene ring structure) cystine crystals: cystinuria

  - Fine, needlelike crystals: tyrosinosis

PROTEINURIA

Definition and Epidemiology

- Normal protein excretion <4 mg/m^2/hr.

- Severe proteinuria >1 g/day.

- Nephrotic range proteinuria >40 mg/m^2/hr.

- Protein excretion highest in infants (due to immaturity of renal function) and decreases slowly until it reaches adult levels in late adolescence.

- Asymptomatic proteinuria range is 0.6–6.3% in childhood and is usually transient and intermittent; of those who have it, 10% have proteinuria after 6–12 mos.

Mechanisms

- Glomerular capillary wall/adjacent structures (endothelial cells lining capillary loops, glomerular basement membrane, visceral epithelial cells) limit passage of macromolecules based on size.

- Negatively charged glomerular capillary wall (secondary to heparin sulfate proteoglycans): repels negatively charged macromolecules.

  - Both "size" and "charge" filters are changed by inflammation in glomerular disease.

- Low molecular weight particles (<40 kD) freely filtered through the glomerulus and reabsorbed by proximal tubules. Injury to the proximal tubules leads to a defect in resorption.

- Hemodynamic alterations in glomerular blood flow (through a decrease in the number of functioning nephrons, exercise, fever, seizures, epinephrine, emotional stress).

- Overflow proteinuria: Concentration of protein overwhelms the ability to reabsorb (multiple myeloma, hemoglobinuria).

Measurement

- Dipstick: Proteinuria defined as ≥1+.

  - False-positive: concentrated urine (specific gravity >1.030), alkaline urine, heavy mucus/blood/pus/semen/vaginal secretions

  - False-negative: dilute urine (specific gravity <1.010), acidic urine, other proteins besides albumin (dipsticks are preferential to albumin)

- Sulfosalicylic acid turbidometry: Add 3 drops of 20% sulfosalicylic acid to 5 cc urine to cause precipitation of proteins in an acid environment and note turbidity by inspection.

  - Advantage: not limited to albumin

- Disadvantage: needs urine with specific gravity >1.015
- False-positives: radiographic contrast, high doses of penicillin or cephalosporin, or sulfonamides
- Timed urine collection over 12 or 24 hrs (difficult to obtain).
- Urine protein/creatinine ratio.
  - Total urine protein $(g/m^2/day) = 0.63 \times (U_{(Pr)}/U_{(Cr)})$
  - Normal ratio for adults and children aged >2 yrs: $U_{(Pr)}/U_{(Cr)} <0.2$
  - Normal ratio for children aged 6 mos–2 yrs: $U_{(Pr)}/U_{(Cr)} <0.5$
  - Proteinuria: $U_{(Pr)}/U_{(Cr)} >3$
  - Not valid in severe malnutrition and significant reductions of GFR

Workup of Proteinuria
History of Present Illness

- Age of onset (the younger the age, the more likely to find a significant cause)
- Associated symptoms or diseases:
  - Inflammation/irritation around urethra or bladder: urethral dysuria
  - Suprapubic tenderness: bladder
  - Flank/unilateral back pain: kidney
  - Dysuria, frequency, incontinence, foul-smelling urine, purulent urethral discharge: urethritis
  - Hemoptysis: Goodpasture's, Wegener's, TB
  - Lower-extremity bruising, arthritis, abdominal pain, testicular swelling/discomfort: HSP
  - Bloody diarrhea: HUS
  - Arthritis, Raynaud's phenomenon, alopecia, photosensitivity, weight loss, malar rash: SLE or other rheumatologic disorder

Past Medical History

- Recurrent pyelonephritis/unexplained fever in infancy: scarred kidney
- Recent streptococcal infection: poststrep acute glomerulonephritis
- Recent viral infection: postinfectious glomerulonephritis
- History of hepatitis or TB
- Presence of hematuria and URI symptoms: IgA nephropathy, hereditary nephritis, thin membrane disease, membranoproliferative glomerulonephritis

- Right-sided congestive heart failure or pericarditis: renal vein congestion syndrome

- Infant of diabetic mother, nephrotic syndrome, severe dehydration: renal vein thrombosis

- Congenital heart disease: proliferative glomerulonephritis associated with subacute bacterial endocarditis

- Travel history

- Drug use

Family History

Deafness or visual disorders suggest hereditary nephritis.

Physical Exam

- Weight, height, occipitofrontal circumference (e.g., evidence of growth failure).

- BP and heart rate.

- Edema (periorbital, presacral, genital, ankle areas).

- Large bladder: urethral obstruction.

- Polythelia, preauricular sinus, single umbilical artery, low-set/malformed ear may point to a congenital urinary problem such as hydronephrosis or cystic/dysplastic kidneys.

Lab Evaluation

- First morning UA and another UA later in day (to rule out orthostatic proteinuria; need multiple samples)

- Microscopic exam: looking at color, stones, WBC, eosinophils, WBC casts, RBC casts, dysmorphic RBC, lipid bodies/casts

- Quantitative protein excretion measurement (or $U_{(Pr)}/U_{(Cr)}$ ratio)

  - Protein excretion >1 g/24 hrs implies glomerular dysfunction; <1 g/24 hrs implies tubular dysfunction.

- CBC, BMP, ESR

- Other labs depending on differential diagnosis (C3 if suspecting glomerulonephritis, antistreptolysin-O/deoxyribonuclease B if the patient had a recent strep infection, double-stranded DNA if suspecting SLE)

Imaging

- U/S of urinary tract with Doppler of renal veins to rule out anatomical abnormalities

- If small or scarred kidneys or a history of pyelonephritis, get voiding cystourethrogram

- If renal scarring present, obtain dimercaptosuccinic acid scan

Renal Biopsy Indications

- Symptoms accompanied by hematuria, HTN, low complement, persistently depressed GFR, signs or symptoms of collagen vascular disease, chronic renal failure, or a family history of chronic renal failure

- Debatable: proteinuria with a later stage of onset, not responsive to therapy, or proteinuria lasting >6 mos–1 yr

- Proteinuria >1 g/m^2/day

- Nephrotic syndrome presenting in patients aged <1 yr or >8 yrs; patients unresponsive to an 8-wk course of prednisone

Differential Diagnosis

- Functional (or transient) proteinuria: cold exposure, congestive heart failure, epinephrine, fever, seizures, abdominal surgery, extreme exercise

- Overflow proteinuria: excessive albumin transfusion, intravascular hemolysis, rhabdomyolysis

- Orthostatic proteinuria

- Glomerular disease: nephrotic syndrome, glomerulonephritis

- Interstitial nephritis:

  - Primary/isolated: infection, drug exposure, immunologic disease, idiopathic

  - Associated with glomerulonephritis

  - Associated with structural renal disease: vesicoureteral reflux, obstruction, cystic disease

  - Hereditary/metabolic: idiopathic familiar interstitial nephritis, cystinosis, Wilson's syndrome, sickle cell, hypercalcemia, hyperuricemia, Lesch-Nyhan syndrome, hyperoxaluria, hypokalemia

  - Neoplastic disease

  - Miscellaneous: allograft rejection, heavy metals, radiation, Balkan nephropathy, idiopathic

  - Associated with chronic progressive renal disease of any etiology

- Renal tubular disorders:

  - Primary renal tubular disorders: isolated tubular proteinuria, Fanconi's syndrome

- Tubular toxins: medications: aminoglycosides, penicillin, polymyxins, cephalosporin, phenacetin, naproxen, allopurinol, phenindione; heavy metals

- Ischemic tubular injury

- Miscellaneous: reflux nephropathy, polycystic kidney disease, renal transplant rejection

Treatment

- Treat the cause if known.

- One suggested method for treating nephrotic syndrome

  - Prednisone (Deltasone), 60 mg/m^2/day in divided doses × 6 wks, followed by 40 mg/m^2/day in a single dose qod × 6 wks.

  - Relapse: defined as proteinuria >2+ × 3 consecutive days.

    - Treat with 60 mg/m^2/day in divided doses until resolved × 3 days, followed by single dose of 40 mg/m^2/day × 1 mo. Taper by 10 mg/m^2/wk until off.

    - If >4 relapses/yr, consider chlorambucil (Leukeran) or cyclophosphamide (Cytoxan, Neosar) with tapered prednisone qod.

HEMATURIA
Epidemiology and Definition

- Prevalance: 1.5% in pediatrics (0.5–1% have microhematuria lasting >1 mo).

- Mostly transient or intermittent.

- Defined as >5 RBCs/high-power field.

- Isolated hematuria: hematuria without proteinuria.

- Refer hematuria associated with *persistent* proteinuria [>1+] to a pediatric nephrologist.

Etiology and Differential Diagnosis (Divided by Source of Bleeding)

- **Glomerular:** postinfectious glomerulonephritis (most common and may last up to 1 yr), IgA nephropathy, lupus nephritis, nephritis of anaphylactoid purpura, Alport's syndrome, benign familiar hematuria, focal segmental glomerulosclerosis, minimal change nephritic syndrome, membranoproliferative glomerulonephritis, and membranous nephropathy

- **Nonglomerular:**

  - Tubulointerstitial: infectious, metabolic, allergic vasculitis, drug or poison induced, and acute tubular necrosis

- Vascular: renal venous thrombosis, sickle cell nephropathy, and malformations

- Proliferative: Wilms' tumor, renal cell carcinoma, polycystic kidney disease, and simple cyst

- **Renal pelvis and ureter:** stones, trauma, vascular malformations, papillary necrosis, hydronephrosis, infections, and vasculitis

- **Bladder:** infection/inflammation, stones, drugs (cyclophosphamide), trauma, tumors, vascular malformations

- **Urethra:** infection/inflammation, trauma

- **Undefined:** hypercalciuria, exercise-induced hematuria

Workup and Evaluation

- Repeat UA 2–3× every few days; work up hematuria if there is microscopic hematuria for >1 mo.

- **History**

  - Characteristics of hematuria to elicit: timing, onset, duration

  - Associated signs and symptoms: concurrent illnesses, joint pains, dysuria, edema, flank pain, rash, abdominal pain, vigorous exercise, drug ingestion

  - Past medical history: cystic kidney disease, sickle cell, skin and throat infections, SLE, malignancy, neonatal course

  - Family history: cystic kidney disease, deafness, hematuria, renal failure, sickle cell disease/trait, nephrolithiasis

- **Exam:** ear abnormalities and hearing (Alport's syndrome), palpate abdomen for masses (polycystic kidney disease, Wilms'), costovertebral/flank tenderness, external genitalia (trauma), edema (periorbital or pedal), skin lesions (malar rash, purpuric lesions in HSP, impetigo).

- **Lab evaluation**

  - Careful urine analysis

    - Many other things can cause discolored urine, whether heme positive or negative. Heme-negative causes include beets, blackberries, ibuprofen, iron sorbitol, methyldopa, metronidazole, nitrofurantoin, rifampin, and sulfasalazine.

    - Dipstick detects heme moiety so is positive for hemoglobinuria or myoglobinuria ± true hematuria. If dipstick is positive for heme, you must follow up with a microscopic exam to determine presence of true hematuria.

TABLE 18-2.
GLOMERULAR VS NONGLOMERULAR
CAUSES OF HEMATURIA

Glomerular	Nonglomerular
Brown or "tea"-colored urine	Red or pink urine
RBC casts, cellular casts, tubular cells	Blood clots
Dysmorphic RBCs	Isomorphic RBCs
>2+ proteinuria	No proteinuria

- UA can give you a hint of the location of the bleeding; glomerular hematuria will require more extensive evaluation (renal U/S, CBC, complement levels, ANA, IgA, antistreptolysin-O titers, hepatitis B screen, ANCA titers, and possibly renal biopsy) (Table 18-2).

- Urine culture.

- Sickle cell prep for black patients (sickle cell trait can cause hematuria).

- Urine calcium and urine calcium/creatinine ratio.

- Idiopathic hypercalciuria is defined as a ratio of >0.21 or a 24-hr urine calcium excretion >4 mg/kg/day).

- Electrolytes, BUN, creatinine.

- Renal U/S.

- C3.

- Antistreptolysin-O (especially with recent strep infection).

- If the workup points to isolated hematuria without a serious pathologic cause, follow up q6mos to 1 yr without further workup. Follow growth pattern, BP, and UA.

HYPERTENSION

Epidemiology

- Prevalence: 0.8–5% in pediatric patients overall.

- Only half of severely hypertensive patients will have symptoms. In first year of life, may present with failure to thrive, irritability, feeding problems, cyanosis, respiratory distress, heart failure, or seizures, but is often silent after 1 yr of age.

Definition

- Normotensive is defined as BP ≤90th percentile for sex and age

- Hypertension is defined as BP ≥95th percentile on three separate occasions.

Etiology and Differential Diagnosis

- Can be divided into transient and sustained.

  - Transient: Usually cause is more likely to be drug induced, from acute renal injury with recovery, hypervolemia from volume overload, postsurgical (e.g., renal transplants, genitourinary, or orthopedic surgery), Guillain-Barré, increased ICP, lead poisoning).

  - Sustained

    - Primary/essential (12–18%)

    - Renal disease: chronic pyelonephritis/reflux nephropathy, chronic glomerulonephritis, chronic renal failure, HUS, polycystic kidney disease, Wilms' tumor

    - Renovascular disease: fibromuscular dysplasia, congenital renal arterial stenosis, neurofibromatosis, renal transplant arterial stenosis

    - Cardiovascular: coarctation of the aorta, Takayasu's arteritis:

    - Endocrine: catecholamine-secreting tumors (pheochromocytoma or neuroblastoma), enzymatic defects in adrenal steroid synthesis

    - Miscellaneous: sickle cell anemia, Williams syndrome, idiopathic arterial calcification of infancy, obesity, closure of abdominal wall defects in neonates

- Age often helps in the differential diagnosis (Table 18-3).

TABLE 18-3.
DIFFERENTIAL DIAGNOSIS OF HTN

Age group	Causes
Neonates	Renal artery thrombosis, renal artery stenosis, congenital renal malformations, coarctation of the aorta, bronchopulmonary dysplasia, patent ductus arteriosus, intraventricular hemorrhage
Infancy–10 yrs	Renal parenchymal disease, coarctation of the aorta
	Less common: renal artery stenosis, hypercalcemia, neurofibromatosis, pheochromocytoma, mineralocorticoid excess, hyperthyroidism, transient HTN status post genitourinary surgery or immobilization, essential HTN
Adolescence	Primary HTN, renal parenchymal disease
	Less common: same as above

Workup

Screening

- Measure annual BP starting at 3 yrs of age.
- If BP is high normal and weight is >90th percentile, encourage weight loss and continue monitoring BP regularly; if weight is OK, then monitor BP q6mos.

History

- Family history of HTN, neonatal history (e.g., umbilical artery catheterization in infancy)
- Abdominal pain, dysuria, frequency, nocturia, enuresis: may suggest underlying renal disease
- Joint pain/swelling, edema: may suggest connective tissues disease and/or nephritis
- Weight loss, failure to gain weight, sweating, flushing, fevers, palpitations: may suggest pheochromocytoma
- Muscle cramps, weakness, constipation: may suggest hypokalemia or hyperaldosteronism
- Age of onset of menarche and sexual development: may suggest hydroxylase deficiencies
- Medications (over the counter, oral contraceptive pills, illegal drugs): may suggest drug-induced HTN

Physical Exam

- **General exam:** Examine skin for pallor, flushing, increased sweating, pale mucous membranes. Note any edema, cushingoid features, dysmorphic features (Turner's or Williams syndrome), thyroid enlargement, and birth marks such as café au lait spots or neurofibromas.
- **Cardiovascular:** Note femoral pulses if absent or delayed or any discrepancy between upper and lower extremity BPs. Examine heart size, rate, rhythm, murmurs, work of breathing, hepatomegaly, bruits over major vessels. Obtain BPs of all four extremities.
- **Abdomen:** Palpate for masses (unilateral or bilateral) or epigastric bruits.
- **Neurologic:** Examine fundi and note any neurologic deficits.

Lab Evaluation and Imaging

- Suspected essential HTN: CBC, UA, BUN, creatinine, uric acid, fasting cholesterol, triglycerides, HDL, LDL, and echocardiogram.

- Suspected secondary etiology: Tailor evaluation depending on suspected cause. Good studies to begin with include CBC, UA (and culture if renal pathology suspected), electrolytes with BUN, creatinine and uric acid, echocardiogram. Other studies to consider, depending on suspected etiology: renal U/S and radionuclide studies, abdominal CT (looking at kidneys and adrenals), urine and plasma catecholamines, plasma renin and aldosterone.

Treatment

- General counseling about cardiovascular risk factors (obesity, exercise, smoking).

- Treatment should begin with nonpharmacologic therapy and lifestyle modification (especially with primary HTN). Weight loss, dietary modifications, and exercise should continue whether or not medications are needed.

- Pharmacologic therapy indicated for patients with symptomatic HTN, severe HTN (defined as ≥99th percentile), end-organ damage secondary to HTN, or HTN refractory to nonpharmacologic treatment.

  - Use a "stepped care" approach. Begin one medication at a low dose and increase until BP controlled, maximum dose is reached, or side effects occur. If this does not provide adequate control, switch to or add a second agent and proceed as above. Consult a specialist before adding a third medication.

  - The same classes of antihypertensives used in adults (including diuretics, beta-blockers, ACE inhibitors, and calcium channel antagonists) are used in children, but there is less information about efficacy and long-term safety.

SUGGESTED READING

Barratt TM, Avner ED, Harmon WE, eds. *Pediatric nephrology*, 4th ed. Baltimore: Williams & Wilkins, 1999:317–329.

Cruz CC, Spitzer A. When you find protein or blood in the urine. *Contemp Pediatr* 1998;15(9):89–109.

Fernandes E, McCrindle BW. Diagnosis and treatment of hypertension in children and adolescents. *Can J Cardiol* 2000;16(6):801–811.

Flynn JT. Neonatal hypertension: diagnosis and management. *Pediatr Nephrol* 2000:14:332–341.

Kher K, Makker S, eds. *Clinical pediatric nephrology*. New York: McGraw Hill, 1992:3–41.

Leung AKC, Robson WL. Evaluating the child with proteinuria. *J Royal Soc Promotion Health* 2000;120(1):16–22.

Loghman-Adham M. Evaluating proteinuria in children. *Am Fam Physician* 1998;58(5):1145–1159.

Roy S. Proteinuria. *Pediatr Ann* 1997;25(5):277–282.

Roy S III. Hematuria. *Pediatr Rev* 1998;19(6):209–212.

19

Neurology

A head game.

NEUROLOGIC EXAM

Although not a complete description, listed are helpful portions that are often overlooked.

Head Circumference

Always document in children aged <2 yrs and with first-time visits. The rule of 3s and 9s is helpful to remember approximate appropriate occipitofrontal circumference (birth, 35 cm; 3 mos, 40 cm; 9 mos, 45 cm; 3 yrs, 50 cm; 9 yrs–adult, 55 cm). Document parental OFCs if there is concern for macro- or microcephaly.

Developmental Milestones

See Table 14-1.

Eye Exam

- **Extraocular movements:** Pay particular attention to nystagmus and palsies of cranial nerves VI (lateral rectus) and III (affects pupil)—often early signs of increased ICP.

- **Conjugate gaze:** Examine whether light reflects identically from each iris; does an alternating cover test uncover a latent esophoria (inward deviation) or an exophoria (outward)?

- **Relative afferent pupillary defect:** brought out by the swinging flashlight test, this documents abnormality in the afferent arc of pupillary light response proximal to the dorsal midbrain (e.g., lesion in macula, retina, optic nerve or tract, brainstem; generally not seen with cataract).

- **Red reflex:** Hold ophthalmoscope at arm's length in a darkened room; examine for equivalence in color, intensity, clarity, absence of opacities or white spots. If abnormal, examine dilated pupils or refer to ophthalmology.

- **Fundoscopic exam:** Evaluate for papilledema (not always present acutely), hemorrhage (easier to demonstrate with pupillary dilation), and venous pulsations (present when ICP is <180 mm).

- **Visual fields.**

Coma Exam

- **Pupillary reactivity:** may need to use ophthalmoscope to see poorly reactive pupils. Response is resistant to metabolic disturbances with the following exceptions:

  - Opiates: pinpoint but may be fixed and dilated

  - Anticholinergics: pinpoint

  - Cholinergics, barbiturates, hypoxia, hypothermia: dilated and fixed

- **Extraocular movements:** Doll's or cold water calorics (20 cc in each ear) to activate vestibuloocular reflex. Be sure there is no wax in the ears.

- **Corneal reflexes:** Tests cranial nerves V and VII.

- **Facial grimace to noxious stimuli:** Nail bed pressure or nasal swab are preferable to sternal rub.

- **Cough/gag.**

- **Respiratory pattern** and effort over ventilator.

- **Response to pain:** purposeful withdrawal, triple flexion (stereotyped response), decerebrate (extensor) or decorticate (flexor) posturing, none.

- **Stretch reflexes and Babinski's sign:** Hyperreflexia often indicates structural lesion, whereas hyporeflexia often indicates metabolic or spinal cord injury. However, uremia, hypoglycemia, and hepatic coma may give focal signs with hyperreflexia.

- **Mental status:** Document response to commands, regard, speech.

INTRACRANIAL HYPERTENSION

Clinical Signs and Symptoms

- Bulging fontanelle in infants

- Early morning headache and nausea

- Cushing's response (increased BP, decreased pulse, irregular respirations)

- Meningismus

- Asymmetric or sluggish pupillary response

- Absent venous pulsations

- Papilledema

- Extraocular nerve palsies such as cranial nerve VI palsy or setting-sun sign with paralysis of upgaze

Management

- Do not lower BP acutely (cerebral perfusion pressure = mean arterial pressure – ICP).
- Elevate head of bed 30 degrees.
- STAT head CT scan with neurosurgery consult.
- Check electrolytes, CBC, glucose.
- Cardiac monitor.
- Avoid hyposmolar IV solutions (prefer NS).
- Acute management hyperventilation (PCO_2 30–35) as a temporizing measure.
- Mannitol works for vasogenic edema (e.g., tumor, diabetic ketoacidosis [DKA]) but not well for cytotoxic edema (e.g., stroke).
- Treat hyperthermia aggressively.

SPINAL CORD COMPRESSION

Consider an extensive differential diagnosis: trauma, tumor, transverse myelitis, infarct, vascular malformation, epidural abscess or hematoma, infection, disk protrusion, and atlantoaxial subluxation.

Symptoms

- Back pain
- Lower extremity and/or upper extremity weakness depending on lesion
- Paresthesias, numbness
- Constipation
- Change in urinary function

Early Signs

- Loss of pinprick; look for a sensory level.
- Position sense or vibration loss in feet.
- Changes in deep tendon reflexes (decreased early).

Late Signs

- Hyperreflexia with extensor plantar responses
- Loss of anal sphincter tone, absent abdominal reflexes
- Urinary retention

Management

- Stabilize airway but avoid hyperextension of neck.

- Immobilize neck.

- Consider plain films of spine.

- If symptoms and signs are acute in onset (<3 days) or rapidly progressive, STAT MRI of spine to evaluate for cord compression.

- Foley catheter.

- Consult trauma/neurosurgery for trauma.

- Methylprednisolone (Medrol) within 8 hrs of injury: 30 mg/kg load over first 15–30 mins followed by 5.4 mg/kg/hr for next 23 hrs. Be aware that steroids may make a diagnosis more difficult, but do not delay administration for this reason.

ACUTE GENERALIZED WEAKNESS IN OLDER CHILDREN OR ADULTS

Principles of Characterizing Weakness

- Consider region: hemiplegia, diplegia, quadriplegia, facial involvement.

- Time course: acute, subacute, or chronic.

- Attempt to localize: central, spinal cord, neuron, neuromuscular junction, muscle.

- *Upper* motor neuron signs are hyperreflexia, spasticity, Babinski's sign; weakness may be more prominent in the upper extremity extensors and lower extremity flexors.

- *Lower* motor neuron signs are hyporeflexia, hypotonicity, fasciculations, weakness, atrophy.

Localize the Lesion

- **Central:** hemiplegia typical (arm > face = leg in middle cerebral artery infarct); bilateral cortical involvement nearly always depresses mental status; brainstem—neighborhood signs nearly always present (i.e., cranial nerve involvement), upper motor neuron signs.

- **Spinal cord:** back or neck pain, sensory level, bowel or bladder changes:

  - Corticospinal tract involvement results in upper motor neuron signs (may not be present in acute injury).

  - Anterior horn cell involvement or nerve root results in lower motor neuron signs.

- **Neuropathy:** *distal weakness greater than proximal*, areflexia.
- **Neuromuscular junction:** There is often facial involvement with bulbar symptoms.
- **Myopathy:** flaccid weakness, *proximal weakness is greater than distal*, depressed or absent reflexes; may have elevation of serum creatine kinase, hypertrophy, or myotonia.

Differential Diagnosis Based on Localization

- **Central:** metabolic abnormality, hypoxic ischemic injury (i.e., watershed infarct involving bilateral hemispheres), infection
- **Spinal cord:** trauma, tumor, transverse myelitis, multiple sclerosis, infarct, vascular malformation, epidural abscess or hematoma, infection (e.g., enteroviral infection such as poliomyelitis), disk protrusion, and atlantoaxial subluxation (see Spinal Cord Compression)
- **Neuropathy:** Guillain-Barré syndrome, acute intermittent porphyria
- **Neuromuscular junction:** myasthenia gravis, botulism, tick paralysis
- **Myopathy:** polymyositis, dermatomyositis, periodic paralysis

Evaluation

- **Central and spinal cord:** MRI imaging study
- **Neuropathy:** nerve conduction studies, EMG, lumbar puncture to evaluate for albuminocytologic dissociation, peripheral neuropathy antibody panel, nerve biopsy
- **Neuromuscular junction:** repetitive nerve stimulation studies, EMG, acetylcholine receptor antibodies, Tensilon test, or trial of anticholinesterase inhibitor
- **Myopathy:** serum creatine kinase, nerve conduction studies, EMG, muscle biopsy

Selected Disorders

Guillain-Barré Syndrome

- Also called *acute inflammatory demyelinating polyradiculoneuropathy*. Antecedent viral infection in many patients (e.g., Epstein-Barr virus [EBV], CMV, *Campylobacter jejuni*). Ascending weakness, nadir of weakness by 2 wks in 50% of patients, symmetric, areflexia, autonomic dysfunction, respiratory weakness may require intubation.
- Diagnosis suggested by CSF albuminocytologic dissociation (protein elevated, cell count typically normal). Nerve conduction studies should show signs of demyelination, serum for EBV and CMV

antibodies, loose stools for culture (for *C. jejuni*), serum for peripheral neuropathy antibody panel (prior to giving IV immunoglobulin [IVIG]).

- Treatment is recommended for patients who are too weak to ambulate independently: IVIG, 1 g/kg/day for 2 doses 24 hrs apart. Pretreat with acetaminophen and diphenhydramine. IVIG may cause anaphylaxis in individuals with IgA deficiency; consider sending immunoglobulin levels before treatment. Plasma exchange is also effective. Follow respiratory function closely, particularly if presenting within the first few days of illness when weakness may progress most rapidly.

- Intubation may be necessary if vital capacity falls to 50% of normal or if negative inspiratory function is low. Monitor for vasomotor instability (i.e., labile BP) but treat cautiously.

Botulism

- Infantile form results from ingestion and colonization of *Clostridium botulinum* organism, whereas all others result from ingestion of the toxin.

- Diplopia, dysarthria, dysphagia, vertigo; may be associated with flaccid weakness.

- Ophthalmoplegia spares pupils.

- Repetitive nerve stimulation gives incremental response.

- Treatment is supportive.

Tick Paralysis

- Caused by a toxin exuded from tick.

- Ocular and pupillary abnormalities common.

- Areflexia.

- Respiratory paralysis frequently requires assisted ventilation.

- Treatment requires removal of the tick.

Transverse Myelitis

- Sudden demyelination of spinal cord (often thoracic) with maximal weakness within days.

- In adolescents, consider multiple sclerosis.

- May be asymmetric and painful.

- Sensory level.

- Areflexia or hyperreflexia.

- Bowel and bladder involvement.
- MRI may show area of demyelination.
- Lumbar puncture may show elevated CSF protein.
- Treat with IV methylprednisolone followed by oral steroid taper.

THE HYPOTONIC INFANT

Principles

Recall that tone increases with gestational age (before 28 wks' gestation extremities held in extension, by term all held in flexion).

Localize the Lesion

- **Central:** often with depressed mental status, poor initial feeding, upper motor neuron findings such as weakness, hyperreflexia, spasticity (may evolve with time), differential involvement of axial and appendicular muscle, and seizures common.
- **Spinal cord:** upper or lower motor neuron findings; with anterior horn cell involvement, fasciculations, and atrophy.
- **Neuropathy:** lower motor neuron findings.
- **Neuromuscular junction:** facial involvement common.
- **Myopathy:** Diffuse weakness may involve face.

Differential Diagnosis Based on Localization

- **Central:** hypoxic-ischemic encephalopathy, kernicterus, hypothyroidism, CNS malformation, congenital infection, metabolic abnormality, mitochondrial disorder, chromosomal abnormality (i.e., trisomy 21), Angelman's, and Prader-Willi
- **Spinal cord:** spinal muscular atrophy (anterior horn cell)
- **Neuropathy:** congenital demyelinating neuropathy
- **Neuromuscular junction:** botulism, familial neonatal myasthenia, and congenital myasthenia
- **Myopathy:** congenital muscular dystrophy, congenital myopathy, and myotonic dystrophy

Evaluation

- **Central:** MRI of the brain, chromosomes, serum lactate, pyruvate, methylation studies for Prader-Willi and Angelman's; TSH and free T_4
- **Spinal cord:** Survival of Motor Neuron gene (SMN gene) test
- **Neuropathy:** nerve conduction studies, EMG

- **Neuromuscular junction:** repetitive nerve stimulation, acetylcholine receptor antibodies, and trial of anticholinesterase inhibitor

- **Myopathy:** serum creatine kinase, nerve conduction studies, EMG, muscle biopsy, gene test for myotonic dystrophy or other specific muscle disorder

Specific Disorders

Spinal Muscular Atrophy

- Progressive loss of anterior horn cells in the spinal cord and brainstem.

- Type is based on maximal ability: Type I is unable to ever sit independently, type II is unable to stand or walk, type III is able to stand. Type I presents earlier in infancy.

- Characteristic signs are fasciculations of tongue, fine hand tremor, generalized hypotonia, and bright alert infant with relative preservation of facial strength. Course can be complicated by poor feeding and respiratory weakness with death by age 2. Diagnosis is made by a test for deletions in the SMN gene. Supportive treatment.

Familial Infantile Myasthenia

- Inherited defect of synaptic transmission

- Not associated with acetylcholine receptor antibodies

- Respiratory insufficiency and feeding difficulty

- Diagnosed by response to acetylcholinesterase inhibitor

Transitory Neonatal Myasthenia

- Observed in 10–15% of mothers with myasthenia gravis

- Generalized hypotonia and feeding difficulties

- Diagnosed by identification of acetylcholine receptor antibodies and response to acetylcholinesterase inhibitor

- Treated with supportive care and exchange transfusion if severe

Prader-Willi Syndrome

- Hypotonia and hypogonadism

- Feeding problems in infancy (followed by obesity in adulthood)

- Diagnosed by methylation study for chromosome 15 (deletion or maternal disomy)

Myotonic Dystrophy

- Results from amplification of trinucleotide repeat with anticipation.

- Mothers of severely affected infants generally have myotonia (prolonged muscle relaxation), abnormal facies, and cataracts.

- Infants have hypotonia and generalized weakness (often affecting respiratory and swallowing ability in severely affected infants).

- Diagnosis is by EMG showing myotonia and gene test for expansion of trinucleotide repeats.

PAROXYSMAL DISORDERS OR "SPELLS"

- Most spells are not seizures.

- Sudden, recurrent, stereotypic episodes of neurologic dysfunction with complete resolution to previous level of function are most commonly:

  - Seizure

  - Migraine

  - Transient cerebral hypoperfusion: syncope/TIAs

- Disorders that mimic seizures:

  - "Breath-holding" spells: disturbance in the central autonomic regulation in response to adverse stimuli. Cyanotic and pallid types have been described. 20% of children have both. Associated with loss of consciousness in 5% of infants. This term is a misnomer, as breathing stops at expiration.

  - Benign nocturnal myoclonus.

  - Jitteriness.

  - Apnea.

  - Syncope.

  - Night terrors.

  - Narcolepsy: cataplexy.

  - Startle responses.

  - Shuddering.

  - Paroxysmal dystonias, movement disorders.

SEIZURES

- A seizure is a symptom. It occurs with excessive electrical discharge of cerebral neurons, manifested as transient impairment of function: motor, sensory, cognitive.

- Classification of epileptic seizures is according to clinical type (see following sections).

Partial (Focal) Seizures

- Simple partial seizures (*consciousness is not impaired*):
  - With motor symptoms
  - With somatosensory or special sensory symptoms (e.g., tingling, flashes, buzzing)
  - With autonomic symptoms or signs (e.g., epigastric sensation, piloerection, mydriasis)
  - With psychic symptoms (e.g., fear, déjà vu)
- Complex partial seizures (*impairment of consciousness and often automatisms*):
  - Unimpaired consciousness at onset followed by impairment of consciousness
  - Impaired consciousness at onset
- Partial onset with secondary generalization:
  - Simple partial seizures evolving to generalized seizures
  - Complex partial seizures evolving to generalized seizures
  - Simple partial seizures evolving to complex partial and further evolving to generalized seizures

Other Types of Seizures

- Generalized seizures (convulsive or nonconvulsive)
- Absence seizures (impairment of consciousness alone or with mild clonic, atonic, or tonic component and automatisms)
- Myoclonic
- Clonic
- Tonic
- Tonic-clonic
- Atonic

FEBRILE SEIZURES

- Most common form of seizures.
- Most common age: 6 mos–3 yrs. More common in boys.
- Overall risk 2–5% of children; if one parent or one sibling with febrile seizures, risk is 10–20%.
- Overall risk of recurrent febrile seizure is 25–30%; 40% after two seizures. Two-thirds recur within the first year.

- Febrile static epilepticus accounts for 5% of febrile seizures, 25% of all status epilepticus.

- Most febrile seizures have no adverse effects on behavior, scholastic performance, or neurocognitive attention.

- Parents may be encouraged that at least one study demonstrated significantly better control of distractibility and attention in school-age children with a history of febrile seizures compared to healthy controls.

Definitions

- Febrile seizure: epileptic seizure occurring in childhood after 1 mo of age, associated with a febrile illness not caused by an infection of CNS, without previous neonatal seizures or a previous unprovoked seizure, and not meeting criteria for other acute symptomatic seizure.

- *Simple* febrile seizures are generalized, last <10–15 mins, **and** do not recur within 24 hrs. These comprise 85% of all febrile seizures.

- *Complex* febrile seizures are focal in nature **or** last >10–15 mins **or** recur within a day.

Etiology

- Lowered seizure threshold in the immature brain.

- Genetic predisposition noted, although a mode of inheritance has not been established. Autosomal dominant or polygenic transmission appears most likely.

Risk Factors
For First Febrile Seizure Occurrence

- Patient age (6 mos–3 yrs)
- Degree of temperature elevation
- Febrile seizures in first- or second-degree relatives
- Family history of afebrile seizures
- Neonatal discharge at 28 days or later
- Developmental delay
- Attendance at day care
- Maternal smoking and drinking during pregnancy

For Febrile Seizure Recurrence

- First febrile seizure before 1 yr.
- Family history of febrile seizures.
- Febrile seizures following low-grade fevers.

- Febrile seizures following brief fevers.

- Attendance in day care.

- Possible risk factors for recurrence include epilepsy in first-degree relatives, complex febrile seizures, and neurodevelopmental abnormalities in the child.

For Later Epilepsy

- Complex partial seizures

- Neurodevelopmental abnormalities in the child

- Afebrile seizures in first-degree relatives

- Recurrent febrile seizures, especially if complex

- Seizures that follow brief fevers

- Family history of mental retardation

- Abnormal neonatal history

To Treat or Not to Treat?

- Evaluate the risk of recurrence with or without therapy, the side effects of therapy, and the consequences of recurrence with or without therapy before making a decision.

- Treatment options for febrile seizure management:

  - No treatment

  - Intermittent prophylaxis (medication only with fever):

INEFFECTIVE	HIGHLY EFFECTIVE	POTENTIALLY EFFECTIVE
Antipyretics	Diazepam (PR)	Nitrazepam (PO)
	Diazepam (PO)	Clobazam (PO)

  - Continuous prophylaxis (daily oral medication):

INEFFECTIVE	OFTEN EFFECTIVE
Phenytoin	Phenobarbital
	Primidone
	Valproic acid

- Consider prophylaxis if

  - Intermittent treatment proves to be ineffective.

  - Child typically experiences sudden elevation of body temperature without premonitory signs of illness.

- Prophylactic agent of choice has unacceptable side effects.

- There is substantially increased risk of further epilepsy.

- Parents are highly anxious.

- *Note*: Prolonged and focal febrile seizures can occasionally cause mesial temporal sclerosis with later development of epilepsy. Whether preventing febrile seizures can lower risk of later epilepsy is still unclear.

Management of an Ongoing Seizure

- Do your best to appear calm if there is no immediate risk for the patient from an ongoing seizure.

- Major threats to life are from aspiration of upper airways content, head injury, or status epilepticus.

  - Quick look test

    - Remember: "A" is for "airway"; proceed with the usual ABC assessment.

    - What is patient's level of consciousness?

    - Are there signs of trauma? Prevent subsequent injury from sharp objects and bed rails.

    - Is the patient still seizing? Look at the clock and time the seizure. Most seizures will stop without intervention within 2–5 mins. Any patient who is seizing on arrival to the ER should be considered in status epilepticus unless the seizure onset or recurrence (after complete resolution of previous seizure) was witnessed and timed en route.

  - Establish IV access

  - If previous history of seizures unknown, or level of consciousness is still altered and/or etiology of current event is unclear:

    - Save 2–5 cc of blood in red-topped tube and a urine sample: may turn out to be crucial for diagnosis later.

    - Obtain blood samples for bedside glucose test (AccuCheck, Dextrostix), calcium, magnesium, CBC (optional).

    - Administer 10 cc/kg D5 NS bolus. For adults at risk for Wernicke's encephalopathy, administer 100 mg thiamin IV before a glucose infusion.

    - Consider LP; perform when in doubt. Children with history of epilepsy, febrile seizures, inborn errors of metabolism, and others are not protected from meningitis/encephalitis.

- Administer: lorazepam (Ativan) IV/IO 0.05–0.1 mg/kg, max 4 mg; **or** diazepam (Valium) IV 0.1–0.3 mg/kg or PR (rectal gel) 0.5 mg/kg, 2–6 yrs; 0.3 mg/kg, 6–11 yrs; >12 yrs, 0.2 mg/kg; **or** midazolam (Versed), 0.5 mg/kg PO, buccal, IN.

- If seizures continue: Proceed to the treatment of status epilepticus (Fig. 19-1).

- Consult neurology if history and physical exam suggest:

  - A chronic neurologic insult/condition not previously evaluated

  - New symptoms (e.g., different type of seizures) or physical findings not consistent with previously established neurologic insult

  - Transient symptoms or physical findings not clearly explained by migraine or syncope

- Instruct caregivers to exercise seizure precautions: Prevent child from staying unattended in a setting that could potentially put his or her life in danger should a seizure occur (e.g., bathtubs, water pools, utility areas in playgrounds).

STATUS EPILEPTICUS

General Principles

- Although defined as any seizure (or group of seizures without recovery to baseline) lasting >30 mins, pharmacologic treatment of seizures is typically required for any seizure >5 mins in duration.

- Status epilepticus is an **emergency.** All medications are more effective when used early. Order the next anticipated medication immediately after giving the first.

- Prognosis is generally related to underlying medical diagnosis. Overall mortality is 1–3%.

Treatment

See Fig. 19-1.

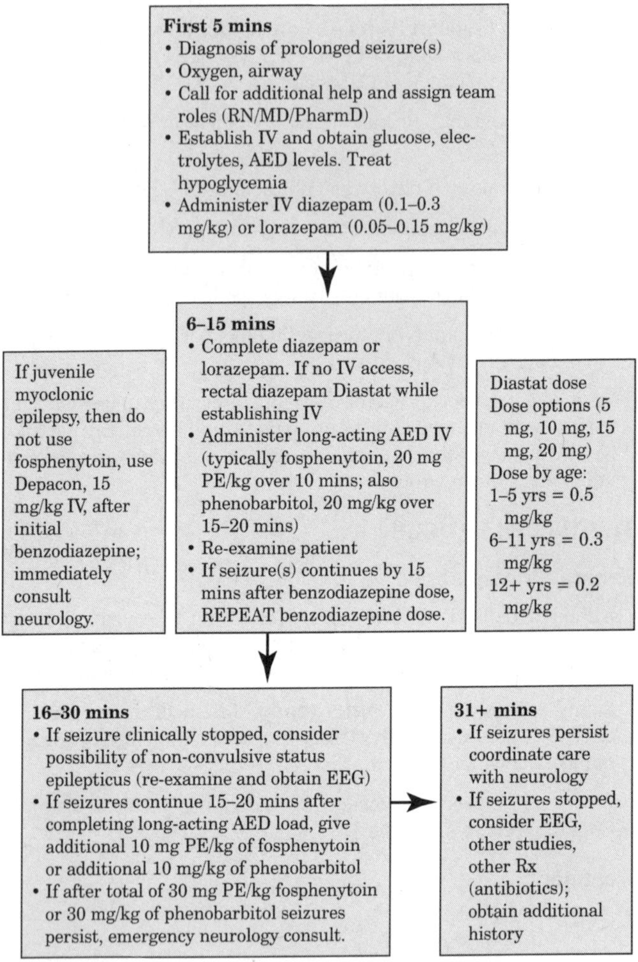

First 5 mins
- Diagnosis of prolonged seizure(s)
- Oxygen, airway
- Call for additional help and assign team roles (RN/MD/PharmD)
- Establish IV and obtain glucose, electrolytes, AED levels. Treat hypoglycemia
- Administer IV diazepam (0.1–0.3 mg/kg) or lorazepam (0.05–0.15 mg/kg)

6–15 mins
- Complete diazepam or lorazepam. If no IV access, rectal diazepam Diastat while establishing IV
- Administer long-acting AED IV (typically fosphenytoin, 20 mg PE/kg over 10 mins; also phenobarbitol, 20 mg/kg over 15–20 mins)
- Re-examine patient
- If seizure(s) continues by 15 mins after benzodiazepine dose, REPEAT benzodiazepine dose.

If juvenile myoclonic epilepsy, then do not use fosphenytoin, use Depacon, 15 mg/kg IV, after initial benzodiazepine; immediately consult neurology.

Diastat dose
Dose options (5 mg, 10 mg, 15 mg, 20 mg)
Dose by age:
1–5 yrs = 0.5 mg/kg
6–11 yrs = 0.3 mg/kg
12+ yrs = 0.2 mg/kg

16–30 mins
- If seizure clinically stopped, consider possibility of non-convulsive status epilepticus (re-examine and obtain EEG)
- If seizures continue 15–20 mins after completing long-acting AED load, give additional 10 mg PE/kg of fosphenytoin or additional 10 mg/kg of phenobarbitol
- If after total of 30 mg PE/kg fosphenytoin or 30 mg/kg of phenobarbitol seizures persist, emergency neurology consult.

31+ mins
- If seizures persist coordinate care with neurology
- If seizures stopped, consider EEG, other studies, other Rx (antibiotics); obtain additional history

FIG. 19-1.
Treatment of status epilepticus in children. AED, antiepileptic drug. (From St. Louis Children's Hospital, Neurology and Pharmacy Departments, with permission.)

SUGGESTED READING

Berg AT, Shinnar S. Unprovoked seizures in children with febrile seizures: short-term outcome. *Neurology* 1996;47(2):562–568.

Berg AT, Shinnar S, Darefsky AS, et al. Predictors of recurrent febrile seizures: a prospective cohort study. *Arch Pediatr Adolesc Med* 1997;151(4):371–379.

Fenichel GM. *Clinical pediatric neurology: a signs and symptoms approach*, 4th ed. Philadelphia: WB Saunders, 2001.

Freeman JM, Vining PG, Pillas DJ. *Seizures and epilepsy in childhood: a guide for parents*. Baltimore: Johns Hopkins University Press, 1990.

Menkes JH, Sarnat HB. *Child neurology*, 6th ed. Philadelphia: Lippincott Williams & Wilkins, 2000.

Pellock JM, Dodson WE, Bourgeois BFD, eds. *Pediatric epilepsy: diagnosis and therapy*, 2nd ed. New York: DEMOS, 2001.

Verity CM, Greenwood R, Golding J. Long-term intellectual and behavioral outcomes of children with febrile convulsions. *N Engl J Med* 1998;338(24):1723–1728.

20 Orthopedics

Them bones, them bones, them dry bones.

DEVELOPMENTAL HIP DYSPLASIA

- Hip can be unstable: malformed, subluxated, or dislocated.
- Etiology: mechanical (abnormal in utero positioning), primary acetabular dysplasia, ligamentous laxity.

Risk Factors

- Breech
- Oligohydramnios
- Postnatal positioning
- Females > males
- Left hip > right hip
- Whites > blacks
- Family history

Associations

- Torticollis
- Clubfoot (metatarsus adductus)
- Scoliosis
- Plagiocephaly
- Low-set ears

Diagnostic Features

- Ortholani's and Barlow's signs (up to 12 wks old) (Fig. 20-1)
- Asymmetry of gluteal and thigh folds
- Leg-length discrepancy (see Fig. 20-1)
- In older child (>3 mos): limited abduction
- Present on U/S of the hips at birth up to 4 mos
- Present on AP x-rays of the hips after 3–4 mos

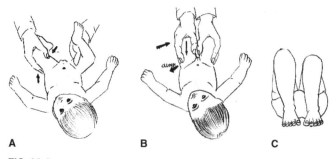

FIG. 20-1.
A: Ortholani's sign (hip is dislocated). **B:** Barlow's sign (hip is dislocatable). **C:** Allis' or Galeazzi sign (leg-length discrepancy).

American Academy of Pediatrics Recommendations

- Screen all newborns.
- If positive Ortholani's or Barlow's, refer to orthopedics.
- If exam is equivocal, reexamine in 2 wks. Keep risk factors in consideration.

Management

- 0–6 mos: Pavlik harness. Hip spica cast. Triple diapering is *not* recommended.
- 6–18 mos: traction for 3 wks followed by attempt at closed reduction and spica cast. Open reduction.
- >18 mos: open reduction, osteotomy.

FRACTURES

Suspicions of nonaccidental trauma: fractures in infants <18 mos or with an unclear mechanism of injury.

Evaluation

- Point of tenderness
- Pulse distally
- Pallor
- Paresthesia distally
- Paralysis distally

General Management

- NPO in case of surgery; cover open wounds with sterile dressing; splint and x-ray.

- Open fractures require tetanus prophylaxis, antibiotics, immediate debridement, and surgery.

- Any physeal fracture needs reduction by an orthopedist.

- Children <8 yrs: Fracture angulation up to 30 degrees is acceptable. If angulation >30 degrees, reduction is needed.

- Open reduction is indicated in a failed closed reduction, displaced intraarticular fracture, displaced Salter-Harris fractures III and IV, unstable fractures in head trauma, or open fractures.

FREQUENT INJURIES

Clavicular Fracture

- Frequent in newborns due to difficult deliveries. In older children, it may be due to falling on an outstretched arm or shoulder.

- Management: Use sling or swathe to bind arm to trunk for few days to 3 wks. Union at 2–4 wks.

- Surgery only if there is an open fracture or neurovascular injury.

Nursemaid's Elbow: Radial Head Luxation

- Secondary to excessive axial traction with an extended elbow of a <5-yr-old child.

- Child is usually unwilling to move that arm and has tenderness on the radial head. Arm is held slightly flexed with hand pronated.

- X-rays are normal. It is reduced by fully extending the elbow while firmly supinating the forearm followed by full flexion of the elbow. Patient will start to use that arm immediately.

Colles' Fracture

- Fracture of the distal radius with displacement resulting in a classic dinner fork deformity of the wrist

- Secondary to falling with a pronated hand outstretched and the wrist dorsiflexed

- Management: reduction and short arm cast

Boxer Fracture

Fracture of the fifth metacarpal with apical dorsal angulation. Reduction usually needs pin fixation.

Scaphoid Fracture

- Characterized by snuff box tenderness or pain on supination with resistance. Most common fracture is of the carpal bone (has a high risk of malunion or avascular necrosis).

- X-rays may be normal; request scaphoid views. Repeat x-ray in 2–3 wks.

Slipped Capital Femoral Epiphysis

- Displacement with external rotation of the femoral head relative to the femoral neck at the epiphyseal plate. Onset usually insidious; limp is present with lack of internal rotation and limited abduction and flexion of the hip.

- 25–50% are bilateral. Males 3:1. More frequent in pubertal black and obese children, as well as in those with endocrinopathies and in those patients receiving growth hormone therapy.

- Diagnosis: AP and frog-leg x-rays.

- Management: no weight bearing, orthopedic consult, and surgical repair.

Osgood-Schlatter Disease

- Painful chronic stress fracture of the tibial tuberosity as a result of a vigorous quadriceps pull in a growing child.

- Pain at the patellar tendon insertion. Activity-related pain may last 1–2 yrs.

- Symptoms are self-limited.

- X-ray: enlargement of the tibial tubercle. X-ray is unnecessary if the presentation is classic.

- Management: rest, quadriceps and hamstring stretches, and NSAIDs.

Ligament Injuries of the Knee

See Table 20-1.

Toddler's Fracture

- Oblique nondisplaced fracture of the distal tibia in a child 9 mos–3 yrs due to low-energy forces.

- Usually spiral and nondisplaced.

- If x-rays are nonrevealing: Obtain an oblique view of tibia.

- Child will present with an antalgic gait and a refusal to bear weight.

- Cast for 3 wks.

TABLE 20-1.
LIGAMENT INJURIES OF THE KNEE

Liga-ment	Mechanism of injury	Physical exam	Management
Medial collat-eral	Twisting or a lateral blow to the knee	Joint effusion and limitation of motion	Ice, elevation, NSAIDs, no weight bearing; once swelling is improved, orthopedic consult
Ante-rior cruciate	Hyperexten-sion with foot planted	Anterior drawer test, hamarthro-sis and avulsion fracture	Urgent orthopedic consult
Poste-rior cruciate	Direct blow to the tibia while knee is flexed	Posterior knee tenderness and small effusion	Ice, elevation, NSAIDs, no weight bearing; once swelling is improved, orthopedic consult

Ankle Sprains

- Inversion during plantar flexion. Talofibular ligament disruption is the most common.

- Presents with pain anterior to the lateral malleolus, swelling, ecchymosis.

- Normal x-rays.

- Difficult to exclude a Salter I fracture (see below).

- Management

  - Grade I: elastic wrap or air cast, ice, elevation, NSAIDs, weight bearing as tolerated

  - Grades II and III: cast or posterior splint for 3 wks

  - If suspicion of Salter I: cast or splint, elevation, and orthopedic consult in 1 wk

GROWTH PLATE INJURIES

- See Fig. 20-2.

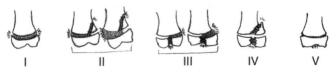

FIG. 20-2.
Salter-Harris fractures types I to V.

Salter-Harris Fractures

- I: Fracture along the growth plate
  - Rarely associated with growth disturbance.
  - If not displaced, difficult to diagnose.
  - Immobilize for 10–14 days.
- II: Fracture along the growth plate with metaphyseal extension
  - Most common.
  - Rarely associated with growth disturbance.
  - Closed reduction.
  - Cast 3–6 wks.
- III: Fracture along growth plate with epiphyseal extension
  - Higher risk of growth disturbance and posttrauma arthritis
  - May require open reduction if displaced
- IV: Fracture across growth plate, including metaphysis and epiphysis
  - High risk of growth disturbance
  - May require open reduction and internal fixation
- V: Crush injury to growth plate without obvious fracture
  - Difficult to diagnose
  - Usually diagnosed when growth disturbance manifested

CASTS

- After placement of a cast, it is very important to pay close attention to signs and symptoms of compartment syndrome. These include severe pain, marked swelling, cyanosis or pallor of the extremity, and the inability to move the fingers.
- See Fig. 20-3 for different types of casts.

IN-TOEING

On exam determine: foot progression angle, range of internal and external hip rotation, thigh-foot angle, and the degree of metatarsus varus. See Table 20-2.

OUT-TOEING

Almost all infants have out-toeing due to external femoral torsion. This usually corrects itself as the patient starts to roll over and bear weight.

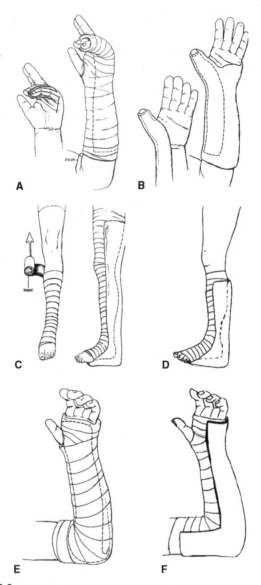

FIG. 20-3.
Cast types according to injury. **A:** Boxer's fracture. **B:** Scaphoid and thumb fracture. **C:** Knee injuries, spiral fractures. **D:** Ankle sprains; foot, ankle, or distal fibula fractures. **E:** Distal radius and wrist fracture. **F:** Elbow and wrist injuries.

TABLE 20-2.
IN-TOEING

Condition	History	Physical exam	Therapy
Metatarsus adductus (5–10%)	Diagnosis: newborn Associated with hip dysplasia; family history	Forefoot in varus, C shape	Flexible: Observe 3–9 mos. Rigid: Refer for casting. If age >2 yrs: surgery.
Internal tibial torsion (5–10%)	Diagnosis: 1.5–4 yrs Increased frequency when sitting or sleeping on feet with feet turned in	Abnormal thigh-foot angle (normal: 0–20 degrees at birth; 20 degrees by age 2–3; 0–40 degrees as an adult)	Growth corrects the majority of cases by 3–4 yrs. Refer to specialist if no improvement over first yr of walking. Surgery if severe or age >8–10 yrs.
Femoral anteversion (80–90%)	Diagnosis: 3–8 yrs	Femoral neck rotated anteriorly from femoral shaft; internal rotation > external rotation up to 90 degrees	Discourage sitting in the W position. Usually resolves by 8–12 yrs. Surgery if internal rotation ≥80 degrees or external rotation ≤15 degrees, severe gait disturbance, persists >8 yrs.

BOW LEGS (GENU VARUM)

- Differential diagnosis: physiologic varus (corrects by 2 yrs), Blount's disease, rickets, familial bow legs, and traumatic growth disturbance.

- Blount's disease: nontraumatic growth disturbance of the medial epiphysis of the tibia, often resulting in progressive bow legs.

  - Two types:

    - Infantile: in early walkers, obese, 1–2 yrs old, 50–75% are bilateral, females > males

    - Adolescent: males > females, obese, 50% are bilateral

- Diagnosis: x-rays: Look for characteristic changes in the films of the proximal tibial epiphysis, growth plate, and metaphysis.

KNOCK KNEES (GENU VALGUM)

- Caused by physiologic valgus, rickets, or other dysplasias.

- Physiologic genu valgum begins at 2–3 yrs, progresses for 1–2 yrs, and spontaneously corrects at 3–4 yrs.

LEGG-CALVÉ-PERTHES DISEASE

- Idiopathic avascular necrosis of the femoral head.
- More frequent in boys. Age: 4–8 yrs.
- Patient presents with a limp, referred knee pain, and limited hip internal rotation and abduction.
- Diagnosis: AP and frog-leg x-ray.
- All patients must be referred to orthopedics for evaluation.

SCOLIOSIS

- Definition: structural lateral and axial rotation of the spine.
- 80% are idiopathic adolescent (occurring during growth spurts), but there are also congenital and neuromuscular causes.
- 2–3% of population has scoliosis ($\geq$10 degrees).
- Girls are more commonly affected than boys.
- Screening should begin at 6–7 yrs.
- Exam: Look for body asymmetry (hips, shoulders, scapulae, spine) when looking from behind. Leg length differences when palpating iliac crests. Forward bend test with hands together. Posterior ribs are prominent on the convex side; scoliometer reading of 5–7 degrees correlated with a curve of 15–20 degrees.
- Classification depends on magnitude, location, direction, etiology.
- No greater incidence of back pain except in thoracolumbar curve area. Pulmonary functions are abnormal in severe thoracic curves ($\geq$90 degrees). Mortality is the same as general population.
- Curve progression: curves $\geq$30–40 degrees can be seen; the younger the patient, the more likely it is to progress.
- Who to refer: angle of trunk rotation >6 degrees or if vertebral angulation >20–25 degrees.
- Treatment: Bracing: a skeletally immature patient with a curve of 25–40 degrees. Surgery: curves $\geq$45 degrees.

SUGGESTED READING

American Academy of Pediatrics. Clinical practice guidelines: early detection of developmental dysplasia of the hip. *Pediatrics* 2000;105:896–905.

Baronciani D, Andiloro F, Bartesaghi A, Gagliardi L, et al. Screening for developmental dysplasia of the hip: from theory to practice. *Pediatrics* 1997;99:E5.

Craig C, Goldberg M. Foot and leg problems. *Pediatr Rev* 1993;14:395.

Marsh J. Screening for scoliosis. *Pediatr Rev* 1993;14:297.

McMillan JA, ed. *Oski's pediatrics: principles and practice*, 3rd ed. Philadelphia: Lippincott Williams & Wilkins, 1999.

All that wheezes is not asthma.

ASTHMA
Definition

Reversible obstructive lung disease. Characterized by a combination of airway obstruction, inflammation, and hyperreactivity, with airway mucosal edema, bronchospasm, and mucus plugging.

History

- Age: age at time of diagnosis.
- Baseline symptoms: daytime symptoms, nighttime symptoms, exercise symptoms. Determine severity.
- Course over time: previous hospitalizations/admissions, PICU admissions, intubations, and ER visits.
- Triggers.
- Environment: housing type, heat/air conditioning, carpet, pets, smoke, etc.
- Usual symptoms and collateral symptoms.
- List of all medications: When was the last course of steroids?
- Previous evaluation: sweat test, CXR, pulmonary function tests, best peak flow.
- Family history and social history. Any barriers to care?
- Duration: Is an action plan available?
- Course and precipitating factors of the present attack.

Physical Exam

- Vital signs
- O_2 saturation
- Pulmonary score (see page 215)
- Adequacy of air exchange
- Mental status
- Peak flow
- SC emphysema
- Pulsus paradoxus

Emergency Unit Pulmonary Score

	RESPIRATORY RATE			ACCESSORY
SCORE	<6 YRS	>6 YRS	WHEEZING	MUSCLE USE
0	<30	<20	None	No apparent activity
1	31–45	21–35	Terminal expiration	Questionable increase
2	46–60	36–50	Entire expiration	Increase apparent
3	>60	>50	Inspiratory and expiratory without stethoscope	Maximal activity

- If no wheezing due to minimal air exchange, score = 3.
- An abrupt decline in respiratory rate may indicate impending respiratory failure.

ER Management of an Acute Asthma Exacerbation: Asthma Algorithm

- See Table 21-1.

Short Albuterol Treatments[a]

WEIGHT (KG)	ALBUTEROL (MG)	ALBUTEROL (CC)	IPRATROPIUM BROMIDE (500-µG VIAL)[b]	TOTAL VOLUME (CC)
10–30	2.5	0.5	1	3
30–50	5	1	1	3.5
>50	10	2	1	4.5

[a]O_2: 7 L/min, may increase to keep saturations >95%.
[b]Give only in first 2 treatments.

Continuous Albuterol Treatments[a]

WEIGHT (KG)	ALBUTEROL (MG)	ALBUTEROL (CC)	NS (CC)	TOTAL VOLUME (CC)
10–30	10	2	6	8
30–50	15	3	5	8
>50	20	4	4	8

[a]O_2: 5 L/min, may increase to keep saturations >95%.

TABLE 21-1.
ER MANAGEMENT OF AN ACUTE ASTHMA EXACERBATION

Pathway	Beta-agonists	Steroids	Other therapies
Mild exacerbation (peak flow >70% or PS ≤3; O$_2$ saturation ≥95%)	MDI with spacer q15mins × 3. <6 yrs: 2 puffs. ≥6 yrs: 4 puffs or short albuterol treatment q15mins × 3	2 mg/kg prednisone (max. 60 mg); give ASAP	Ipratropium bromide (Atrovent) can be given with first albuterol short treatment. Discharge if peak flow >80% or PS <2. If worsening/no improvement, go to moderate pathway.
Moderate exacerbation (peak flow 40–70% or PS 4–6)	Short albuterol treatment × 1, then continuous albuterol treatment × 1, or for child <24 mos: short albuterol treatment q15mins × 3	2 mg/kg prednisone (max. 60 mg); give ASAP	Atrovent can be given with first albuterol short treatment. If worsening/no improvement, go to severe pathway; consider admission and alert attending. Discharge if peak flow >80% or PS <2.
Severe exacerbation (peak flow <40% or PS >6); alert attending	Short albuterol treatment × 1, then continuous albuterol treatment × 1 or for child <24 mos: short albuterol treatment q15mins × 3	2 mg/kg IV/PO/IM prednisone (max. 60 mg); give ASAP	Atrovent can be given with first albuterol short treatment. If worsening/no improvement, alert attending and give another continuous treatment. Consider starting an IV with NS. Consider: Epinephrine: 0.01 mL/kg SC (1:1000, max. dose, 0.3 mL) q15mins, up to 3 doses. Magnesium: 25–75 mg/kg/dose IV/IM (max. dose, 2 g) infused over 20 min q4–6h, up to 3–4 doses. Terbutaline: 0.01 mg/kg SC (max. dose, 0.4 mg) q15min, up to 3 doses.

PS, pulmonary score. See page 215 for short and continuous albuterol treatment dosing. (From St. Louis Children's Hospital, Emergency and Pulmonary Departments, with permission.)

Hospital Management of an Asthma Exacerbation: Asthma Pathway

- An asthma pathway allows patients to progress from one level of care to the next by following the patient's response to treatment, peak flow, O_2 requirement, oral intake, and exercise tolerance.

- The asthma pathway can be used in addition to other orders (i.e., antibiotics for pneumonia).

- Asthma pathway

  - Level 1: Poor to fair air movement, inspiratory and expiratory wheezing, moderate to severe retractions, peak flow >50%: give systemic steroids, albuterol nebulizers q1–2h, ipratropium bromide (Atrovent) q6h. In severe cases, limited air movement results in no wheezing.

  - Level 2: Fair to moderate air movement, expiratory wheezing, mild to moderate retractions, peak flow >60%, tolerates room air: give systemic steroids, albuterol nebulizers q3h, discontinue Atrovent.

  - Level 3: Good air movement, end expiratory wheezing, no retractions, peak flow >70%, tolerates normal activity and PO: give PO steroids, albuterol q4h.

Therapy Practice Tips
Steroids

- Oral: 2 mg/kg/day up to 60–80 mg/day qd. Encourage qam dosing even if P.M. emergency unit dose was given.

- Must tolerate PO steroids before discharge.

- At discharge, prescribe extra dose(s) for future use.

- Rinse mouth after inhaled steroids.

Albuterol

- Usually 0.5 cc/nebulizer regardless of age. Consider 1 cc for older children or when symptoms not improving.

- If no home nebulizer: Change to MDI/spacer when albuterol treatments are q3h to assess tolerance.

- At discharge, prescribe one of the following q4h × 24 hrs, then q6h × 1 wk, then prn following the asthma action plan:

  - 2 puffs albuterol MDI with spacer
  - prediluted 0.083% albuterol vial
  - 0.5 cc albuterol in 2 cc normal saline (from 0.5% multidose albuterol nebulizer solution)

Atrovent

- Usually q6h via nebulizer for the first 24 hrs only

Oxygen

- Continuous pulse oximetry of no benefit for most asthmatics. Spot-check O_2 saturation if respiratory status worsens or q4h if on O_2.
- Consider O_2 if room air saturation <90% or if increased work of breathing.

Metered-Dose Inhaler

- Always use appropriate spacer.
- Always use aerochambers.

Peak Flow (Usually for Children ≥7 yrs)

- Predicted peak flow is based on height.
- If known, personal best peak flow is preferred over predicted peak flow.
- Encourage good effort and technique.
- Give peak flow meters to patients.

Discharge Teaching Tips

Use an asthma action plan on discharge.

Asthma Action Plan

- Every family should receive an asthma action plan before discharge.
- See Fig. 21-1.
- Emphasis should be placed on prompt recognition and correlation of symptoms with recommended actions.
  - Green zone: what families should do every day
  - Yellow zone: use of albuterol with early signs; may double inhaled corticosteroid dose (not Advair) or add oral steroids
    - Family to call primary care physician if albuterol does not work within 15–30 mins or if patient requires albuterol more frequently than q4h or if patient requires albuterol q4h for >24 hrs
  - Red zone: emergency action

After Discharge

- If you anticipate a need, order a nebulizer early in the hospital stay and deliver on discharge. Consider a home RT/RN visit to reinforce education and assess compliance.
- School/day care note:

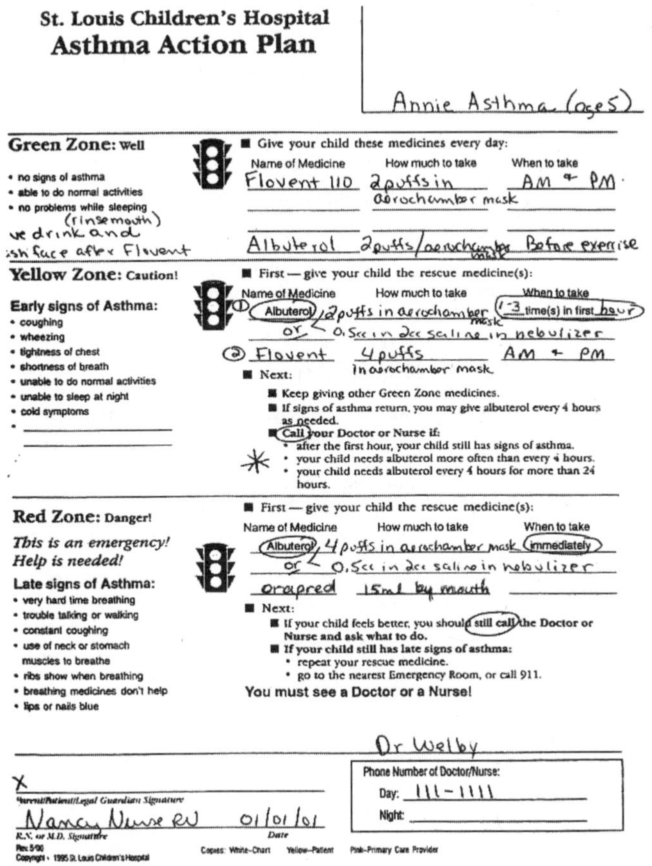

St. Louis Children's Hospital
Asthma Action Plan

Annie Asthma (age 5)

Green Zone: Well

- no signs of asthma
- able to do normal activities
- no problems while sleeping

(rinse mouth) ve drink and ish face after Flovent

■ Give your child these medicines every day:

Name of Medicine	How much to take	When to take
Flovent 110	2 puffs in aerochamber mask	AM + PM
Albuterol	2 puffs/aerochamber mask	Before exercise

Yellow Zone: Caution!

Early signs of Asthma:

- coughing
- wheezing
- tightness of chest
- shortness of breath
- unable to do normal activities
- unable to sleep at night
- cold symptoms

■ First — give your child the rescue medicine(s):

Name of Medicine	How much to take	When to take
① Albuterol	2 puffs in aerochamber mask or 0.5cc in 2cc saline in nebulizer	1-3 time(s) in first hour
② Flovent	4 puffs in aerochamber mask	AM + PM

■ Next:

■ Keep giving other Green Zone medicines.

■ If signs of asthma return, you may give albuterol every 4 hours as needed.

■ Call your Doctor or Nurse if:

- after the first hour, your child still has signs of asthma.
- your child needs albuterol more often than every 4 hours.
- your child needs albuterol every 4 hours for more than 24 hours.

Red Zone: Danger!

This is an emergency! Help is needed!

Late signs of Asthma:

- very hard time breathing
- trouble talking or walking
- constant coughing
- use of neck or stomach muscles to breathe
- ribs show when breathing
- breathing medicines don't help
- lips or nails blue

■ First — give your child the rescue medicine(s):

Name of Medicine	How much to take	When to take
Albuterol	4 puffs in aerochamber mask or 0.5cc in 2cc saline in nebulizer	immediately
orapred	15ml by mouth	

■ Next:

■ If your child feels better, you should still call the Doctor or Nurse and ask what to do.

■ If your child still has late signs of asthma:

- repeat your rescue medicine.
- go to the nearest Emergency Room, or call 911.

You must see a Doctor or a Nurse!

Dr Welby

Phone Number of Doctor/Nurse:
Day: 111-1111
Night:

X
Parent/Patient/Legal Guardian Signature

Nancy Nurse RN 01/01/01
R.N. or M.D. Signature Date

Rev. 5/00
Copyright © 1995 St. Louis Children's Hospital

Copies: White-Chart Yellow-Patient Pink-Primary Care Provider

FIG. 21-1.
Sample asthma action plan.

- Usually no gym/exercise for 1 wk.
- Attach a copy of the asthma action plan to the note.

Long-Term Management of Asthma

Environmental

Avoid specific respiratory irritants, dust mite exposure, in-house pets, and smoking. Use air conditioning to reduce exposure to outdoor allergens.

Pharmacologic

- See Table 21-2.

TABLE 21-2.
LONG-TERM PHARMACOLOGIC MANAGEMENT
OF ASTHMA

Severity and clinical features	Daily medications	Follow-up
Mild intermittent (symptoms ≤2 days/wk, nighttime cough ≤2 days/mo; FEV_1 ≥80%)	No daily medications Short-acting bronchodilators prn Intensity of treatment depends on severity of exacerbation	q6mos
Mild persistent (symptoms 3–6 days/wk; nighttime cough 3–4 days/mo; FEV_1 ≥80%)	Daily medications needed: Low-dose inhaled steroids, cromolyn, or nedocromil Leukotriene modifiers	q6mos
Moderate persistent (symptoms daily; nighttime cough ≥5/mo; FEV_1 >60–80%)	Moderate-dose inhaled steroids **OR** Low-dose inhaled steroids + long-acting bronchodilator and/or leukotriene modifiers	q4mos Specialist if age <5 yrs
Severe persistent (symptoms continuous; nighttime cough frequent; FEV_1 ≥60%)	High-dose inhaled steroids **OR** Medium- to high-dose inhaled steroids + long-acting bronchodilator and/or leukotriene modifier Oral steroids	q1–2mos All patients should see a specialist

For dosages of medications mentioned in this table, please see Appendix B.

- The presence of even one of the features of severity is sufficient to place patient in that category. A child should be assigned to the most severe grade in which any feature occurs.

BRONCHIOLITIS

An acute infectious disease of the lower respiratory tract preceded by fever, rhinitis, or both. It is also characterized by tachypnea, wheezing, hyperinflation, and increased respiratory effort.

Etiology

Usually viral, most common RSV.

History

Should include presence or absence of apnea and the evaluation of hydration status, including ability to take oral fluids and the number of wet diapers.

TABLE 21-3.
ASSESSMENT OF BRONCHIOLITIS

Score	Wheezing	Accessory muscle use
0	None[a]	No apparent activity
1	Terminal expiration	Minimal increase (mild intercostal retraction)
2	Entire expiration	Increase apparent (intercostal and tracheosternal retractions)
3	Inspiration and expiration	Maximum activity (retractions and nasal flaring)

[a]If no wheezing due to minimal air exchange, score 3.

Diagnosis

- Based on clinical presentation. RSV nasopharyngeal swab is **not** routinely needed.

- Routine x-rays are not recommended.

Assessment

See Table 21-3.

Treatment

- Begin O_2 if room air saturations are <95%.

- Treatment is based on score (Table 21-3).

  - If score 0–2 and no risk factors: may observe and treat at home.

  - If score 3–4 and there are no risk factors, begin supportive therapy: adequate hydration, humidified O_2.

  - If score >5, consider hospitalization.

- Discuss all sick patients with your attending (if there is a history of apnea and score >4, O_2 required).

- Do **not** treat with steroids. Dexamethasone use is controversial.

Conservative Treatment

- Preferred for most infants: hydration and O_2.

- Discuss natural history of the disease with the family.

Other Treatment Options

- No pharmacologic therapy has been proven to be effective.

- There is good evidence-based data supporting the use of racemic epinephrine nebulizer treatment (0.5 mL/dose q3–4h).

- The benefit of albuterol is unclear.
- Obtain a score 15–20 mins after an albuterol treatment; if there is improvement, discharge with an albuterol MDI.
- Ribavirin is suggested only in patients with underlying cardiopulmonary disease or immunosuppression.
- Consider admission if:
  - Apnea or history of apnea
  - Resting respiratory rate >70
  - Room air O_2 saturations <95%
  - Infants <8 wks of age
  - Score ≥5
  - History of chronic lung or heart disease
  - Infant not feeding well

CROUP OR VIRAL LARYNGOTRACHEOBRONCHITIS

Definition

- Acute inflammation of the entire airway, but mainly in the glottis and subglottic area, resulting in airway narrowing, obstruction, and voice loss.
- It affects younger children (<3 yrs) in the fall and winter.
- Most common pathogens: parainfluenza, respiratory syncytial virus, influenza, and less commonly an adenovirus, *Mycoplasma pneumoniae*.

Clinical Presentation

- A coryzal prodrome is common, followed by barking cough, hoarseness, stridor, and low-grade fever.
- Usually occurs at nighttime.

Physical Exam

- The goal is to determine the severity of airway narrowing.
- Stridor at rest, tachypnea, retractions, and decreased breath sounds indicate critical narrowing.

Diagnosis

- Is clinical, but an AP x-ray of neck showing "steeple sign" may be helpful.
- Obtain arterial blood gas and O_2 saturation if patient has signs of hypoxia (i.e., restlessness, altered mental status, cyanosis).

Differential Diagnosis

This includes epiglottitis (patient is toxic looking), spasmodic croup (no prodrome), bacterial tracheitis, and laryngitis.

Therapy

- If stridor is present at rest:

  - Racemic epinephrine, 0.25–0.5 mL/3 mL normal saline nebulized, humidified O_2, and dexamethasone, 0.6 mg/kg/dose IV/IM/PO.

  - Patients may have rebound symptoms up to 3–4 hrs after racemic epinephrine treatment. Observe in an emergency unit for 2–3 hrs before discharge for this reason.

  - If the patient's stridor and work of breathing continue to improve 3–4 hrs after these therapies, patient may be discharged.

  - If there is **no** response, repeat racemic epinephrine.

  - Admit patient for further observation and management if two or more racemic epinephrine treatments are given and there is no improvement.

  - If respiratory failure is imminent or present, admit patient to PICU and intubate under controlled situation.

  - If wheezing is present, also give albuterol.

- If no stridor is present at rest:

  - May observe for 1 hr; if the patient is stable, reassure the parents and management can be done as an outpatient.

  - Can give dexamethasone, 0.6 mg/kg/dose IV/IM/PO.

  - Cool-mist vaporizer, increase fluid intake, decrease agitation, careful observation.

  - Instruct parents to call or return to medical care if respiratory distress worsens.

EPIGLOTTITIS
Introduction

- Defined as an acute infectious supraglottic obstruction that may rapidly lead to respiratory distress and failure.

- **A true pediatric emergency.**

- May affect all ages; peak 3–6 yrs.

Etiology

- *Haemophilus influenzae* type B. Rarely group A streptococci, pneumococci.

- Incidence has declined significantly since *H. influenzae* type B immunization became available.

Clinical Presentation

- Rapid onset.
- Patient usually anxious and appears toxic.
- Symptoms include high fever, muffled or absent voice, sore throat, drooling, inspiratory stridor, dysphagia, protruded jaw, and extended neck. The patient will prefer a sitting position.

Diagnosis

- Presumptive diagnosis should be made on clinical grounds.
- If patient is in little distress and the diagnosis is unclear, obtain a lateral neck x-ray: A thumb sign may be present, but the x-ray is normal in 20% of patients.

Therapy

- Airway stabilization and maintenance must be done quickly and early in the course of the illness. Call otolaryngology or anesthesia for airway assistance.
- Administer O_2 at minimal signs of distress.
- Minimize stimulation and disturbance of the patient to avoid complete obstruction.
- If diagnosis suspected, do not attempt to visualize the epiglottis.
- Always have an artificial airway ready next to the patient.
- Antibotics: ampicillin (Unasyn), ceftriaxone (Rocephin), cefotaxime (Claforan).

UPPER AIRWAY OBSTRUCTION

See Table 21-4.

CYSTIC FIBROSIS
Introduction

- Autosomal recessive disorder caused by mutations of both alleles of the CF gene. This results in abnormalities in the production of the gene product, cystic fibrosis transmembrane regulator (CFTR) gene. The CFTR gene allows chloride to be transported out of the cell to the epithelial surface and determines hydration of the mucous gel.
- Inadequate hydration is believed to cause inspissated secretions and organ damage in the pancreas and biliary tree.
- In the lungs, it impairs ciliary clearance, promoting bacterial infection.

TABLE 21-4.
UPPER AIRWAY OBSTRUCTION

	Epiglottitis	Croup	Bacterial tracheitis	Foreign body
Onset	Rapid: hours	Prodrome, 1–7 days	Prodrome, 3 days, then hrs	Acute or chronic
Age	1–6 yrs	3 mos–3 yrs	3 mos–2 yrs	Any
Season	None	October–May	None	None
Etiology	*H. influenzae*	Parainfluenza	*Staphylococcus*	Many
Pathology	Inflammatory edema of epiglottis and supraglottis	Edema and inflammation of trachea and bronchial tree	Tracheal-bronchial edema	Localized tracheitis
Dysphagia	Yes	No	No	Rare
Difficulty swallowing	Yes	No	Rare	No
Drooling	Yes	No	Rare	No
Stridor	Inspiratory	Inspiratory and expiratory	Inspiratory	Variable
Voice	Muffled	Hoarse	Normal	Variable
Cough	No	Barking	Variable	Yes
Temperature	High	Minimal	Moderate	Normal
Position	Erect, anxious, worse when supine	No effect on airway obstruction	No effect	No effect
Respiratory rate	Increased early	Increased late	Normal	Variable

Adapted from Scruggs K. *Pediatrics 5-minute review*, 1998–1999 ed. Laguna Hills, CA: Current Clinical Strategies Publishing, Inc., 1999.

Epidemiology

- Occurs in 1:2500 live births.
- It is the most common genetic lethal disease in whites.
- Occurs more often in Northern Europeans and Ashkenazi Jews. Occurs in blacks and Hispanics but seldom in the Asian population.
- Mean survival age is ±31 yrs.

Presenting Features

Pulmonary

- First year of life: recurrent respiratory tract disease, cough, wheezing, pneumonia

- Later presentation: clubbing, wheezing/asthma, recurrent pneumonia, chronic sinusitis

GI

- Early in life: meconium ileus: 10% of newborns; *pathognomonic* of CF

- Also a failure to thrive, steatorrhea, obstructive jaundice, rectal prolapse, and hypoproteinemia

Less Common Presenting Features

- Neonatal: delayed passage of meconium (>24–48 hrs after birth), meconium plug syndrome. Prolonged cholestasis.

- Respiratory: nasal polyps, chronic sinusitis, allergic bronchopulmonary aspergillosis, and *Pseudomonas* bronchitis.

- GI: meconium plug syndrome/distal intestinal obstruction: most do not have CF. Differential diagnosis includes Hirschprung's, hypothyroidism. Recurrent/chronic pancreatitis.

- Salt depletion: hyponatremic dehydration and hypochloremic metabolic alkalosis.

- Male infertility: congenital bilateral absence of the vas deferens.

Diagnosis

- Clinical findings and family history **AND**

    Neonatal screening: increased circulating levels of immunoreactive trypsinogen, **OR**

    Sweat test: chloride ≥60 mmol/L on ≥2 occasions (40–60 borderline), **OR**

  - Genotyping for CFTR mutations (2 mutations confirms the diagnosis)

  - Obstructive azoospermia in males

- False-positive sweat test results can occur in adrenal insufficiency, nephrogenic diabetes insipidus, type I glycogen storage disease, hypothyroidism, hypoparathyroidism, familial cholestasis, and malnutrition.

Treatment Goals

- Delay and/or prevent lung disease.

- Promote good nutrition and growth.
- Treat any complications and maximize quality of life.

Characteristics and Antibiotic Therapy of Pulmonary Exacerbations in Cystic Fibrosis

- See Table 21-5.

TABLE 21-5.
CHARACTERISTICS AND ANTIBIOTIC THERAPY OF PULMONARY EXACERBATIONS IN CF

Severity	Therapy[a]
Mild	Amoxicillin or amoxicillin/clavulanate (Augmentin)
Mild decreased lung function (change in FEV_1 <10%)	**OR**
No change in CXR	TMP/SMX (Bactrim, Septra)
Cough and congestion for a few days	**OR**
Can be treated orally	Cephalexin or cefaclor
Moderate	Ciprofloxacin (Cipro) or ofloxacin (Floxin) (>18 yrs)
Decreased lung function (change in FEV_1 >10%)	**OR**
Minimal changes on CXR	Inhaled gentamicin (Garamycin), tobramycin (Tobrex), or colistin (Colimycin)
Increased cough or sputum >2 wks	
Treat orally, inhaled, or parenterally	IV: see Severe
Severe	Gentamicin[b] or tobramycin[b] or amikacin[b] (Amikin)
Worsening lung function	
Pneumothorax or hemoptysis	**OR**
Increased cough and sputum	Ticarcillin (Ticar) or piperacillin (Pipracil) or oxacillin (Bactocill, Prostaphlin)
Fever and weight loss	
Treat parenterally	**OR**
	Aztreonam or imipenem (Primaxin)
	OR
	Ceftazidime (Fortaz)

[a]Always base your antibiotic choice on sputum cultures and prior therapies and sensitivities.
[b]Follow levels closely at initiation of therapy and 1 wk after.

- Adequate therapy should always include intensive chest physiotherapy 4×/day and good nutritional support.
- Treat all patients for a minimum of 14 days of systemic and, if indicated, inhaled antibiotics.
- All CF patients should be hospitalized in separate rooms.
- Always consult the pulmonary service.

Lab Tests

Pulmonary exacerbations: CXR; sputum cultures, pulmonary function tests on admission and qwk, BMP, serum transaminases, gamma-glutamyltransferase, alkaline phosphatase, bilirubin, CBC with differential, IgE, PT, PTT, fasting glucose.

Complications

Hemoptysis, pneumothorax, nasal polyps, sinusitis, allergic bronchopulmonary aspergillosis, meconium ileus, distal intestinal obstructive syndrome, rectal prolapse, pancreatitis, biliary cirrhosis, insulin deficiency, infertility, pancreatic exocrine function deficiency.

Outpatient Monitoring

Spirometry, sputum cultures when cough increases, electrolyte monitoring, adjustment of pancreatic enzyme replacement.

Admission

The length of admission depends on the severity of the exacerbation, but hospitalize the patient for a minimum 5 days or until

- Clinical improvement is seen.
- There is improvement in pulmonary function studies.

SUGGESTED READING

Colin AA, et al. Cystic fibrosis. *Pediatr Rev* 1994;15:192–200.
Expert Panel Report 2: guidelines for the diagnosis and management of Asthma, May 1997. U.S. Department of Health and Human Services. National Institutes of Health publication No. 97–4051A.
McMillan JA, ed. *Oski's pediatrics: principles and practice*, 3rd ed. Philadelphia: Lippincott Williams & Wilkins, 1999.
Stern RC. The diagnosis of cystic fibrosis. *N Engl J Med* 1997;336:487–491.

22 **Radiology**

Say cheese.

ORDERING A RADIOLOGY EXAM

The radiologist may customize the exam or even suggest a different one to answer the specific clinical question. Key information to provide:

- Exam requested
- Specific clinical question and/or clinical situation
- Relevant medical diagnoses and surgeries
- In cancer patients: date of last chemotherapy or radiation therapy
- Allergy to iodinated IV contrast
- Renal function (serum creatinine)
- IV access: location and gauge
- Exam to be portable or in radiology department
- Patient factors such as NPO status, mechanical ventilation, cooperativeness, and need for sedation

Safety Considerations

- For young patients who cannot stay still or are uncooperative, monitor conscious sedation with pentobarbital (Nembutal) and midazolam (Versed).
- For potentially painful procedures, add morphine or fentanyl.
- Keep patient NPO.
- See Appendix B (Formulary) for dosages.

Radiation Considerations

Although it may be minimal, x-rays, fluoroscopy, and CT scans do expose the patient to ionizing radiation, whereas U/S and MRI do not.

GI Contrast Considerations

- The radiologist chooses between barium and water-soluble contrast. Barium is usually the GI contrast of choice but should not be used if a leak is suspected or surgery is imminent because barium can cause peritonitis or mediastinitis. Also, barium can limit future abdominal CT imaging due to scatter artifact from retained material.

- Water-soluble contrast (Hypaque, Gastroview) is used when barium is contraindicated. Its advantage over barium is that it reabsorbs into body cavities. However, it produces poorer image quality. It is hyperosmolar and causes fluid shifts into the GI tract, although this usually is tolerated by the patient. It should not be used when large-volume aspiration is a possibility. In the lungs, it causes pulmonary edema.

MRI Considerations

- Contraindicated in patients with programmable implanted devices (such as pacemakers and cochlear implants), non–MRI-compatible aneurysm clips, and metallic fragments in the eye.

- Some stents, filters, coils, and prosthetic valves require 6–8 wks to allow tissue in-growth before an MRI may be performed.

- Magnetic resonance compatibility must be considered for other implants, prostheses, metal objects, and some dark tattoos. Closed-loop wires tend to heat up during the exam. Skin staples are usually tolerated if taped securely.

- Patients must be able to lie flat for 30–90 mins. They are relatively unmonitored and must be cooperative enough to lie still (or be sedated). Consider claustrophobia a potential limitation to obtaining an optimal study.

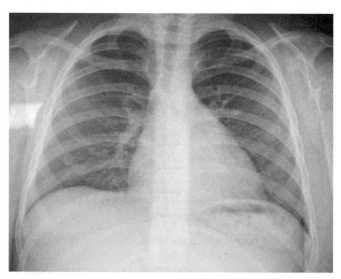

FIG. 22-1.
Normal chest x-ray.

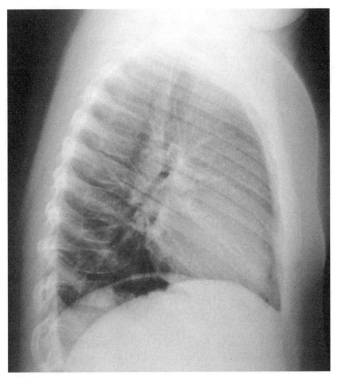

FIG. 22-2.
Normal lateral chest x-ray.

CHEST X-RAY

- Check for infiltrates, thickened bronchial walls, pulmonary edema, enlarged or decreased pulmonary vascularity, pleural effusions, heart size, midline trachea, rib fractures, and septal lines (Kerley B lines).

- Check aeration: Flattened or inverted diaphragm on the lateral view suggests air trapping and hyperinflation.

- Check for anomalies: Check on which side (left or right) lie the cardiac apex, aortic arch, stomach bubble, and liver shadow.

- Normal PA and lateral chest x-rays are shown in Figs. 22-1 and 22-2.

Evaluation of NICU Chest X-Rays

- Check on every line and tube position.

- Check for pneumothorax.

Evaluation for Infiltrates

Check for subtle infiltrates behind the diaphragm and heart on the frontal view. Normally, the borders of heart and diaphragm are sharp, and the right and left heart shadows should be similar in density. Right middle lobe and lingular infiltrates project over the heart on the lateral. Infiltrates are present if the lung projecting over the spine does not become increasingly dark as you look down the spine; however, note that normal posterior lower-lobe vessels are often mistaken for infiltrates. The normal thymus, which can be large and triangular in young children, is sometimes confused for upper-lobe infiltrates.

Classic Appearances

- *Respiratory syncytial virus*: hyperinflation, perihilar infiltrates, and thickened bronchial walls.

- *Pneumonia*: focal infiltrates, especially lobar consolidation.

- *Atelectasis*: linear opacities and volume loss.

- Often, *infiltrates* and *atelectasis* have similar appearances, especially in infants.

Newborn Chest X-Ray

- *Transient tachypnea of the newborn*: infiltrates that resolve in <2 days, usually with normal lung volumes.

- *Hyaline membrane disease*: in a premature neonate, ground glass opacities, small lung volumes, and typically no pleural effusions. May progress to pulmonary interstitial emphysema or bronchopulmonary dysplasia.

- *Meconium pneumonia*: usually in a term or postterm newborn; hyperinflated lungs with patchy, coarse infiltrates.

- *Neonatal pneumonia*: variable appearance including asymmetric infiltrates, often with pleural effusions. Group B streptococcal pneumonia is the most common etiology.

Evaluation for Pneumothorax

- Classic appearance: thin, sharp, white line representing pleural surface; no vessels beyond the pleura; air present beyond the pleura (air is dark, lucent) (Fig. 22-3).

- Also look for:

  - Deep sulcus sign: lateral costophrenic angle deepened with increased lucency (basilar pneumothorax)

  - Increased lucency over one lung (anterior pneumothorax)

  - Increased sharpness of the cardiomediastinal border (medial pneumothorax)

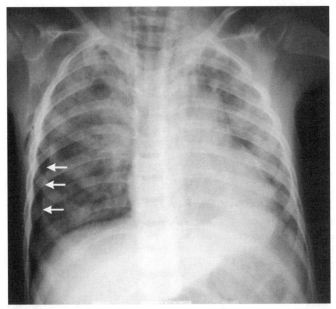

FIG. 22-3.
Right pneumothorax. Notice sharp pleural line and absence of pulmonary vessel beyond. This trauma patient also has lung contusions and SC air in the chest wall soft tissue.

- If uncertain, for cooperative patients, order an upright or expiratory film. For the uncooperative or intubated patient, order a cross table lateral or lateral decubitus (opposite side down) film.

- Tension pneumothorax is suggested by a mediastinal shift away from the pneumothorax or if the hemidiaphragm is depressed on the side of pneumothorax. These radiographic findings of tension pneumothorax may not be seen with PEEP ventilation or diseased noncompliant lung.

Evaluation for Foreign Body

In young children, aspirated foreign bodies most often cause ipsilateral air trapping and hyperinflation. Thus, to evaluate for radiolucent foreign bodies, expiratory or ipsilateral lateral decubitus CXRs may be helpful. Real-time fluoroscopy or even CT may be performed if x-rays are equivocal.

CHEST CT

IV contrast optimizes the evaluation of vessels, mediastinum, chest trauma, empyema, and hilar masses. Noncontrast CT is adequate for evaluating peripheral pulmonary nodules and lung parenchymal disease. High-resolution imaging may be performed to further characterize subtle lung parenchymal disease.

ABDOMINAL IMAGING
Abdominal X-Ray

- Abdomen one view is synonymous with kidneys, ureters, and bladder (KUB); abdominal flat plate; and supine abdomen x-ray.

- Obstructive series: abdomen two view (supine and either upright or left lateral decubitus) and may include an upright chest. The supine film is used to evaluate bowel gas pattern and abnormal calcifications (such as renal calculi and appendicolithiasis), whereas the upright or left lateral decubitus additional allows evaluation for pneumoperitoneum and gas-fluid levels.

Evaluation of Bowel Gas Pattern

- **Normal bowel gas pattern:** typically includes nondilated colon with stool and gas, gas in the rectum, a few loops of nondilated gas-

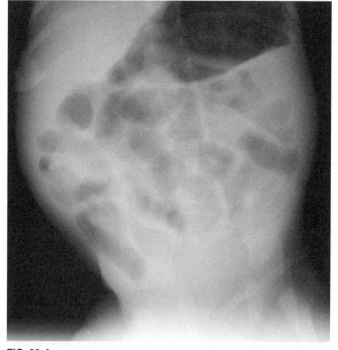

FIG. 22-4.
Small bowel obstruction. Numerous loops of dilated small bowel. Also, there is an absence of gas in the rectum and sigmoid colon in the pelvis.

filled small bowel, and a gastric bubble. Crying babies often swallow air and have many loops of gas-filled nondilated proximal small bowel loops. *Remember*: Small bowel folds completely encircle bowel and colonic folds (haustra) only partially encircle bowel.

- **Complete small bowel obstruction:** Most important sign is dilated small bowel. The colon usually has little or no gas. Gas is usually not seen in rectum. The more loops of dilated small bowel, the more distal the obstruction (Fig. 22-4).

- **Partial or early small bowel obstruction:** dilated small bowel with some gas and stool still seen in the colon and rectum.

- **Ileus:** dilated small and large bowel with large bowel dilated more prominently than small bowel. Usually postop.

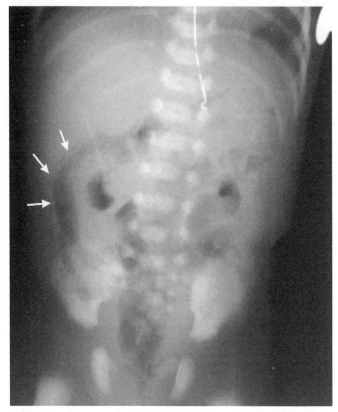

FIG. 22-5.
Pneumatosis of the right colon.

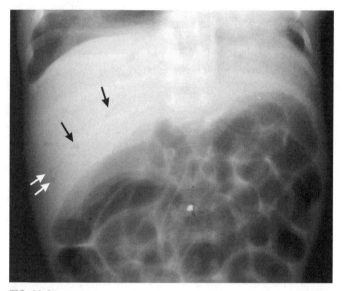

FIG. 22-6.
Portal venous gas. Branching gas pattern within the liver.

- **Intussusception:** small bowel obstruction pattern. Classic sign of a right upper quadrant soft tissue mass sometimes seen. May have a normal bowel gas pattern.

- **Necrotizing enteritis:** Look for pneumatosis (Fig. 22-5), portal venous gas (Fig. 22-6), and pneumoperitoneum (Fig. 22-7).

- **Nonspecific bowel gas pattern:** not normal but not clearly obstructed. Usually a few loops of mildly dilated small bowel or a gasless abdomen (Fig. 22-8). May be seen in many abdominal diseases such as gastroenteritis or pancreatitis.

- Remember, if dilated bowel loops are fluid filled they may not be seen. Hence, a **paucity of bowel gas** may suggest a small bowel obstruction in the appropriate clinical setting.

Evaluation of Pneumoperitoneum

- On upright film: Look for subdiaphragmatic gas.

- On left lateral decubitus film: Look for gas between the liver and body wall. Adequate exams must include the superior liver border/ entire right hemidiaphragm (Fig. 22-7).

- On supine: often subtle. The inferior liver edge appears sharp; there is increased lucency, especially over liver; the falciform ligament is

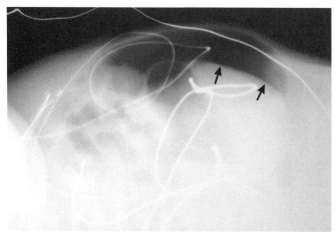

FIG. 22-7.
Pneumoperitoneum (free air), left lateral decubitus (left side of patient down). Peritoneal air seen lateral to edge of liver. Peritoneal air also demarcates the outer border of the bowel wall in the loop of bowel inferior to the liver.

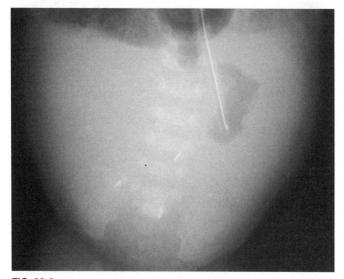

FIG. 22-8.
Gasless abdomen. Considerations include an inflammatory process such as enteritis or pancreatitis, bowel obstruction (atypical appearance), or abdominal mass.

237

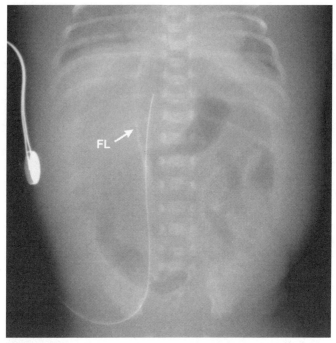

FIG. 22-9.
Pneumoperitoneum (free air), supine abdomen. Large amount of air outside the confines of bowel. The falciform ligament (FL, thin white line projecting over the liver lateral to the umbilical venous catheter) is visualized because it is outlined by gas.

outlined by air; the inner and outer margins of bowel wall are well delineated; or there is air not conforming to typical bowel appearance such as in the subhepatic space (Fig. 22-9). These changes are often subtle.

Evaluation of NICU Abdominal Films

- **Check all line positions!**

- Umbilical arterial catheter: from the umbilicus, courses caudally to the internal iliac arteries and then cranially to the aorta. There are two preferred positions:

  - Between the mid-descending thoracic aorta (below ductus arteriosus) and above vertebral body T10 (above the celiac artery)

  - At the level of the vertebral body L3 or L4 (below the renal arteries and above the aortic bifurcation)

- Umbilical venous catheter: from umbilicus, courses cranially through umbilical vein to ductus venosus to intrahepatic IVC. The preferred position is at the IVC/right atrial junction. Check for mal-positioned catheters with tip projecting over or below the liver (in a hepatic, portal, or umbilical vein).

Abdominal U/S

- Assesses abdominal organs: liver, gallbladder, bile ducts, pancreas, spleen, and kidney. Unable to assess gas-filled structures such as intestines. Can be performed at the patient's bedside. Keep patient NPO.

  - Hypertrophic pyloric stenosis: With an experienced sonographer, U/S is a fast, comfortable exam. (Fluoroscopic upper GI exam is also first-line option.)

  - Ascites: U/S can diagnose and localize it for drainage.

  - Appendicitis: with an experienced sonographer, fast exam for thin, young children.

  - Gallstones: sensitive exam for diagnosis.

Abdominal/Pelvic CT

- Assesses abdominal solid organs, intestines, mesentery, and retro-peritoneum very well. Keep patient NPO.

- U/S is better for characterizing adnexal and uterine pathology. CT is preferred for appendicitis evaluation in teenagers or larger children and when U/S results are equivocal.

- CT typically performed with oral and IV contrast. Without oral con-trast, differentiation of small bowel from masses or fluid collections may be limited. Without IV contrast, evaluation of solid abdominal organs and vessels is limited.

Abdominal/Pelvic MRI

Usually reserved for characterizing atypical lesions first seen by other imaging.

GI FLUOROSCOPIC EXAMS

- Fluoroscopic exams can be performed with barium or water soluble-contrast (Gastroview, Hypaque).

- Exams involve a radiologist at the patient's side performing a real-time fluoroscopic exam.

- Keep patient NPO.

Speech Swallow Study

- Multiple food and liquid consistencies given with real-time fluoroscopic evaluation to assess which foods can be tolerated without aspiration

- Exam performed in conjunction with trained speech therapist

Barium Swallow/Upper GI Exam

- Assesses pharynx, esophagus, stomach, and duodenum.

- Upper GI is the exam of choice to evaluate for malrotation and midgut volvulus (additional small follow-through not needed).

- When evaluating for hypertrophic pyloric stenosis, upper GI can reveal other GI pathology if hypertrophic pyloric stenosis is not present. (U/S is also a first-line option for hypertrophic pyloric stenosis.)

Small Bowel Follow-Through

- Evaluation of small intestines.

- Administered oral contrast is fluoroscopically evaluated periodically as peristalsis carries it through the entire small intestine.

- Often performed in conjunction with the upper GI exam.

- Assesses for Crohn's disease, strictures, masses, and sometimes obstruction. Small bowel obstruction can usually be diagnosed and managed with abdominal x-rays.

Contrast Enema

- Assesses the colon for strictures, obstruction, masses, and fistulas.

- Enema is the exam of choice for intussusception, Hirshsprung's disease, microcolon, and meconium ileus.

- With intussusception, therapeutic reduction (with air, water-soluble contrast, or barium) may be performed.

- Therapeutic reduction carries the small risk of perforation, so IV access and a surgical consult before the exam are needed. Active colitis is a relative contraindication.

GENITOURINARY IMAGING

Voiding Cystourethrogram

- After the bladder is catheterized, fluoroscopy is performed during bladder filling and spontaneous or voluntary voiding.

- Exam of choice to diagnose and grade vescicoureteral reflex or posterior urethral valves. Urine must be clear of infection.

Renal U/S

- Evaluate for age-appropriate kidney size, cystic masses, and hydronephrosis.
- CT is more sensitive for small solid masses and tiny calculi.

Scrotal U/S

- Exam of choice to evaluate for testicular or scrotal pathology, including testicular torsion, trauma, masses, and infection
- Doppler evaluation performed to assess blood flow

Pelvic U/S

- Exam of choice for ovarian and uterine pathology.
- Pediatric pelvic U/S performed transabdominally. Full bladder required.
- Doppler evaluation performed to assess blood flow.
- Common indications include ovarian torsion, tuboovarian abscess, pregnancy, ectopic pregnancy, and adnexal masses.

Renal Stone Protocol

- CT performed without oral contrast and usually without IV contrast to assess for renal and ureteral calculi and associated obstruction.
- IV contrast can be administered to opacify the ureters when their course is uncertain.

IV Pyelography

- Reserved for situations in which other imaging modalities are unable to answer a clinical question or detect pathology.
- Exam consists of a series of abdominal x-rays taken after administering IV contrast.
- Excellent for assessing ureters. Screening for renal or ureteral calculi usually performed by CT or U/S.

EXTREMITY IMAGING

- X-rays are used predominately for bone evaluation.
- CT provides excellent bone detail and some soft tissue detail.
- U/S and MRI can be used for better soft tissue (muscle and tendon) evaluation.

Skeletal Survey

- X-rays of skull, chest, abdomen, and extremities for indications such as child abuse, skeletal dysplasias, and, rarely, histiocytosis X.

- In infants, a skeletal survey may be more sensitive than bone scan for multifocal osteomyelitis and metastatic neuroblastoma.

Hip U/S

One of two indications may be requested:

- Assess for dislocation (congenital).
- Check for effusion.

Bone Age

One of two methods chosen by radiologists to assess if skeletal age is advanced or delayed relative to chronological age.

- A single left-hand x-ray compared with an atlas of normal standard examples
- Multiple films of one side of the patient to count the ossification centers throughout skeleton (for ages <2 yrs)

NEUROIMAGING

Neonatal Head U/S

Assesses for hemorrhage, hydrocephalus, large arterial-venous shunts, and gross brain maturity.

Head CT

- After the neonatal period, noncontrast head CT is the usual *screening* modality of choice, including for trauma.
- Contrast may be used to assess for tumors but MRI is preferred for greater sensitivity.

Head MRI

- Excellent for further characterizing CT findings such as tumors, congenital anomalies, and strokes
- Also a screening tool for seizure focus

Cerebral Magnetic Resonance Arteriogram

Screening exam for cerebral arterial pathology

Spine CT

Excellent for evaluating vertebral bodies

Spine MRI

- Excellent for overall spine imaging, including spinal cord, intervertebral disks, subarachnoid, and epidural pathology. MRI is the exam of choice for tumors, tumor extension into spinal canal such as neuroblastoma, congenital anomalies, and epidural abscesses.

NUCLEAR MEDICINE

- Nuclear medicine exams can provide functional information that other imaging modalities cannot. Anatomic detail, however, is usually decreased compared with that of other imaging modalities.
- Most nuclear medicine exams can be performed portably.

Bone Scan

More sensitive than x-rays for bone pathology (exceptions include histiocytosis X and osteomyelitis and metastatic neuroblastoma in infants). MRI is also excellent for bone pathology. The radiologist chooses between these exams:

- Three-phase bone scan consists of blood flow, immediate uptake, and delay retention (about 2–4 hrs after injection) imaging of a technetium-radiolabeled agent injected IV. The imaging of the first two phases is limited to the primary region of concern. Delayed imaging is often of the whole body. Usual indication is osteomyelitis (which can be multifocal in children via hematogenous spread) or an occult fracture.
- Delayed whole-body imaging only: usually for a skeletal metastasis survey or for follow-up.

Renal Scan

- Technetium-radiolabeled agent injected by IV and kidneys are imaged to assess for the relative contribution to function for each kidney and to assess for urinary obstruction.
- Furosemide (Lasix) is sometimes helpful in the setting of prior or chronic obstruction.

Hepatoiminodiacetic Acid (HIDA Scan)

- Technetium-radiolabeled agent that is excreted into the biliary system.
- Useful for differentiating congenital biliary atresia from neonatal hepatitis.
- Some pediatricians administer phenobarbital for a few days before imaging to improve sensitivity for biliary atresia.
- Also useful for the diagnosis of acute or chronic cholecystitis.
- Keep patient NPO.

Gastric Emptying

- Technetium-radiolabeled solid meal is given and stomach imaged to assess emptying.

• Keep patient NPO.

GI Bleeding

• Technetium-radiolabeled (tagged) RBCs injected IV to evaluate for bleeding over 60–90 mins of imaging.

• Patient must be actively bleeding for a positive exam.

• Because GI bleeding is episodic, evacuation of bloody stools does not directly correlate with the timing of active bleeding.

Meckel's Scan

• Technetium compound injected IV and abdomen imaged

• Does not require active bleeding

• Highly specific exam for Meckels's diverticulum containing ectopic gastric mucosa

Lung Scan

• Usually a two-part exam

• Ventilation imaging with inhaled xenon gas or technetium-radiolabeled particles

• Perfusion imaging with technetium-labeled, IV-injected particles, which are trapped in small arterial branches

• Used to evaluate for pulmonary embolism and for lung transplantation surveillance

SUGGESTED READING

Burton E, Brody A. *Essentials of pediatric radiology*. New York: Thieme Medical Publishers, 1999.

Donnelly, LF. *Fundamentals of pediatric radiology*. Philadelphia: WB Saunders, 2001.

Seigel M, ed. *Pediatric sonography*, 3rd ed. Philadelphia: Lippincott Williams & Wilkins, 2001.

23 Rheumatology

Chasing away the evil humors.

APPROACH TO THE CHILD WITH JOINT PAIN AND SWELLING

Joint pain is common in children. It is generally transient, secondary to trauma and/or increased activity. It is important to determine if it is secondary to muscular, ligament, bone, or referred pain.

History

- Age and gender

- History of sexual activity (e.g., gonococcus)

- Onset characteristics (e.g., trauma, immunizations, infections, and travel history)

- Other associated symptoms:

  - Morning stiffness: juvenile rheumatoid arthritis (JRA), ankylosing spondylitis

  - Migratory: acute rheumatic fever

  - Hematuria: HSP

  - GI bleeding: HSP, *Yersinia*, and inflammatory bowel disease

  - Rash: JRA, HSP, serum sickness, Lyme disease, gonococcus, Kawasaki's disease, parvovirus, and inflammatory conditions

- Family history: SLE

Number and Type of Joints Involved

- **Monoarticular:** infectious (e.g., septic arthritis, toxic synovitis, osteomyelitis, psoas abscess, TB), fracture, hemarthrosis, avascular necrosis (e.g., Calvé-Perthes disease, sickle cell disease. slipped capital femoral epiphysis), tumors (e.g., osteosarcoma, Ewing's sarcoma, osteoid osteoma, leukemia, rhabdomyosarcoma, JRA)

- **Pauciarticular:** inflammatory (e.g., JRA, Reiter's syndrome, juvenile ankylosing spondylitis, psoriasis), infectious (e.g., Lyme disease)

- **Polyarticular:** inflammatory (e.g., polyarticular and systemic JRA, HSP, serum sickness, dermatomyositis, SLE, scleroderma, sarcoid, Kawasaki's), malignancy, leukemia, rickets, infectious (e.g., gonococcus, parvovirus)

TABLE 23-1.
JOINT FLUID ANALYSIS

	Normal	Reactive arthritis	Inflammatory	Infectious
Color	Colorless/clear	Colorless/clear	Yellow/clear	Variable/turbid
WBC	<200/mm³	3000–10,000/mm³	5000–100,000/mm³	>100,000/mm³
Neutrophils (%)	<25	<25	>50	>75
Glucose	± Serum glucose	± Serum glucose	<2.8 mmol/L	> 2.8 mmol/L
Culture	Negative	Negative	Negative	Positive

- **Large joints:** gonococcus, Lyme disease, septic arthritis, HSP, leukemia, solid tumors, Calvé-Perthes, slipped capital femoral epiphysis, parvovirus
- **Small joints:** JRA, SLE, dermatomyositis, mixed connective tissue disease, scleroderma, Reiter's, psoriatic arthritis, gonococcus

Physical Exam

- Assess gait, muscle strength, muscle wasting, and tenderness.
- Do a careful joint exam noting any effusions, warmth, painful range of motion, tenderness, and fever.
- Examine for any associated skin or extraarticular findings.

Labs

- CBC: increased WBC in infection, inflammatory and hematologic disorders.
- ESR and C-reactive protein: not increased in trauma, mechanical problems, or viral infection.
- ANA: increased in SLE (ANA occurs in low titer in 5% of healthy children), mixed connective tissue disease, myositis, and scleroderma.
- Joint fluid analysis: See Table 23-1.

JUVENILE RHEUMATOID ARTHRITIS

- Etiology unknown.
- Increased incidence in females.
- Arthritis in ≥1 joint for at least 6 wks, often painless.

- Onset peak 1–3 or 2–8 yrs.

- Exclusion of other causes of joint inflammation.

- Increased susceptibility in children with HLA-DR5, HLA-DR8.

- There are five major forms of JRA (Table 23-2).

Treatment

- NSAIDs: naproxen, 20 mg/kg/day bid PO; or ibuprofen, 40 mg/kg/day q6h PO. Patients with polyarticular and systemic onset disease often fail to respond to NSAIDs.

- ASA: start 80 mg/kg/day; titrate to obtain a salicylate level 20–30 mg/dL.

- Second-line agents: methotrexate (Folex, Rheumatrex, Trexall) (7.5 mg/m^2 weekly), etanercept (Enbrel).

- Short course of prednisone (Deltasone) (2 mg/kg) used for severe systemic manifestations and carditis.

- Physical therapy, occupational therapy, and psychological support are essential for good long-term outcome.

SYSTEMIC LUPUS ERYTHEMATOSUS

- Autoimmune disorder affecting multiple tissues mediated by auto-antibodies and immune complexes.

- More frequent in females.

- Can develop at any age >5 yrs.

- Common features in children are skin rash and arthritis.

- Constitutional symptoms are common before the onset of organ-specific disease.

Diagnosis

- ≥4 criteria, serially or simultaneously (MD SOAP BRAIN):
  - **M**alar rash: spares nasolabial folds and eyelids
  - **D**iscoid rash
  - **S**erositis
    - Pleuritis
    - Pericarditis
  - **O**ral ulcers: painless
  - **A**rthritis: ≥2 peripheral joints; nonerosive arthritis
  - **P**hotosensitivity

TABLE 23-2.
FIVE MAJOR FORMS OF JUVENILE RHEUMATOID ARTHRITIS

	Pauciarticular I	Pauciarticular II	Polyarticular (RF negative)	Polyarticular (RF positive)	Systemic onset
Frequency (%)	30–40	10–15	25	10	5–10
Population	Females 80%; <5 yrs	Males 90%; >10 yrs	Females 90%; any age	Females 80%; >10 yrs	Males = females; any age
Joints	Large joints (hip and sacroiliac spared)	Large joints (hip and sacroiliac involvement)	Symmetric, any joint, no sacroiliitis	Symmetric, any joint, rare sacroiliitis	Any joint, >5 joints, no sacroiliitis
Extraarticular manifestations	Fever and rash are rare; painless chronic iridocyclitis	Fever and rash are rare; painful acute iridocyclitis, psoriasis, colitis, sausage digits, mouth ulcers, urethritis	Low-grade fever, malaise, growth retardation, rare eye involvement	Low-grade fever, malaise, rheumatoid nodules, no eye involvement	High fever, rash, organomegaly, polyserositis, growth retardation, no eye involvement, lymphadenopathy, carditis
Labs	ANA positive: 30% (risk factor for eye involvement); RF negative: ESR normal or increased	ANA negative, RF negative	ANA positive: 25%; RF negative: mild anemia	ANA positive: 75%; RF positive: 100%, anemia	ANA negative, RF negative, leukocytosis, anemia, thrombocytosis, hypoalbuminemia, increased ferritin
Prognosis	Very good; 10–20% ocular damage	Good, could progress to spondyloarthropathy	Severe arthritis: 10–15%	Severe arthritis: >50%	Severe arthritis: 25–50%

RF, rheumatoid factor.

- **B**lood
  - Hemolytic anemia (Coombs' positive)
  - Leukopenia (<4000 mm^3) on ≥2 occasions
  - Lymphopenia (<1500 mm^3) on ≥2 occasions
  - Thrombocytopenia (<100,000/mm^3)
- **R**enal disorder
  - Persistent proteinuria (> 0.5 g/dL)
  - Cellular casts: RBC, hemoglobin, granular, tubular, and mixed casts
- **A**NA: >1:80
- **I**mmunologic: positive anti–double-stranded DNA antibody has high sensitivity and specificity for diagnosis, anti-Sm has high specificity 99%; false-positive VDRL, presence of antiphospholipid antibody
- **N**eurologic
  - Seizure
  - Psychosis

Treatment

- Supportive: Avoid triggering factors (e.g., sun exposure, infections, cold exposure).
- Pharmacologic:
  - ASA, NSAIDs (helps with symptoms of arthritis but can decrease renal blood flow)
  - Corticosteroids
    - Topical: for skin disease
    - Oral: prednisone, 0.5–2 mg/kg/day; taper until inflammation is controlled (ESR decreased and complement increased)
  - Pulse therapy: methylprednisolone (Medrol), 30 mg/kg/day PO × 3–5 days for CNS and renal disease
- Cytotoxic therapy: cyclophosphamide (Cytoxan, Neosar), chlorambucil (Leukeran), and azathioprine for diffuse proliferative glomerulonephritis and life-threatening disease.

HENOCH-SCHÖNLEIN PURPURA

- Hypersensitivity vasculitis
- Occurs after viral respiratory illness, gastroenteritis, or streptococcal pharyngitis

- Onset before 10 yrs of age in 75% of cases; peak of onset: 5 yrs
- Males > females

Clinical Manifestations

- Palpable purpuric rash on dependent portions of the body (legs and buttocks)
- Arthritis/arthralgia
- Abdominal pain and GI hemorrhage
- Renal disease: hematuria ± proteinuria

Lab

- Elevated serum IgA titers and ESR
- Normal platelets
- Normal PT, PTT

Diagnosis

- Should be clinical.
- Tissue biopsy may reveal perivascular deposits of IgA.

Treatment

- Supportive and symptomatic.
- Corticosteroids have been used for bowel involvement or severe arthritis. They have not shown to change the course of nephritis.

Prognosis

- 70% of patients recover within 4 wks.
- Some patients may have intermittent hematuria without renal compromise.
- <1% progress to renal failure.

DERMATOMYOSITIS

- An autoimmune vasculopathy of muscle, skin, and GI tract.
- It occurs frequently after a viral infection.
- Onset occurs throughout childhood; peak at 10 yrs.
- It may present acutely or insidiously.

Clinical Features

- Erythematous dermatitis over the dorsum of the metacarpophalangeal and proximal interphalangeal joints (Gottron's papules);

lichenified rash over medial malleoli, knees, and elbows; photosensitivity; or heliotrope rash **in addition to** three of the following criteria are diagnostic of childhood dermatomyositis:

- Symmetric proximal muscle weakness
- Elevated serum enzymes in muscle (creatine kinase, aldolase, LDH, AST)
- Abnormal EMG
- Characteristic muscle biopsy: perifascicular atrophy
- SC calcification, muscle atrophy and pain, arthritis, and GI vasculitis are some potential complications.

Diagnosis

- Increased levels of serum muscle enzymes.
- MRI: edema of inflamed proximal muscle; appears bright on T_2 images.
- Muscle-specific antibodies, myositis-associated antibodies.
- Biopsy is confirmatory but not necessary if pathognomonic rash is present.

Therapy

- Supportive: physical and occupational therapy.
- Corticosteroids: prednisone, 2 mg/kg/day, until clinical improvement and decreased muscle enzymes.
- Maintenance steroids may be required for years.
- Methotrexate, 5–15 mg/wk, maintenance therapy.
- NSAIDs/ASA.
- IV immunoglobulin or cytotoxic agents, cyclosporin A (Neoral, Sandimmune) may be beneficial.

RHEUMATIC FEVER

- An inflammatory disease that follows infection with group A streptococci.
- Treating or eradicating carriers of streptococcal infection can prevent primary and secondary exacerbations.
- Rare in children aged <5 yrs.

Jones Criteria

Major

- **A**rthritis: generally migratory, affecting knees, elbows, and wrists

- **C**arditis: pancarditis; mitral insufficiency; aortic insufficiency
- **C**horea, Sydenham's: sudden writhing movements of extremities
- **N**odules, subcutaneous: painless, 0.5–1 cm on extensor joint surfaces
- **E**rythema marginatum: serpiginous erythematous and with clear center rash

Minor

- Clinical: fever (rarely >40°C)
- Arthralgias
- Lab and data findings:
  - Increased ESR
  - CRP increased
  - Leukocytosis
- Prolonged PR interval

Accessory Criteria

- Previous evidence of streptococcal infection:
  - Rising antistreptolysin-O titer
  - Antistreptolysin-O titer ≥333 in children or ≥250 in adults
- Positive rapid streptococcal test or throat culture
- History of scarlet fever or previous rheumatic fever

Diagnosis

High probability:

- Two major criteria with evidence of previous streptococcal infection.
- One major and two minor criteria.
- Exceptions to the above: Rheumatic carditis or Sydenham's chorea alone is sufficient for diagnosis.

Treatment

- Eradication of group A beta hemolytic streptococcus infection
  - Patients who meet diagnostic criteria should be treated despite negative group A streptococcal cultures.
  - Benzathine penicillin (Bicillin L-A), 1.2 million U IM × 1.
  - Penicillin V: 25–50 mg/kg/day divided tid–qid × 10 days.
  - Erythromycin (E-Mycin, E.E.S., Ery-Tab, Eryc, EryPed, Ilosone), 20–40 mg PO divided qid × 10 days.

- Other alternatives are amoxicillin, azithromycin, or cephalosporins.
- Arthritis
  - ASA is usually used 80–100 mg/kg/day × 2 wks in the management of associated arthritis.
  - NSAIDs.
- Carditis
  - Mild: ASA
  - Moderate to severe: prednisone, 2 mg/kg/day

Prophylaxis for Recurrences

- Benzathine penicillin, 1.2–2.4 million U IM q3wks.
- Penicillin V or erythromycin.
- Treatment is up to 18 yrs of age or indefinite.

KAWASAKI'S DISEASE

Diagnosis: fever (38–41°C) × 5 days or longer **and** 4 out of 5 of the following:

- Bilateral conjunctivitis
- Mucositis (e.g., erythema of the lips, strawberry tongue, oropharyngeal erythema)
- Cervical lymphadenopathy, usually a solitary node
- Polymorphic erythematous rash
- Swelling of hands or feet

Associated Symptoms

- CNS involvement: irritability, lethargy, aseptic meningitis
- Urethritis
- Cardiac abnormalities: pericarditis, gallop, congestive heart failure
- Liver dysfunction
- Arthritis
- Abdominal pain/diarrhea
- Coronary artery abnormalities
- Gallbladder hydrops
- Jaundice

Labs

- Elevated ESR, elevated IgE, elevated alpha$_1$-antitrypsin, elevated WBC with left shift, elevated CRP, negative blood culture, elevated platelet count, mild to moderate anemia, elevated bilirubin, elevated liver enzymes, pyuria

Echocardiography

Perform at onset of symptoms and 3–6 wks after onset of fever to evaluate for coronary artery aneurysm. If cardiac involvement, consult a pediatric cardiologist.

Treatment

- Gamma globulin, 2 g/kg over 10–12 hrs. Monitor heart rate and BP at beginning of infusion and at 30 mins, 1 hr, and q2h after infusion begun.
- Patients given steroids in combination with IV immunoglobulin may have a better outcome.
- ASA, 100 mg/kg/d PO divided qid until afebrile × 14 days, then 3–10 mg/kg/day until cardiac abnormalities, platelet count, and ESR return to normal.

Follow-Up

Monthly × 6 mos, then q3–6mos. Risk of sudden death is highest 12–30 days after onset of symptoms.

SUGGESTED READING

McMillan JA, ed. *Oski's pediatrics: principles and practice*, 3rd ed. Philadelphia: Lippincott Williams & Wilkins, 1999.

24 **Procedures**

Time for some hands-on activities.

INTRODUCTION

The most important aspect of beginning a procedure is to make yourself comfortable. If you are uncomfortable, the procedure will be more uncomfortable for the patient, will take longer, and is less likely to be successful. So take a few extra minutes to make sure you are as comfortable as possible and have all the supplies close by and ready: It will save time and frustration in the end.

UMBILICAL ARTERY CATHETERIZATION

- Complications: hemorrhage (from perforation of an artery or line displacement); thrombosis; infection; ischemia/infarction of lower extremities, bowel, or kidney; arrhythmias.
- Line placement
  - Low line: The tip of the catheter should lie just above the aortic bifurcation between L3 and L5, avoiding the renal and mesenteric arteries, but this type of line is at increased risk for being accidentally pulled out.
  - High line: The tip of the catheter should be above the diaphragm, between T6 and T9 (above the renal and mesenteric arteries).
- Catheter length
  - Birth weight (BW) regression formula:
    - Low line: umbilical artery catheter (UAC) length in cm = BW (kg) + 7
    - High line: UAC length in cm = $[3 \times BW (kg)] + 9$
- **Procedure**
  - Determine catheter length.
  - Restrain infant. Using sterile technique, prep and drape umbilical cord and adjacent skin.
  - Flush catheter with sterile saline before insertion.
  - Place sterile umbilical tape around base of cord. Cut through cord horizontally about 1.5–2.0 cm above the skin. Tighten umbilical tape to stop bleeding.

- Identify the one large, thin-walled vein and the two smaller, thicker-walled arteries. Use the curved tip forceps to gently open and dilate one of the arteries.

- Grasp catheter approximately 1 cm from the tip with toothless forceps and insert catheter into artery to the desired length. Feed catheter into the artery using gentle pressure. Do not force the catheter. If resistance is met, loosen the umbilical tape, manipulate the angle of the umbilical stump to skin, or apply firm, gentle pressure. Forcing the catheter may create a false luminal tract.

- Secure the catheter with a suture through the cord and around the catheter.

- Confirm catheter position with x-ray. Catheter may be pulled back but not advanced once the sterile field is broken.

UMBILICAL VEIN CATHETERIZATION

- Complications: hemorrhage from line displacement or vessel perforation; infection, air embolism, arrhythmias.

- Line placement: Umbilical vein catheters should be placed in the IVC above the level of the ductus venosus and the hepatic veins and below the level of the left atrium.

- Catheter length
  - Regression formula: umbilical vein catheter length (cm) = [$0.5 \times$ UAC (cm)] + 1

- **Procedure**
  - Follow procedure steps for UAC placement up to the step identifying the artery. In this case, identify the thin-walled vein and insert catheter. Gently advance catheter to desired distance. Do not force, as this may cause a false luminal tract. Again, if resistance is met, try the same maneuvers as with the UAC before advancing.

- Secure catheter as in UAC placement.

- Confirm catheter placement with x-ray.

LUMBAR PUNCTURE

- Complications: headache, acquired epidermal spinal cord tumor caused by implantation of epidermal material into spinal canal if no stylet used on skin entry, local back pain, infection, bleeding, herniation associated with increased ICP.

- Contraindications:
  - Increased ICP: if signs or symptoms of increased ICP are present (papilledema, retinal hemorrhage, trauma with associated head injury), perform fundoscopic exam and CT before LP.

- Bleeding diathesis: Platelet count >50,000/mm^3 is preferred before LP. Correction of clotting factor deficiencies before LP prevents spinal cord hemorrhage and potential paralysis.

- Overlying skin infections may inoculate CSF.

- **Procedure**

  - Position the child in the sitting position or lateral recumbent position with the hips, knees, and neck flexed. Be careful not to compromise cardiorespiratory status.

  - Locate either the L3–L4 or L4–L5 interspace by drawing an imaginary line between the two iliac crests.

  - Clean the skin with povidone-iodine (Betadine) and drape the child in sterile fashion.

  - Use a 20- to 22-gauge spinal needle with stylet of desired length.

  - Anesthetize overlying skin and SC tissue with lidocaine.

  - Puncture midline just caudal to palpated spinous process, angling the needle slightly caudal and toward the umbilicus. Advance the needle slowly, withdrawing the stylet every few millimeters to check for CSF flow.

  - If resistance is met (i.e., you hit bone), withdraw the needle to the skin and redirect the angle of the needle.

  - Send CSF for appropriate studies. (Tube 1 for culture and Gram's stain, tube 2 for glucose and protein, tube 3 for cell count and differential, tube 4 for saved serum or any additional specialized studies.)

  - To measure CSF pressure, patient must be lying on his or her side in an unflexed position. Once free flow of CSF is established, attach the manometer and measure CSF pressure.

CHEST TUBE PLACEMENT AND THORACENTESIS

- Complications: pneumothorax or hemothorax; bleeding or infection; pulmonary contusion or laceration; puncture of diaphragm, liver, or spleen

- **Procedure: needle decompression**

  - For tension pneumothorax, decompress by sterilely inserting a 23-gauge butterfly or 22-gauge angiocatheter at the second intercostal space in the midclavicular line.

  - Attach to a three-way stopcock and syringe and aspirate air.

- **Procedure: chest tube placement**

  - Position child supine or with affected side up.

  - Entry point is the third to fifth intercostal space in the mid- to anterior axillary line, usually at the level of the nipple. (Be careful to avoid breast tissue.)

  - Prep and drape sterilely with Betadine.

  - Locally anesthetize skin, SC tissue, rib periosteum, chest wall muscles, and pleura with lidocaine.

  - Make a sterile incision one intercostal space below the desired insertion point and bluntly dissect through tissue layers until the superior portion of the rib is reached. (This avoids the neurovascular bundle on the inferior portion of each rib.)

  - Push hemostat over top of rib, through the pleura, and into the pleural space. Enter the pleural space cautiously. Spread hemostat to open, place chest tube in clamp, and guide into entry point.

  - For a pneumothorax, insert the tube anteriorly toward the apex. For a pleural effusion, direct the tube inferiorly and posteriorly.

  - Secure the tube with purse-string sutures.

  - Attach the tube to the drainage system with −20 to −30 cm of water pressure.

  - Apply sterile occlusive dressing.

  - Confirm position with CXR.

- **Procedure: Thoracentesis**

  - Confirm fluid in the pleural space with clinical exam, CXR, or sonography.

  - Place child in sitting position leaning over a table if possible. Otherwise place child supine.

  - Point of entry is in the seventh intercostal space and posterior axillary line.

  - Sterilely prep and drape area.

  - Anesthetize the skin, SC tissue, rib periosteum, chest wall, and pleura with lidocaine.

  - Advance an 18- to 22-gauge IV catheter or large-bore needle attached to a syringe onto rib and then walk needle over top of rib into pleural space while providing steady negative pressure.

- Attach syringe and stopcock device to remove fluid.

- After removing needle or catheter, place occlusive dressing and obtain CXR to rule out pneumothorax.

SUTURING

- General information:

  - Lacerations to be sutured should be <6 hrs old (12 hrs on the face).

  - Usually, bite wounds should not be sutured.

  - The longer sutures are left in place, the bigger the potential for scarring and infection. (See page 260 for suture selection.)

- When should you involve plastic surgery?

  - Consider with any laceration involving the face, lips, hands, genitalia, mouth, or orbital area

  - Deep lacerations with nerve damage

  - Stellate lacerations

  - Flap lacerations

  - Lacerations involving the vermilion border

  - Lacerations with questionable tissue viability

  - Large complex lacerations

- Anesthesia

  - If there is no end artery supply: 1% lidocaine with 1% epinephrine (without epinephrine if there is end artery supply or cartilage); max. dose: 3–5 mg/kg without epinephrine, 7 mg/kg with epinephrine

  - Topical: lidocaine, tetracaine, ELA-Max (topical lidocaine)

- Technique

  - Remove foreign bodies.

  - Examine the area for exposed nerves, tendons, and bone.

  - Perform a neurovascular exam.

  - Remember to ask about tetanus status and immunize if needed (see page 261).

  - Irrigate wound with copious amounts of sterile saline to clean area. (*This is the most important step to prevent infection.*)

  - Prep and drape the patient.

CH. 24: PROCEDURES

- Apply anesthetic.
- Débride any necessary areas.
- Begin suturing.
- Apply antibiotic ointment and sterile dressing.

Suture Material, Size, and Removal

LOCATION	MONOFILAMENT (FOR SUPERFICIAL LACERATIONS)	ABSORBABLE (FOR DEEP LACERATIONS)	REMOVAL (DAYS)
Face	6-0	5-0	3–5
Scalp	4-0 or 5-0, consider staples	4-0	5–7
Eyelid	6-0 or 7-0	—	3–5
Eyebrow	5-0 or 6-0	5-0	3–5
Trunk	4-0 or 5-0	3-0	5–7
Extremities	4-0 or 5-0	4-0	7
Joint surface	4-0	—	10–14
Hand	5-0	5-0	7
Sole of foot	3-0 or 4-0	4-0	7–10

SKIN ADHESIVES

- Appropriate uses: low-tension areas.
- Inappropriate uses: high-tension areas, contaminated wounds, wounds across mucocutaneous junctions, animal or human bites, or wounds with evidence of infection.
- Application: clean and dry area. Achieve hemostasis. Approximate wound edges. Squeeze adhesive onto wound edges then apply in a circular motion around wound. Apply at least three layers, allowing each layer to dry between applications.
- Postapplication: no dressing needed, adhesive falls off in 5–10 days, avoid topical ointments, no scrubbing or submersion of the area.

TETANUS PROPHYLAXIS

CLINICAL SCENARIO	CLEAN WOUND	TETANUS-PRONE WOUND
Fully immunized and <5 yrs since last booster	None	None
Fully immunized 5–10 yrs since last booster	None	Td
Fully immunized and >10 yrs since last booster	Td	Td
Incompletely immunized or unknown	Td	Td and tetanus immunoglobulin

Td, tetanus-diphtheria.

SUGGESTED READING

Dieckman RA, Fisher DH, Selbst SM. *Pediatric emergency and critical care procedures.* St. Louis: Mosby–Year Book, 1997.

Appendixes

Algorithms

Pediatric Tachycardia with Poor Perfusion

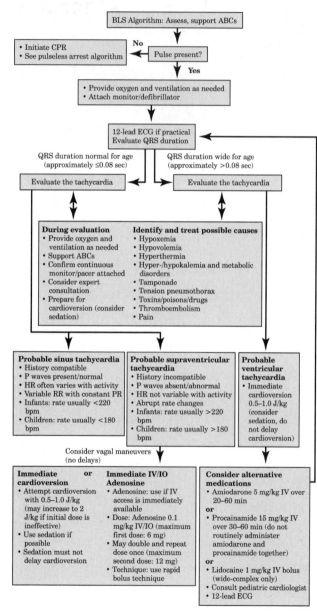

FIG. A-1.
Algorithm for pediatric tachycardia with poor perfusion.

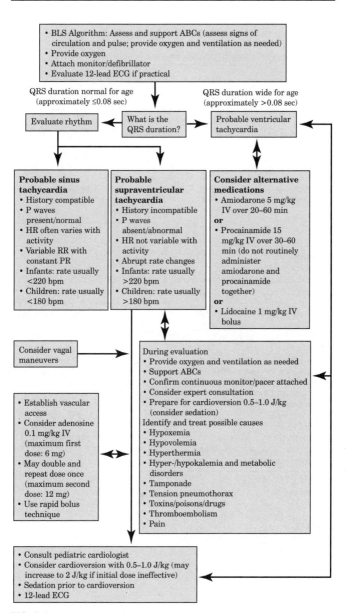

FIG. A-2.
Algorithm for pediatric tachycardia with adequate perfusion.

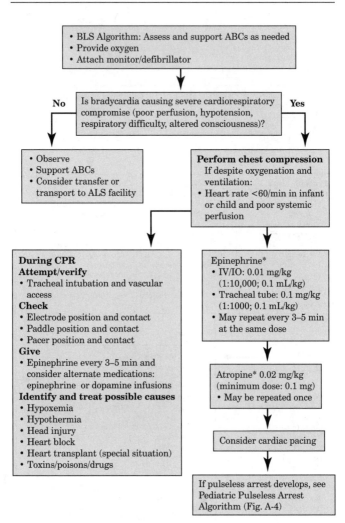

FIG. A-3.
Pediatric bradycardia algorithm.
*Give atropine first for bradycardia due to suspected increased vagal tone or primary AV block.

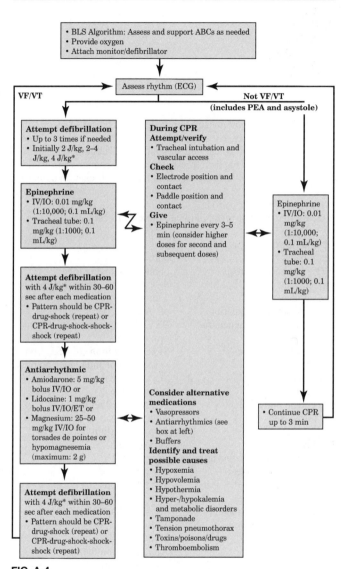

FIG. A-4.
Pediatric pulseless arrest algorithm.
*Alternative waveforms and higher doses are class indeterminate for children.

B | Formulary

FORMULARY

This formulary is by no means comprehensive. Classes of medications that change frequently (e.g., anti-HIV medications) or that should only be administered with the aid of a specialist (e.g., antiarrhythmics) have not been included. This list represents the most common medications prescribed by general pediatricians as well as pediatricians in training.

Day refers to a 24-hr period.
R means that an adjustment in renal failure is necessary.

Abbreviations:

A, alopecia
AVN, avascular necrosis
cap, capsule
div, divided
DPI, dry powder inhalation
EDTA, ethylenediaminetetra-
    acetic acid
ER, extended release
F, fever
fxn, function
HA, headache
IBW, ideal body weight
IN, intranasal
inh, inhaler
IT, intrathecal
JRA, juvenile rheumatoid arthritis
LFT, liver function test
maint, maintenance
max, maximum
MDI, metered-dose inhaler
MS, myelosuppression
MT, microtubules
Muc, mucositis
N, nausea

oint, ointment
ophtho, ophthalmologic
PCP, pneumocystis carinii pneu-
    monia
pt, patient
RSV, respiratory syncytial virus
rxn, reaction
SIADH, syndrome of inappropriate
    secretion of antidiuretic hormone
SL, sublingual
sol, solution
SR, sustained release
supp, suppository
susp, suspension
sx, symptom
sz, seizure
tab, tablet
TB, tuberculosis
TBL, total body load
Topo, topoisomerase
V, emesis
VS, vital signs
XRT, radiation therapy
yo, year(s) old

ANTIRHEUMATIC AGENTS

Name	Oral or topical forms	Dosage	Comments
Azathioprine (Imuran)	Susp: 50 mg/mL Tab: 50 mg	Initial: 2–5 mg/kg/day IV/PO qd. Maint: 1–2.5 mg/kg/day IV/PO qd. Max: 2.5 mg/kg/day.	R. Hematologic toxicities.
Etanercept (Enbrel)		4–17 yo: 0.4 mg/kg/dose SC 2×/wk 72–96h apart. Max: 25 mg/dose.	Contraindicated in serious infections. Do not administer live vaccines concurrently. Onset of action is 1–4 wks.
Hydroxychloroquine sulfate (Plaquenil)	Tab: 200 mg	JRA: 3–5 mg/kg/day PO div qd–bid. Max: 400 mg/day.	Bone marrow suppression.
Methotrexate (Rheumatrex)	Tab: 2.5, 5, 7.5, 15 mg	JRA: 5–15 mg/m²/wk PO/SC/IM as a single dose or in 3 divided doses given 12 h apart.	R. Give folate replacement while on therapy.
Sulfasalazine (Azulfidine, Azulfidine EN-tabs, Salazopyrin EN-tabs)	Tab: 500 mg	JRA: >6 yo: Start with 10 mg/kg/day div bid PO and increase by 10 mg/kg/day q7days until maint of 30–50 mg/kg/day div bid. Max: 2 g/day.	R. Contraindicated in sulfa allergy, porphyria, GI obstruction. May cause orange-yellow discoloration of the skin and mucous membranes.

MUSCLE RELAXANTS

Name	Oral or topical forms	Dosage	Comments
Baclofen (Lioresal)	Tab: 10, 20 mg Susp: 5, 10 mg/mL	>2 yo: 10–15 mg/day PO div q 8h. Titrate dose q3days by increments of 5–15 mg/day to max of 40 mg/day if <8 yo and max of 60 mg/day if >8 yo.	R. May cause drowsiness. Do not abruptly withdraw drug.
Diazepam (Valium, Diastat)	Tab: 2, 5, 10 mg Sol: 1, 5 mg/mL	IV/IM: 0.04–0.3 mg/kg/dose q2–4h. Max: 0.6 mg/kg within 8h. PO: 0.12–0.8 mg/kg/day div q6–8h.	May cause hypotension and respiratory depression.

NONSTEROIDAL ANTIINFLAMMATORIES

Name	Oral or topical forms	Dosage	Comments
Aspirin (Ecotrin, Bayer)	Tab: 325, 500 mg Tab, enteric coated: 81, 165, 325, 500, 650 mg Tab, buffered: 325, 500 mg Tab, chewable: 81 mg Supp: 60, 120, 125, 200, 300, 325, 600, 650 mg	Antiinflammatory: 60–90 mg/kg/day PO div q6–8h. Kawasaki disease: 80–100 mg/kg/day PO div qid during febrile phase then 3–5 mg/kg/day qam after defervescence. Give until ESR and platelet count are normal.	R. Do not use if <16 yo if patient has flu or varicella due to risk of Reye's syndrome.

Drug	Formulations	Dosing	
Ibuprofen (Motrin, Advil)	Susp: 100 mg/5 mL Drops: 40 mg/mL Chewable tab: 50, 100 mg Cap: 100, 200 mg Tab: 100, 200, 300, 400, 600, 800 mg	Analgesic, antipyretic: 5–10 mg/kg/dose PO q6–8h. Max: 40 mg/kg/day. JRA: 30–50 mg/kg/day PO div q6h. Max: 2400 mg/day.	R. Contraindicated with GI bleeding and ulcer disease. Inhibits platelet aggregation.
Indomethacin (Indocin)	Cap: 25, 50 mg Cap, ER: 75 mg Supp: 50 mg Susp: 25 mg/5 mL	Antiinflammatory: >14 y: 1–3 mg/kg/day PO div tid–qid. Max: 200 mg/day. Closure of ductus: 0.1–0.2 mg/kg/dose IV q12–24 hr × 3 total doses.	R. Contraindicated in bleeding, NEC, coagulopathies. Monitor urine output and platelet count during therapy. Do not give subsequent doses if either falls too low.
Ketorolac (Toradol)	Tab: 10 mg	IM/IV: 0.5 mg/kg/dose q6h. Max: 30 mg q6h or 120 mg/day. PO: >50 kg: 10 mg prn q6h. Max: 40 mg/day.	R. Do not exceed 5 days of therapy.
Naproxen/naproxen sodium (Naprosyn, Aleve, Anaprox)	Tab (Naproxen): 250, 375, 500 mg Tab (Naproxen sodium): Anaprox: 275 mg (250 mg base), 550 mg (500 mg base), Aleve: 220 mg (200 mg base) Susp (Naproxen): 125 mg/5 mL	>2 yo: Analgesic: 5–7 mg/kg/dose PO q8–12h. JRA: 10–20 mg/kg/day PO div q12h. Max: 1000 mg/day.	R. May cause GI bleeding, thrombocytopenia.

OPIOIDS

See Pain Service Medication Dosing Guide.

OTHER ANALGESICS

Name	Oral or topical forms	Dosage	Comments
Acetaminophen (Tylenol)	Drops: 80 mg/0.8 mL Susp: 160 mg/5 mL Elixir: 120 mg, 160 mg/5 mL Cap: 325, 500, 650 mg Gelcap: 500 mg Chewable tab: 80, 160 mg Supp: 80, 120, 325, 650 mg	Neonate dosing: See Neonatal Drug Recommendations. Children: 10–15 mg/kg/dose PO/PR q4-6h. Max: 4 g/day.	R. Does not possess antiinflammatory properties. Hepatotoxicity in overdose. See Figure 11-3 for details.

ANESTHETICS AND SEDATIVES
See Sedation Agents.

ANTIMICROBIALS

Aminoglycosides

Name	Oral or topical forms	Dosage	Comments
Amikacin (Amikin)		Neonates: See Neonatal Drug Recommendations. Infants/Peds: 15 mg/kg/day div q8h IV/IM. Initial max dose 1.5 g/day, then monitor levels.	R. Check peak and trough with 3rd dose.

Name	Oral or topical forms	Dosage	Comments
Gentamicin (Garamycin)		Neonates: See Neonatal Drug Recommendations. 1 mo–<14 yo: 7.5 mg/kg/dose IV qd. >14 yo: 6.5 mg/kg/dose IV qd.	R. qd dosing not appropriate in weight >20% IBW, ascites, >20% burns, altered renal function, endocarditis, tularemia, meningitis, osteomyelitis, hemodynamic instability. Dosing may need to be adjusted in patients with cystic fibrosis. Check peak and trough.
Tobramycin (Nebcin, TOBI)		Neonates: See Neonatal Drug Recommendations. 1 mo–<14 yo: 7.5 mg/kg/dose IV qd. >14 yo: 6.5 mg/kg/dose IV qd.	R. qd dosing not appropriate in weight >20% IBW, ascites, >20% burns, altered renal function, endocarditis, tularemia, meningitis, osteomyelitis, hemodynamic instability. Dosing may need to be adjusted in patients with cystic fibrosis. Check peak and trough.

Antifungals

Name	Oral or topical forms	Dosage	Comments
Amphotericin B (Fungizone)		Neonates: See Neonatal Drug Recommendations. IV: test dose: 0.1 mg/kg/dose IV up to max of 1 mg (followed by remaining initial dose). Initial dose: 0.25–0.5 mg/kg/day IV. Increase as tolerated by 0.25–0.5 mg/kg/qd or qd IV. Maint: qd dosing: 0.25 mg–1 mg/kg/dose IV. qod dosing: 1.5 mg/kg/dose IV. Max: 1.5 mg/kg/day.	R. Hypercalciuria, hypokalemia, hypomagnesemia, RTA may occur. Fever, chills, hypotension may occur with infusion. Premedicate with acetaminophen and diphenhydramine. Meperidine can be used for chills.

Name	Oral or topical forms	Dosage	Comments
Amphotericin B lipid formulations (Amphotec, Abelcet)		IV: 2.5–5 mg/kg qd.	Hypokalemia, hypomagnesemia, RTA may occur. Fever, chills, hypotension may occur with infusion. Premedicate with acetaminophen and diphenhydramine. Meperidine can be used for chills.
Clotrimazole (Mycelex, Lotrimin)	Cream: 1% Vaginal supp: 200 mg Vaginal cream: 1%, 2% Oral troche 10 mg	Vaginal candidiasis: 100 mg/dose qhs × 7 days or 200 mg/dose qhs × 3. Thrush: >3 yo: Dissolve one troche 5×/day × 14 days. Topical: Apply bid.	
Fluconazole (Diflucan)	Tab: 50, 100, 150, 200 mg Susp: 10, 40 mg/mL	Neonates: See neonate chart. Children: Load with 10 mg/kg IV/PO then maint: (24 h after load) 3–6 mg/kg qd IV/PO. Max: 12 mg/kg/day. Vaginal candidiasis: 150 mg PO × 1.	R. Do not use concurrently with cisapride, terfenadine, astemizole.
Griseofulvin	Microsize: Tab: 250, 500 mg, Cap: 125, 250 mg, Susp: 125 mg/5 mL, Ultramicrosize: Tab: 125, 165, 250, 330 mg	Microsize: >2 yo: 10–20 mg/kg/day PO div qd–bid. Max: 1 g/day. Ultramicrosize: >2 yo: 5–10 mg/kg/day PO div qd–bid. Max dose: 750 mg/day.	Contraindicated in hepatic disease.

Ketoconazole (Nizoral)	Tab: 200 mg Susp: 100 mg/5 mL Cream: 2% Shampoo: 2%	PO: >2 yo: 3.3–6.6 mg/kg qd. Max: 800 mg/day div bid. Topical: 1–2 applications/day. Shampoo: Twice weekly for 4 wks.	Do not use concurrently with cisapride, terfenadine, astemizole. Monitor LFTs in long-term use.
Miconazole (Monistat)	Cream, lotion, oint, solution: 2%, vaginal supp: 100, 200 mg	*Tinea cruris* or *corporis* or *Candidiasis*: Apply bid. *Tinea versicolor*: Apply qd. Vaginal: 1 applicator full of cream or 100 mg supp qhs × 7 days.	
Nystatin	Tab: 500,000 U Troches: 200,000 U Susp: 100,000 U/mL Cream/oint: 100,000 U/g, Topical powder: 100,000 U/g, Vaginal tab: 100,000 U	Oral: Preterm infants: 0.5 mL to each side of mouth qid. Term infants: 1 mL to each side of mouth qid. Children: Susp: 4–6 mL swish and swallow qid or troche: 200,000–400,000 U 4–5 ×/day. Vaginal: 1 tab qhs × 14 days. Topical: Apply bid–qid.	
Voriconazole	Tab: 50, 200 mg	IV: >12 yo: 6 mg/kg q12h for 2 doses then 4 mg/kg bid. PO: >12 yo and >40 kg: 200 mg bid, <40 kg: 100 mg bid.	R for IV form only.

277

Antimycobacterial Agents

Name	Oral or topical forms	Dosage	Comments
Ethambutol (Myambutol)	Tab: 100, 400 mg	TB: 15–25 mg/kg/dose PO qd or 50 mg/kg/dose PO twice weekly. Max: 2.5 g/day. Non-TB mycobacterial infection: 15–25 mg/kg/day PO. Max: 1 g/day.	R. May cause reversible optic neuritis.
Isoniazid (INH)	Tab: 50, 100, 300 mg Syrup: 50 mg/5 mL	Prophylaxis: 10 mg/kg PO qd. Max dose: 300 mg. After 1 mo of qd, may change to 20–40 mg/kg (max, 900 mg) per dose PO, 2×/wk. Treatment: 10–15 mg/kg (max dose, 300 mg) PO qd or 20–30 mg/kg PO (max, 900 mg) per dose 2×/wk with rifampin.	R. Should not be used alone for treatment. Supplemental pyridoxine recommended.
Rifampin (Rimactane, Rifadin)	Cap: 150, 300 mg Susp: 10, 15 mg/mL	TB: Twice weekly therapy may be used after 1–2 mo of daily therapy. 10–20 mg/kg/day IV/PO div q12–24h then 10–20 mg/kg/day PO twice weekly. Max: 600 mg/day. Neisseria meningitidis prophylaxis: 0–1 mo: 10 mg/kg/day PO div q12h × 2 days. >1 mo: 20 mg/kg/day PO div q12h × 2. Max: 600 mg/day.	R. Causes red discoloration of bodily fluids. Many drug interactions. Give 1 hr before or 2 hrs after meals.

Antiparasitics

Name	Oral or topical forms	Dosage	Comments
Albendazole (Albenza)	Tab: 200 mg	Hydatid disease: >6 yo: 15 mg/kg/day PO div bid with meals. Max: 800 mg/day. Neurocysticercosis: 15 mg/kg/day PO div bid. Max: 800 mg. Cutaneous larva migrans: 400 mg PO × 3days. Roundworm, hookworm, whipworm: 400 mg × 1 PO. Pinworms: 400 mg PO × 1, repeat in 2 wks.	
Ivermectin (Stromectol)	Tab: 3, 6 mg	>15 kg: Strongyloidiasis, scabies: 200 µg/kg PO × 1 dose. Onchocerciasis: 150 µg/kg PO × 1 dose.	
Mebendazole (Vermox)	Chewable: 100 mg	Pinworm: 1 tab PO × 1 dose. Whipworm, common roundworm, hookworm: 1 tab bid PO × 3 days.	
Metronidazole (Flagyl)	Tab: 250, 500 mg Tab, ER: 750 mg Cap: 375 mg Susp: 20, 50 mg/mL Gel, topical: 0.75% Cream, topical: 0.75% Gel, vaginal: 0.75%	Neonates: see Neonatal Drug Recommendations. Amebiasis: 35–50 mg/kg/day PO div tid. Max: 750 mg/dose. *Clostridium difficile*, anaerobic infection: 30 mg/kg/day IV/PO div q6h. Max: 4 g/day. Bacterial vaginosis: 500 mg bid PO × 7 days or 2 g PO × 1 dose or 5 g vaginal gel qd–bid × 5 days. Giardiasis: 15 mg/kg/day PO div tid × 5 d. Max: 250 mg PO tid. Trichomoniasis: see Chap. 7, Adolescent Medicine.	R. Patients should avoid alcohol while taking this medication.

Name	Oral or topical forms	Dosage	Comments
Pentamidine (Pentam)		PCP treatment: 4 mg/kg/day IM/IV qd × 14–21 days. Trypanosomiasis treatment: 4 mg/kg/day IM qd × 10 days. Leishmaniasis: 2–4 mg/kg/dose IM qd or qod for 15 doses. PCP prophylaxis: IM/IV: 4 mg/kg/dose q2–4 wks, Inh (>5 yo): 300 mg in 6 mL water q mo, Trypanosomiasis prophylaxis: 4 mg/kg/day IM q3–6mo. Max single dose: 300 mg.	R. May cause hypoglycemia, hyperglycemia, hypotension.
Permethrin (Elimite, Nix)	Cream: 5% Rinse: 1%	Head lice: Saturate hair and scalp with 1% rinse after shampooing and towel drying hair. Leave on 10 mins then rinse. May repeat in 7–10 days. Scabies: Apply 5% cream from neck to toes, wash off with water in 8–14 h. May repeat in 7 days.	Avoid contact with eyes.
Pyrantel (Pin-X)	Susp: 50 mg/mL Liquid: 50, 144 mg/mL Cap: 180 mg	Roundworm: 11 mg/kg/dose PO × 1; pinworm: 11 mg/kg/dose PO × 1 dose, repeat 2 wks later; hookworm: 11 mg/kg/dose PO qd × 3 days. Max dose: 1 g/dose.	

Anti-CMV Agents

Name	Oral or topical forms	Dosage	Comments
Foscarnet (Foscavir)		Induction: 90 mg/kg/dose IV q12h or 60 mg/kg/dose q8h Maint: 90–120 mg/kg/day IV	R. May cause peripheral neuropathy, bronchospasm.

Ganciclovir (Cytovnene)	Cap: 250 mg	CMV infection or CMV prevention in transplant: >3 mo: Induction therapy: 10 mg/kg/day div q12h IV; Maint: 5 mg/kg/dose qd IV or 6 mg/kg/dose qd for 5 days/wk; PO maint: 3 mg/kg/dose q 8h. Max: 1000 mg tid	R. Common side effects include neutropenia, thrombocytopenia.

Antiherpetic Agents

Name	Oral or topical forms	Dosage	Comments
Acyclovir (Zovirax)	Cap: 200 mg Tab: 400, 800 mg Susp: 200 mg/5 mL	Neonate dosing: see Neonatal Drug Recommendations. Immunocompetent: Mucocutaneous HSV: Initial infection: IV 15 mg/kg/day div q8h × 5–7 days or PO 1200 mg/day div q8h × 7–10 days. Recurrence: PO 1200 mg/day div q8h. Suppressive: PO 800–1000 mg/day div 2–5× day for up to 1 yr. Max: 80 mg/kg/day div q6–8h. Zoster: IV 30 mg/kg/day div q8h × 7–10 days or if >12 yo: PO 4000 mg/day div 5×/day × 5–7 days. Varicella: IV 30 mg/kg/day div q8h × 7–10 days or PO 80 mg/kg/day div qid × 5 days. Max: 3200 mg/day. Dosing for immunocompromised patients is different. Please consult the *AAP Red Book* (see Suggested Reading).	R. Adequate hydration and slow administration are necessary to prevent crystallization in the renal tubules.

Antiviral–Antiinfluenza

Name	Oral or topical forms	Dosage	Comments
Amantadine (Symmetrel)	Tab: 100 mg Susp: 50 mg/5 mL	Influenza A prophylaxis and treatment: 1–9 yo: 5 mg/kg/day PO div qd–bid . Max: 150 mg/day. >9 yo: 5 mg/kg/day PO div qd–bid. Max: 200 mg/day.	R. May cause dizziness, depression, anxiety. Initiate therapy within 2 days of onset of sx.
Oseltamivir (Tamiflu)	Cap: 75 mg Susp: 12 mg/mL	Treatment of influenza (all for 5 days): 1–12 yo based on weight: <15 kg: 30 mg PO bid 15–23 kg: 45 mg PO bid 23–40 kg: 60 mg PO bid >40 kg: 75 mg PO bid >12 yo: 75 mg PO bid	R. Initiate therapy within 2 days of onset of sx.
Rimantadine (Flumadine)	Tab: 100 mg Syrup: 50 mg/5 mL	Influenza A prophylaxis: <10 yo: 5 mg/kg/day PO qd. Max: 150 mg/day. >10 yo: 100 mg PO bid. Treatment: <10 yo or <40 kg: 5 mg/kg/day PO div qd–bid × 5–7 days. Max: 150 mg/day. >10 yo and >40 kg: 100 mg PO bid × 5–7 days.	R. Initiate therapy within 2 days of onset of sx.

RSV Immunoglobulin

Name	Oral or topical forms	Dosage	Comments
Palivizumab (Synagis)		RSV prophylaxis: 15 mg/kg IM q mo during RSV season	

Carbapenems

Name	Oral or topical forms	Dosage	Comments
Meropenem (Merrem IV)		>3 mo: mild to moderate infection: 60 mg/kg/day IV div q8h. Max: 3 g/day. Meningitis and severe infections: 120 mg/kg/day IV div q8h. Max: 6 g/day.	R.

Cephalosporins—1st Generation

Name	Oral or topical forms	Dosage	Comments
Cefazolin (Ancef)		Neonate dosing: See Neonatal Drug Recommendations. >1 mo: 50–100 mg/kg/day div q8h IV/IM. Max: 6 g/day.	R. Does not penetrate into CNS well.
Cephalexin (Keflex)	Cap: 250, 500 mg Susp: 125, 250 mg/5 mL Tab: 250 mg, 500 mg	25–100 mg/kg/day PO div q6h. Max: 4 g/day.	R.

Cephalosporins—2nd Generation

Name	Oral or topical forms	Dosage	Comments
Cefaclor (Ceclor)	Cap: 250, 500 mg Susp: 125, 187, 250, 375 mg/5 mL	20–40 mg/kg/day PO div q8h. Max: 2 g/day.	R.

Name	Oral or topical forms	Dosage	Comments
Cefoxitin (Mefoxin)		80–160 mg/kg/day IM/IV div q4–8h. Max: 12 g/day.	R. Good anaerobic activity.
Cefprozil (Cefzil)	Susp: 125, 250 mg/5 mL Tab: 250, 500 mg	Otitis media: 6 mo–12 yo: 30 mg/kg/day PO div q12h. Pharyngitis: 2–12 yo: 15 mg/kg/day PO div q12h. Acute sinusitis: 6 mo–12 yo: 15–30 mg/kg/day PO div q12–24h. Skin infection: >2: 20 mg/kg/day PO div q24h. Max: 1 g/day.	R.
Cefuroxime (Ceftin)	Tab: 125, 250, 500 mg Susp: 125, 250 mg/5 mL	Neonates: See Neonatal Drug Recommendations. Children: IM/IV: 75–150 mg/kg/day div q8h. Max: 6 g/day. PO: Pharyngitis: Susp: 20 mg/kg/day div q12h. Max: 500 mg/day. Otitis media: Susp: 30 mg/kg/day div q12h. Max: 1 g/day.	R. Tablets and suspension are not bioequivalent. Cannot substitute on a mg/mg basis.

Cephalosporins—3rd Generation

Name	Oral or topical forms	Dosage	Comments
Cefdinir (Omnicef)	Cap: 300 mg Susp: 125 mg/5 mL	6 mo–12 yo: 14 mg/kg/day PO div q12h. Max: 600 mg/day. >12 yo 600 mg/day PO div q12h.	R.
Cefixime (Suprax)	Susp: 100 mg/5 mL Tab: 200, 400 mg	8 mg/kg/day div q12–24h. Max: 400 mg/day.	R.

Name	Dosage	Comments
Cefotaxime (Claforan)	Neonatal dosing: See Neonatal Drug Recommendations. <50 kg: 100–200 mg/kg/day div q6–8h IV/IM. Max: 12 g/day. >50 kg: 1–2 g/dose q6–8h IV/IM. Max: 12 g/day.	R. Good CNS penetration.
Ceftazidime (Fortaz)	IV/IM: Child: 90–150 mg/kg/day div q8h IV/IM. Meningitis or cystic fibrosis: 150 mg/kg/day IV/IM div q8h. Max: 6 g/day.	R. Good *Pseudomonas* coverage and CSF penetration.
Ceftriaxone (Rocephin)	Neonate gonococcal ophthalmia: 25–50 mg/kg/dose IM/IV ×1 with max 125 mg/dose. Children: 50–75 mg/kg/day div q12–24h IM/IV. Meningitis: 100 mg/kg/day IM/IV div q12h. Max: 4 g/day. Otitis media: 50 mg/kg IM × 1. Max: 1 g.	May cause hyperbilirubinemia in neonates; use with caution.

Cephalosporins—4th Generation

Name	Oral or topical forms	Dosage	Comments
Cefepime (Maxipime)		>2 mo: 100 mg/kg/day div q12h IV/IM. Meningitis, fever and neutropenia, cystic fibrosis: 150 mg/kg/day div q8h IV/IM Max: 6 g/day.	R. Good *Pseudomonas* coverage.

Macrolides

Name	Oral or topical forms	Dosage	Comments
Azithromycin (Zithromax)	Susp: 100, 200 mg/5 mL Tab: 250, 600 mg	Otitis media or pneumonia: 10 mg/kg PO day 1 (max, 500 mg) then 5 mg/kg/day. PO (max, 250 mg) qd × 4 more days. Pharyngitis: 12 mg/kg/day PO qd × 5 days (max, 500 mg/day).	R. Can prolong QT interval.
Clarithromycin (Biaxin)	Susp: 125, 250 mg/5 mL Tab: 250, 500 mg	15 mg/kg/day PO div q12h. Max: 1 g/day.	R. Many drug interactions.

Erythromycin preparations: base (E-mycin)	Base: Cap, enteric: 250 mg
	Tab, enteric: 250, 333, 500 mg
	
	Ethyl succinate (EES)
	  Chewable: 200 mg
	  Susp: 200, 400 mg/5 mL
	  Drops: 100 mg/2.5 mL
	  Tab: 400 mg
	
	Estolate
	  Susp: 125, 250 mg/5 mL
	  Drops: 100 mg/mL
	  Chewable: 125, 250 mg
	  Tab: 500 mg
	  Cap: 125, 250 mg
		Chlamydia conjunctivitis and pneumonia: 50 mg/kg/day PO div q6h × 14 days.
		
		Pertussis: Estolate salt: 50 mg/kg/day PO div q6h × 14 days. Other infections: base, estolate and ethylsuccinate: 30–50 mg/kg/day PO div q6–8h. Max: 2 g/day as base or 3.2 g/day as ethylsuccinate.	

Penicillins—1st Generation

Name	Oral or topical forms	Dosage	Comments
Benzathine penicillin G (Bicillin L-A)		Group A strep: 25,000–50,000 U/kg/dose IM × 1. Max: 1.2 million U/dose. Rheumatic fever prophylaxis: 25,000–50,000 U/kg/dose IM q 3–4 wks. Max: 1.2 million U/dose.	Provides sustained levels for 2–4 wks. Do not give IV.
Penicillin G procaine		Newborns: 50,000 U/kg/day IM qd. Children: 25,000–50,000 U/kg/day div q12–24h IM. Max: 4.8 million U/day.	Provides sustained levels for 2–4 days. Do not give IV.
Penicillin V potassium	Susp: 125, 250 mg/mL Tab: 125, 250, 500 mg	25–50 mg/kg/day div q6–8h PO. Max: 3 g/day. Acute group A strep: 250 mg PO bid–tid × 10 days. Rheumatic fever/pneumococcal prophylaxis: <5 yo: 125 mg PO bid, >5 yo: 250 mg PO bid.	R.

Penicillins—2nd Generation—Penicillinase Resistant

Name	Oral or topical forms	Dosage	Comments
Dicloxacillin (Dynapen)	Cap: 125, 250, 500 mg Susp: 62.5 mg/5 mL	<40 kg: 25–50 mg/kg/day PO div q6h. Max: 2 g/day. >40 kg: 125–500 mg/dose PO q6h. Max: 2 g/day.	

Name	Oral or topical forms	Dosage	Comments
Nafcillin (Nallpen)	Tab: 500 mg Cap: 250 mg Sol: 250 mg/5 mL	Neonates: See Neonatal Drug Recommendations. PO: 50–100 mg/kg/day div q6h, IM/IV: mild to moderate infections: 50–100 mg/kg/day div q6h. Severe infection: 100–200 mg/kg/day div q4–6h. Max: 12 g/day.	R.
Oxacillin (Bactocill)	Cap: 250, 500 mg Sol: 250 mg/5 mL	Doses are the same as for nafcillin.	R. Poor CSF penetration.

Penicillins—3rd Generation—Aminopenicillins

Name	Oral or topical forms	Dosage	Comments
Amoxicillin (Amoxil)	Cap: 250, 500 mg Chewable: 125, 200, 250, 400 mg Susp: 125, 200, 250, 400 mg/5 mL Tab: 500, 875 mg Drops: 50 mg/mL	25–50 mg/kg/day div bid–tid PO. High dose: 80–90 mg/kg/day div bid PO. Max: 2–3 g/day. Recurrent otitis media prophylaxis: 20 mg/kg/dose qhs PO.	R.

Amoxicillin clavulanate (Augmentin)	Chewable: 125/31.25 mg, 200/28.5 mg, 250/62.5 mg, 400/57 mg Susp: (per 5 mL): 125/31.25 mg, 200 /28.5 mg, 250/62.5 mg, 400/57 mg Tab: 250/125, 500/125, 875/125 mg, Augmentin ES: 600/42.9 mg/5 mL	Dosage based on amoxicillin component: <3 mo old: 30 mg/kg/day div bid PO. >3 mo old: 20–40 mg/kg/day div tid PO or 25–45 mg/kg/day div bid PO. Augmentin ES: >3 mo old and <40 kg: 90 mg/kg/day div bid PO. Max: 2 g/day.	R.
Ampicillin (Principen)	Cap: 250, 500 mg Susp: 125, 250, 500 mg/5 mL	Neonates: See Neonatal Drug Recommendations. Children: mild–moderate infections: IM/IV: 100–200 mg/kg/day div q6h. PO: 50–100 mg/kg/day div q6h. Max PO: 2–3 g/day. Severe infections: 200–400 mg/kg/day div q4–6h IM/IV. Max IV/IM dose: 12 g/day.	R. CSF penetration only with inflamed meninges.
Ampicillin sulbactam (Unasyn)		Dose based on component: >1 mo infant: mild/moderate infection: 100–150 mg/kg/day div q6h IM/IV. Severe infection: 200–300 mg/kg/day div q6h IM/IV. Children: mild/moderate infection: 100–200 mg/kg/day div q6h IM/IV. Severe infection: 200–400 mg/kg/day div q4–6h IM/IV. Max: 8 g/day.	R.

Penicillins—4th Generation—Extended Spectrum

Name	Oral or topical forms	Dosage	Comments
Piperacillin (Pipracil)		Neonates: See Neonatal Drug Recommendations. Children: 200–300 mg/kg/day IM/IV div q4–6h. Max: 24 g/day. Cystic fibrosis: 350–600 mg/kg/day IM/IV div q4–6h. Max: 24 g/day.	R.
Piperacillin tazobactam (Zosyn)		Dosages based on piperacillin component. <6 mo old: 150–300 mg/kg/day IV div q6–8h. >6 mo old: 200–400 mg/kg/day IV div q6–8h. Cystic fibrosis dosing same as piperacillin.	R.
Ticarcillin (Ticar)		Neonates: See Neonatal Drug Recommendations. Children: 200–300 mg/kg/day IM/IV div q4–6h. Max: 24 g/day. Cystic fibrosis: 300–600 mg/kg/day IM/IV. Max: 24 g/day.	R.
Ticarcillin clavulanate (Timentin)		Dosing same as for ticarcillin.	R.

Quinolones

Name	Oral or topical forms	Dosage	Comments
Ciprofloxacin (Cipro)	Susp: 250, 500 mg/5 mL Tab: 100, 250, 500, 750 mg	PO: 20–30 mg/kg/day div q12h. Max: 1.5 g/day. IV: 10–20 mg/kg/day div q12h. Max: 800 mg/day. Cystic fibrosis: PO: 40 mg/kg/day div q12h. Max: 2 g/day. IV: 30 mg/kg/day div q8h. Max: 1.2 g/day.	R. Use with caution in children <18 yo. Quinolones have caused arthropathy in animals.

Levofloxacin (Levaquin)	Tab: 250, 500 mg	5–10 mg/kg/dose PO/IV qd. Max: 500 mg.	R. Use with caution in children <18 yo. Quinolones have caused arthropathy in animals.

Sulfonamides

Name	Oral or topical forms	Dosage	Comments
Bactrim (trimethoprim/sulfamethoxazole)	Tab: (double strength) 160/800 mg, (single strength) 80/400 mg Susp: 40/200 mg/5 mL	Doses based on TMP component: Minor infections: 8–10 mg/kg/day PO/IV div bid. Max: 320 mg/day. UTI prophylaxis: 2–4 mg/kg/day PO qd. PCP treatment: 20 mg/kg/day PO/IV div q6–8h. PCP prophylaxis: 5–10 mg/kg/day PO/IV div bid or 150 mg/m^2/day div bid × 3 consecutive days/wk.	R. May cause kernicterus in newborns.

Tetracyclines

Name	Oral or topical forms	Dosage	Comments
Doxycycline (Vibramycin)	Cap or Tab: 20, 50, 100 mg Susp: 25 mg/5 mL Syrup: 50 mg/5 mL	2–4 mg/kg/day PO/IV div q12–24h. Max: 200 mg/day.	Use with caution in children <8 yo due to risk of tooth enamel hypoplasia and discoloration.

Name	Oral or topical forms	Dosage	Comments
Minocycline (Mino-cin)	Cap: 50, 75, 100 mg Tab: 50, 100 mg Susp: 50 mg/5 mL	8–12 yo: 4 mg/kg/dose × 1 PO/IV then 2 mg/kg/dose q12h PO/IV. Max: 200 mg/day. >12 yo: 200 mg/dose × 1 PO/IV then 100 mg q12h PO/IV. Acne: 50 mg PO qd–tid.	R. Use with caution in children <8 yo due to risk of tooth enamel hypoplasia and discoloration.
Tetracycline (Achro-mycin, Sumycin, etc.)	Tab: 250, 500 mg Cap: 250, 500 mg Susp: 125 mg/5 mL	>8 yo: 25–50 mg/kg/day PO div q6h. Max: 3 g/day.	R. Use with caution in children <8 yo due to risk of tooth enamel hypoplasia and discoloration.

Other Antimicrobials

Name	Oral or topical forms	Dosage	Comments
Aztreonam (Azactam)		Neonates: See Neonatal Drug Recommendations. Children: 90–120 mg/kg/day IV/IM div q6–8h. Cystic fibrosis: 150–200 mg/kg/day IV/IM div q6–8h. Max: 8 g/day.	R.
Clindamycin (Cleo-cin)	Cap: 75, 150, 300 mg Sol: 75 mg/5 mL	Neonates: See Neonatal Drug Recommendations. Children: PO: 10–30 mg/kg/day div q6–8h. PO max: 1.8 g/day. IM/IV: 25–40 mg/kg/day div q6–8h. IM/IV max: 4.8 g/day.	May cause pseudomembranous colitis.

Linezolid (Zyvox)	Susp: 100 mg/5 mL Tab: 400, 600 mg	10 mg/kg/dose IV/PO q8–12h. Max: 600 mg/dose.	
Nitrofurantoin (Furadantin)	Cap: 25, 50, 100 mg Susp: 25 mg/5 mL	>1 mo old: 5–7 mg/kg/day PO div q6h. Max: 400 mg/day. UTI prophylaxis: 1–2 mg/kg/dose PO qhs. Max: 100 mg/day.	R.
Vancomycin (Vancocin)	Cap: 125, 250 g Sol: 250 mg/5 mL	Neonate: See Neonatal Drug Recommendations. Children: CNS infection: 60 mg/kg/day IV div q6h, other infections: 40 mg/kg/day IV div q6–8h. Max: 1 g/dose. C. difficile colitis: 40–50 mg/kg/day PO div q6h. Max: 500 mg/day.	R. Associated with "red man syndrome." Treat with diphenhydramine and slower vancomycin infusion. Monitor drug levels.

CARDIOVASCULAR

ACE Inhibitors

Name	Oral or topical forms	Dosage	Comments
Captopril (Capoten)	Tab: 12.5, 25, 50, 100 mg Susp: 1 mg/mL	Infants: Initially: 0.15–0.3 mg/kg/dose PO, titrate upward if needed to max of 6 mg/kg/day div qd–qid. Children: Initially: 0.3–0.5 mg/kg/dose PO q8h, titrate upward to max of 6 mg/kg/day div bid–qid.	R. May cause cough.
Enalapril (Vasotec)	Tab: 2.5, 5, 10, 20 mg Susp: 1 mg/mL	Infants and children: PO: 0.1 mg/kg/day div qd–bid, titrate up as needed over 2 wks to max of 0.5 mg/kg/day. IV: 0.005–0.01 mg/kg/dose q8–24h.	R.

Antiadrenergic Agents

Name	Oral or topical forms	Dosage	Comments
Clonidine (Catapres)	Tab: 0.1, 0.2, 0.3 mg Patch: 0.1, 0.2, 0.3 mg	5–7 µg/kg/day PO div q6–12h, titrate up q5–7days to 5–25 µg/kg/day PO div q6h. Max: 0.9 mg/day.	Do not abruptly discontinue.

Inotropes

Name	Oral or topical forms	Dosage	Comments
Digoxin (Lanoxin)	Cap: 50, 100, 200 µg Elixir: 50 µg/mL Tab: 125, 250, 500 µg	1 mo–2 yo: Initial: 35–60 µg/kg PO or 30–50 µg/kg IV/IM. Maint: 10–15 µg/kg/day PO or 7.5–12 µg/kg/day IV/IM. 2–5 yo: Initial: 30–40 µg/kg PO or 25–35 µg/kg IV/IM. Maint: 7.5 µg/kg/day PO or 6–9 µg/kg/day IV/IM. 5–10 yo: Initial: 20–35 µg/kg PO or 15–30 µg/kg IV/IM. Maint: 5–10 µg/kg/day PO or 4–8 µg/kg/day IV/IM. >10 yo: Initial: 10–15 µg/kg PO or 8–12 µg/kg IV/IM. Maint: 2.5–5 µg/kg/day PO or 2–3 µg/kg/day IV/IM.	R. Give one-half of the total initial dose then give one-fourth of the remaining dose in each of the subsequent two doses at 6–12-h intervals. Obtain ECG 6 h after each dose to assess toxicity. Toxicity includes bradycardia, heart block, ventricular arrhythmias, vertigo, hyperkalemia, abdominal pain.
Digoxin immune Fab (Digibind)		To determine dose, calculate the TBL of digoxin: TBL (mg) = serum digoxin level (ng/mL) × 5.6 × body weight (kg) div by 1000. Dose of digoxin immune Fab (mg) IV = TBL × 76.	

Antihypertensives—Miscellaneous

Name	Oral or topical forms	Dosage	Comments
Nitroprusside sodium (Nipride)		IV, continuous infusion: start at 0.3–0.5 μg/kg/min, titrate to effect. Usual dose is 3–4 μg/kg/min. Max: 10 μg/kg/min.	R. Contraindicated in patients with decreased cerebral perfusion. Converted to cyanide, which may produce metabolic acidosis and methemoglobinemia.

Beta Blockers

Name	Oral or topical forms	Dosage	Comments
Atenolol (Tenormin)	Tab: 25, 50, 100 mg Susp: 2 mg/mL	1–1.2 mg/kg/day PO. Max: 2 mg/kg/day.	R. Contraindicated in pulmonary edema and cardiogenic shock.
Propranolol (Inderal)	Cap, ER: 60, 80, 120, 160 mg Sol: 20, 40 mg/5 mL Tab: 10, 20, 40, 60, 80 mg	HTN: PO: initial: 0.5–1 mg/kg/day div q6–12h. Increase q3–5days prn to max of 8 mg/kg/day. Migraine prophylaxis: <35 kg: 10–20 mg PO tid, >35 kg: 20–40 mg PO tid. Tetralogy spells: IV: 0.15– 0.25 mg/kg/dose slow IV push. May repeat in 15 min × 1. PO: initial: 2–4 mg/kg/day div q6h prn with usual dose range of 4–8 mg/kg/day div q6h prn. Thyrotoxicosis: Neonates: See Neonatal Drug Recommendations. Children: IV: 1–3 mg/dose over 10 min. May repeat in 4–6 hr. PO: 10–40 mg/dose PO q6h.	R. Contraindicated in asthma, heart failure, and heart block.

Calcium Channel Blockers

Name	Oral or topical forms	Dosage	Comments
Amlodipine (Norvasc)	Tab: 2.5, 5, 10 mg Susp: 1 mg/mL	Start with 0.1 mg/kg/dose PO qd–bid and titrate up q5–7days to a max of 0.6 mg/kg/day or 20 mg/day.	
Diltiazem (Cardizem)	Cap, ER: 60, 90, 120, 180, 240, 300 mg Cap, SR: 60, 90, 120 mg Tab: 30, 60, 90, 120 mg Elixir: 12 mg/mL	Initial: 1.5–2 mg/kg/day PO div tid–qid. Max: 3.5 mg/kg/day.	Contraindicated in second and third degree heart block
Nifedipine (Procardia)	Cap: 10, 20 mg Tab, ER or SR: 30, 60, 90 mg	HTN: 0.25–0.5 mg/kg/dose q4–6h prn PO/SL. Max: 10 mg/dose or 3 mg/kg/day. Hypertrophic cardiomyopathy: 0.5–0.9 mg/kg/day div q6–8h PO/SL.	

Diuretics—Carbonic Anhydrase Inhibitors

Name	Oral or topical forms	Dosage	Comments
Acetazolamide (Diamox)	Tab: 125, 250 mg Susp: 25, 30, 50 mg/mL Cap, SR: 500 mg	Diuretic: 5 mg/kg/dose PO/IV qd–qod. Glaucoma: 20–40 mg/kg/day IM/IV div q6h or 8–30 mg/kg/day PO div q6–8h. Szs: 8–30 mg/kg/day PO div q6–12h. Max: 1g/day. Urine alkalinization: 5 mg/kg/dose PO bid–tid. Hydrocephalus: Initial: 20 mg/kg/day PO/IV div q8h, titrate to 100 mg/kg/day. Max: 2 g/day.	R.

Diuretics—Loop

Name	Oral or topical forms	Dosage	Comments
Bumetanide (Bumex)	Tab: 0.5, 1, 2 mg	PO/IV/IM: >6 mo: 0.015–0.1 mg/kg/dose qd–qod. Max: 10 mg/day.	R. Contraindicated in anuria and hepatic coma. May cause hypokalemia, alkalosis, hyperuricemia, and hypercalciuria.
Furosemide (Lasix)	Sol: 10 mg/mL, 40 mg/5 mL Tab: 20, 40, 80 mg	Neonates: See Neonatal Drug Recommendations. PO: 1–6 mg/kg/day q6–12h. IV/IM: 1–2 mg/kg/dose q6–12h. Max: 6 mg/kg/dose.	

Diuretics—Potassium Sparing

Name	Oral or topical forms	Dosage	Comments
Spironolactone (Aldactone)	Tab: 25, 50, 100 mg Susp: 1, 2, 5, 25 mg/mL	Diuretic: Neonates: See Neonatal Drug Recommendations. Children: 1–3.3 mg/kg/day PO div qd–qid. Max: 200 mg/day. Primary aldosteronism: 125–375 mg/m²/day PO hr div bid–qid. Max: 400 mg qd.	R. Contraindicated in acute renal failure. May cause hyperkalemia.

Diuretics—Thiazides

Name	Oral or topical forms	Dosage	Comments
Chlorothiazide (Diuril)	Susp: 250 mg/5 mL Tab: 250, 500 mg	<6 mo: PO: 20–40 mg/kg/day div bid. Max: 375 mg/day IV: 2–8 mg/kg/day div bid. >6 mo: PO: 20 mg/kg/day div bid. Max: 1 g/day. IV: 4 mg/kg/day div qd–bid. Max: 500 mg/day.	R. May cause hypercalcemia, alkalosis, hypokalemia, hypomagnesemia.
Hydrochlorothiazide (HCTZ)	Cap: 12.5 mg Sol: 50 mg/5 mL Tab: 25, 50, 100 mg	<6 mo: 2–4 mg/kg/day div bid PO. Max: 37.5 mg/day. >6 mo: 2 mg/kg/day div bid PO. Max: 100 mg/day.	R. May cause hypercalcemia, alkalosis, hypokalemia, hypomagnesemia.
Metolazone (Zaroxolyn)	Tab: 2.5, 5, 10 mg Susp: 1 mg/mL	0.2–0.4 mg/kg/day PO div qd–bid.	Contraindicated in patients with anuria or hepatic coma. May cause electrolyte imbalances, hyperglycemia, marrow suppression.

Thrombolytics

Name	Oral or topical forms	Dosage	Comments
Alteplase (t-PA)		For use in occluded IV catheters: <10 kg: 0.5 mg to each lumen, >10 kg: 1–2 mg to each lumen. Instill into catheter over 1–2 mins and leave in place for 2–4 h before blood withdrawal. May be repeated qd.	Do not infuse into patient.

Volume Expanders

Name	Oral or topical forms	Dosage	Comments
Albumin		0.5–1 g/kg/dose IV over 30–120 mins. Max: 6 g/kg/day.	Contraindicated in CHF or severe anemia. Use 5% albumin in patients with hypovolemia or intravascular volume depletion. Use 25% albumin in fluid or sodium restriction.

Miscellaneous

Name	Oral or topical forms	Dosage	Comments
Alprostadil (PGE1)		0.05–1 µg/kg/min	Apnea, pyrexia, hypotension may occur.

DERMATOLOGY

Acne Preparations

Name	Oral or topical forms	Dosage	Comments
Adapalene (Differin)	Cream, Gel, Sol: 0.1%	Apply to affected area qhs.	
Benzoyl peroxide (Clearasil)	Gel, wash, cream, lotion: 2.5%, 5%, 10%	Apply to affected area qd–bid.	
Clindamycin (Cleocin T)	Gel, Lot, Sol: 1%, 2%	>12 yo: Apply to area bid.	

Erythromycin	Oint, Gel, Sol: 2%	Apply to affected area bid.	
Isotretinoin (Accutane)	Cap: 10, 20, 40 mg	0.5–2 mg/kg/day PO div bid for 15–20 wks.	Known teratogen, contraindicated in pregnancy. May cause hyperlipidemia, pseudotumor cerebri, elevated transaminases.
Tretinoin (Retin-A)	Cream: 0.025%, 0.05%, 0.1% Gel: 0.01%, 0.025%, 0.1% Liquid: 0.05%	Apply to affected area qhs.	Avoid excessive sun exposure while using this medication.

Antibacterials—Topical

Name	Oral or topical forms	Dosage	Comments
Bacitracin	Oint: 500 U/g	Apply small amount qd–tid.	
Mupirocin (Bactroban)	Cream, oint: 2%	Apply bid–tid.	Avoid contact with eyes.
Neosporin Ointment (bacitracin + neomycin + polymyxin)	Oint: 400 U/3.5 mg/5000 U/g	Apply to affected area qd–tid.	
Polysporin (bacitracin + polymyxin)	Oint: 500 U/10,000 U/g	Apply to affected area qd–tid.	
Silver sulfadiazine (Silvadene)	Cream: 1%	Apply qd–bid to thickness of 1/16th in.	Contraindicated in infants <2 mo. May cause bone marrow suppression and interstitial nephritis.

Antipsoriatics

Name	Oral or topical forms	Dosage	Comments
Tazarotene (Tazorac)	Gel: 0.05%, 0.1%	Apply to affected area qpm.	

Antivirals—Topical

Name	Oral or topical forms	Dosage	Comments
Imiquimod (Aldara)	Cream: 5%	Apply 3×/wk. Leave on skin 6–10h then wash off.	
Podofilox (Condylox)	Sol: 0.5% Gel: 0.5%	Apply to intact lesions, leave on for 30 min the first time then 1–4 h. Remove with soap and water.	

Corticosteroid/Antimicrobial Combinations

Name	Oral or topical forms	Dosage	Comments
Cortisporin (neomycin/poly-myxin/hydrocortisone)	Cream: 3.5 mg/10,000 U/5 mg/g Oint: 5 mg/5000 U/10 mg/g (oint also has 400 U of bacitracin)	Apply thin layer to affected area bid–qid.	

Dermatology—Miscellaneous

Name	Oral or topical forms	Dosage	Comments
Calamine	Lotion: 8%	Apply a thin layer to affected area 1–4 × day.	
EMLA (lidocaine + prilocaine)	Cream: 2.5%/2.5%	Total max dose: <5 kg: 1 g (10 cm²), 5–10 kg: 2 g (20 cm²), 10–20 kg: 10 g (100 cm²), >20 kg: 20 g (200 cm²).	Do not use on mucous membranes or eyes.
Pimecrolimus (Elidel)	Cream: 1%	Apply a thin layer to affected areas bid.	May use on face. Do not place over areas of infected skin.
Selenium sulfate (Selsun)	Lotion, shampoo: 1%, 2.5%	Dandruff: Massage 5–10 mL into wet scalp, leave on 5–10 mins then rinse off. *Tinea versicolor*: 2.5% lotion in a thin layer covering body from face to knees, leave on 30 mins then rinse. Apply daily for 7 days then q mo for 3 mo.	
Tacrolimus (Protopic)	Oint: 0.03%, 0.1%	>2 yo: Apply 0.03% oint to affected areas bid. Continue for 1 wk after resolution of symptoms.	

ENDOCRINE

Androgens

Name	Oral or topical forms	Dosage	Comments
Testosterone		IM (cipionate or enanthate ester): Initiation of pubertal growth: 40–50 mg/m²/dose monthly until the growth rate falls to prepubertal levels. Terminal growth phase: 100 mg/m²/dose monthly until growth ceases. Maint virilizing dose: 100 mg/m²/dose twice monthly. Delayed puberty: 40–50 mg/m²/dose monthly for 6 mo.	Contraindicated in severe renal, cardiac, or hepatic disease.

Bisphosphonates

Name	Oral or topical forms	Dosage	Comments
Pamidronate (Aredia)		Hypercalcemia: Mild: 0.5–1 mg/kg/dose IV × 1, may repeat in 7 days. Severe: 1.5–2 mg/kg/dose, may repeat in 7 days.	R. Maintain adequate hydration and urinary output during treatment.

Corticosteroids

Corticosteroid	Dose equivalent (mg)	Relative antiinflammatory potency	Relative mineralocorticoid potency	Biologic half-life (h)
Betamethasone	0.6–0.75	20–30	0	36–54

Name				
Cortisone	25	0.8	2	8–12
Dexamethasone	0.75	20–30	0	35–54
Hydrocortisone	20	1	2	8–12
Methylprednisolone	4	5	0	18–36
Prednisolone	5	4	1	18–36
Prednisone	5	4	1	18–36
Triamcinolone	4	5	0	18–36

Name	Oral or topical forms	Dosage	Comments
Dexamethasone (Decadron)	Tabs: 0.25, 0.5, 0.75, 1, 1.5, 2, 4, 6 mg Elixir: 0.5 mg/5 mL Oral Sol: 1 mg/mL	Physiologic replacement: 0.03–0.15 mg/kg/day div q6–12h IV/IM/PO. Cerebral edema: Loading dose: 1–2 mg/kg/dose IV/IM × 1 then maint: 1–1.5 mg/kg/day div q4–6h. Max: 16 mg/day. Airway edema: 0.5–2 mg/kg/day IV/IM/PO div q6h. Croup: 0.6 mg/kg/dose PO/IV/IM × 1. Antiemetic: Initial: 10 mg/m^2/dose IV with max: 20 mg then 5 mg/m^2/dose q6h IV. Antiinflammatory: 0.08–0.3 mg/kg/day PO/IV/IM div q6–12h. Spinal cord compression: 2 mg/kg/day IV div q6h.	Contraindicated in active, untreated infections. May cause hyperglycemia, mood changes, osteopenia. Taper if given for more than 7 days.

Name	Oral or topical forms	Dosage	Comments
Fludrocortisone (Florinef)	Tab: 0.1 mg	0.05–0.2 mg qd PO.	Contraindicated in CHF and fungal infections.
Hydrocortisone (Cortef)	Tab: 5, 10, 20 mg Susp: 10 mg/5 mL	Acute adrenal insufficiency: 1–2 mg/kg/dose IV bolus then 25–250 mg/day IM/IV div q6–8h. Congenital adrenal hyperplasia: Initial: 10–20 mg/m²/day PO div tid. Maint: 2.5–10 mg/day PO div tid. Physiologic replacement: PO: 0.5–0.75 mg/kg/day div q8h. IM: 0.25–0.35 mg/kg/day qd. Status asthmaticus: 8 mg/kg/day IV div q6h. Antiinflammatory/immunosuppressive: PO: 2.5–10 mg/kg/24h div q6–8h, IM/IV: 1–5 mg/kg/24h div q12–24h.	Contraindicated in active, untreated infections. May cause hyperglycemia, mood changes, osteopenia. Taper if given for more than 7 days.
Methylprednisolone (Solu-Medrol, Medrol)	Tab: 2, 4, 8, 16, 24, 32 mg	Antiinflammatory/immunosuppressive: 0.5–1.7 mg/kg/day PO/IV/IM div q6–12h. Status asthmaticus: 2 mg/kg/day IM/IV div q6h. Acute spinal cord injury: 30 mg/kg IV over 15 min followed in 45 min by a continuous infusion of 5.4 mg/kg/hr × 23h.	Contraindicated in active, untreated infections. May cause hyperglycemia, mood changes, osteopenia. Taper if given for more than 7 days.
Prednisolone (Pediapred, Prelone, Orapred)	Tab: 5 mg Syrup: 5, 15 mg/5 mL	Antiinflammatory/immunosuppressive: 0.5–2 mg/kg/day PO div qd-bid. Acute asthma: 2 mg/kg/day PO div qd-bid with max of 80 mg/day. Nephrotic syndrome: Start at 2 mg/kg/day PO div qd-bid with max of 80 mg/day.	Contraindicated in active, untreated infections. May cause hyperglycemia, mood changes, osteopenia. Taper if given for more than 7 days.

Prednisone	Tab: 1, 2.5, 5, 10, 20, 50 mg Syrup: 1, 5 mg/mL	Antiinflammatory/immunosuppressive: 0.5–2 mg/kg/day PO div qd-bid. Acute asthma: 2 mg/kg/day PO div qd-bid with max of 80 mg/day. Nephrotic syndrome: Start at 2 mg/kg/day PO div qd-tid. Max: 80 mg/day.	Contraindicated in active, untreated infections. May cause hyperglycemia, mood changes, osteopenia. Taper if given for more than 7 days.

DIABETES-RELATED AGENTS

Name	Oral or topical forms	Dosage	Comments
Diazoxide (Proglycem)	Cap: 50 mg Susp: 50 mg/mL	Hyperinsulinemic hypoglycemia: Infants: 8–15 mg/kg/day PO div q8–12h. Children: 3–8 mg/kg/day PO div q8–12h.	May cause hyponatremia, ketoacidosis, hyperuricemia, arrhythmias.
Glucagon (Glucagon)		<20 kg: 0.5 mg/dose IM q20min prn, >20 kg: 1 mg/dose IM q20min prn.	
Metformin (Glucophage)	Tab: 500, 850, 1000 mg Tab, ER: 500 mg	10–16 yo: Initial dose of 500 mg bid PO, increase qwk to max of 2000 mg/day. >17 yo: Same dosing except max is 2500 mg/day.	R. Contraindicated in renal impairment, CHF, metabolic acidosis. Fatal lactic acidosis can occur.

See Chap. 12, Endocrinology, for insulins.

Thyroid Agents

Name	Oral or topical forms	Dosage	Comments
Levothyroxine (Synthroid)	Tab: 25, 50, 75, 88, 100, 112, 125, 137, 150, 175, 200, 300 µg Susp: 25 µg/mL	PO: 0–6 mo: 8–10 µg/kg/dose qd. 6–12 mo: 6–8 µg/kg/dose qd. 1–5 yr: 5–6 µg/kg/dose qd. 6–12 yo: 4–5 µg/kg/dose qd. >12 yo: 2–3 µg/kg/dose qd. IM/IV dose is 50–75% of PO dose.	Contraindicated in acute MI, thyrotoxicosis, uncorrected adrenal insufficiency.
Methimazole (Tapazole)	Tab: 5, 10 mg	Initial: 0.4–0.7 mg/kg/day PO div q8h then maint: 1/3–2/3 of initial dose div q8h. Max: 30 mg/day.	
Propylthiouracil (PTU)	Tab: 50 mg Susp: 5 mg/mL	Neonates: See Neonatal Drug Recommendations. Initial: 5–7 mg/kg/day PO div q8h then maint after 2 mo: 1/3–2/3 of initial dose. Max: 300 mg/day.	R.

Vitamins

Name	Oral or topical forms	Dosage	Comments
Calcitriol (vitamin D, Rocaltrol)	Cap: 0.25, 0.5 µg Sol: 1 µg/mL	Renal failure: PO: 0.01–0.05 µg/kg/day qd. Titrate in 0.005–0.01 µg/kg/day in 1–2 month increments. Max: 0.5 µg/day. IV: 0.01–0.05 µg/kg/kg/dose 3×/wk. Hypoparathyroidism: <1 yo: 0.04–0.08 µg/kg qd PO. 1–5 yr: 0.25–0.75 µg/kg qd PO. >6 yr: 0.5–2 µg qd PO. Vitamin D–dependent rickets: 1 µg qd PO. Vitamin D–resistant rickets: Initial 0.015–0.02 µg/kg PO qd. Maint: 0.03–0.06 µg/kg/day qd. Max: 2 µg qd.	
Dihydrotachysterol (vitamin D)	Sol: 0.2 mg/mL Cap: 0.125 mg Tab: 0.125, 0.2, 0.4 mg	Hypoparathyroidism: infants/young children: initial 1–5 mg/day PO ×4 days then 0.5–1.5 mg/day PO. Older children: initial: 0.75–2.5 mg/day PO × 4 days then 0.2–1.5 mg/day PO. Nutritional rickets: 0.5 mg × 1 PO or 13–50 µg/day PO qd until healing. Renal osteodystrophy: 0.1–0.5 mg/day PO.	Use caution in patients with renal stones, renal failure, heart disease.
Phytonadione (vitamin K)	Tab: 5 mg Susp: 1 mg/mL	Neonatal hemorrhagic disease: Prophylaxis: 0.5–1 mg IM × 1, Treatment: 1–2 mg/day IM/IV/SC. Vitamin K deficiency: PO: 2.5–5 mg/day IM/IV/SC: 1–2 mg/dose × 1.	Monitor PT/PTT. IV/IM dosing may cause flushing, dizziness, hypotension, cardiac arrest.

Other Endocrine Agents

Name	Oral or topical forms	Dosage	Comments
Desmopressin (DDAVP)	Tab: 0.1, 0.2 mg Nasal sol: 100 µg/mL, 1500 µg/mL Nasal spray: 100 µg/mL	Diabetes insipidus: PO: Start with 0.05 mg/dose qd–bid and titrate to effect. IN: 5–30 µg/day div qd–bid with max 40 µg/day. IV/SC: 2–4 µg/day div bid. Hemophilia A and von Willebrand's disease: IN: <50 kg: 150 µg, >50 kg: 300 µg, IV 0.2–0.4 µg/kg/dose over 15–30 mins. Nocturnal enuresis: PO 0.2 mg qhs titrated to max of 0.6 mg, IN 20 µg qhs to max of 40 µg.	
Vasopressin (Pitressin)		Diabetes insipidus: Titrate dose to effect: SC/IM: 2.5–10 U bid–qid. Continuous infusion: Start at 0.5 milliunits/kg/h, double dose q30mins up to max of 10 milliunits/kg/h. GI hemorrhage: IV: Start at 0.002–0.005 U/kg/min and titrate to max of 0.01 U/kg/min.	Use with caution in vascular disease. Do not abruptly stop infusion.

ENT

Antihistamines—Nonsedating

Name	Oral or topical forms	Dosage	Comments
Fexofenadine (Allegra)	Tab: 30, 60, 180 mg Cap: 60 mg ER with pseudoephedrine: 60 mg/120 mg	6–11 yo: 30 mg PO bid >11 yo: 60 mg PO bid or 180 mg PO qd ER: >11 yo: 1 tab PO bid	R.
Loratadine (Claritin)	Tab: 10 mg RediTab: 10 mg Syrup: 1 mg/mL ER with pseudoephedrine: 12 h: 5 mg/120 mg; 24 h: 10 mg/240 mg	2–5 yo: 5 mg PO qd >5 yo: 10 mg PO qd ER >11 yo: 1 tab PO bid for 12h and 1 tab qd for 24h	R.

Antihistamines—Sedating

Name	Oral or topical forms	Dosage	Comments
Cetirizine (Zyrtec)	Syrup: 5 mg/5 mL Tab: 5, 10 mg ER tab with pseudoephedrine: 5 mg/120 mg	2–5 yo: 2.5 mg PO qd >5 yo: 5–10 mg PO qd ER tab >11 yo: 1 tab bid	R.

Name	Oral or topical forms	Dosage	Comments
Chlorpheniramine (Chlor-Trimeton)	Tab: 4 mg Chewable: 2 mg SR tab: 8, 12 mg Syrup: 2 mg/5 mL	2–6 yo: 1 mg/dose PO q4–6h. Max: 6 mg/day. 6–12 yo: 2 mg/dose PO q4–6h. Max: 12 mg/day. >12 yo: 4 mg/dose q4–6h PO. Max: 24 mg/day. SR, 6–12 yo: 8 mg/dose PO q12h, >12 yo: 8–12 mg PO q12h. IV/SC/IM: 5–20 mg × 1. Max: 40 mg/day.	Use with caution in asthma.
Cyproheptadine (Periactin)	Tab: 4 mg Syrup: 2 mg/5 mL	0.25–0.5 mg/kg/day PO div q8–12h. Max in 2–6 yo: 12 mg/day. Max in 7–14 yo: 16 mg/day. Max in adults: 0.5 mg/kg/day.	Contraindicated in neonates, asthma, glaucoma.
Diphenhydramine (Benadryl)	Elixir, syrup, liquid: 12.5 mg/5 mL Cap/tab: 25, 50 mg Chewable: 12.5 mg	5 mg/kg/day div q6h PO/IV/IM. Max: 300 mg/day. For anaphylaxis: 1–2 mg/kg IV slowly.	R. Contraindicated in neonates, acute asthma, GI or urinary obstruction.
Promethazine (Phenergan)	Tab: 12.5, 25, 50 mg Syrup: 6.25 mg/5 mL Supp: 12.5, 25, 50 mg	>2 yo: 0.1 mg/kg/dose PO q6h and 0.5 mg/kg/dose qhs PO prn.	

Antitussives/Expectorants

Name	Oral or topical forms	Dosage	Comments
Codeine	Sol: 15 mg/5 mL Tab: 15, 30, 60 mg	>2 yo: 1–1.5 mg/kg/day PO in div doses q4–6h prn. Max: 120 mg/day.	R. May cause respiratory depression.

Dextromethorphan (Delsym, Vick's)	Vicks: 10 mg/5 mL Delsym (SR): 30 mg/5 mL	1–3 mo: 0.5–1 mg PO q6–8h. 3–6 mo: 1–2 mg PO q6–8h. 7 mo–1 yo: 2–4 mg PO q6–8h. 2–6 yo: 2.5–7.5 mg PO q4–8h, SR: 15 mg/dose PO bid. 7–12 yo: 5–10 mg PO q4h or 15 mg PO q6–8hr, SR: 30 mg/dose PO bid. >12 yo: 10–30 mg PO q4–8h, SR: 60 mg/dose PO bid.
Guaifenesin (Hytuss, Robitussin)	Tab: 100, 200 mg Syrup: 100 mg/5 mL	<2 yo: 12 mg/kg/day PO div q4h. 2–5 yo: 50–100 mg PO q4h. Max: 600 mg/day. 6–11 yo: 100–200 mg PO q4h. Max: 1.2 g/day. >11 yo: 200–400 mg PO q4h. Max: 2.4 g/day.

Decongestants

Name	Oral or topical forms	Dosage	Comments
Pseudoephedrine (Sudafed, Pediacare, Triaminic, etc.)	Tab: 30, 60 mg Syrup: 15, 30 mg/5 mL Tab ER: 120 mg Chewable: 15 mg	<2 yo: 4 mg/kg/day PO div q6h. 2–5 yo: 15 mg PO q6h. Max: 60 mg/day. 6–12 yo: 30 mg PO q6h. Max: 120 mg/day. >12 yo: 60 mg PO q6h. Max: 240 mg/day or ER: 120 mg PO q12h.	R. Contraindicated in severe HTN.

Ear Preparations

Name	Oral or topical forms	Dosage	Comments
Auralgan (benzocaine/antipyrine)	Sol: 1.4%/5.4%	Fill ear canal, place cotton in external ear. May repeat q1–2h prn.	
Carbamide peroxide (Debrox)	Sol: 6.5%	1–5 drops bid for up to 4 days.	
Cipro HC otic (ciprofloxacin/hydrocortisone)	Susp: 0.2%/1%	>1 yo: Instill 3 drops into the affected ear(s) bid for 7 days.	Do not use if tympanic membrane perforated.
Cortisporin Otic (hydrocortisone/polymyxin/neomycin)	Sol and Susp: 10 mg/10,000 units/5 mg/mL	3 drops into affected ear tid–qid.	

Mouth Preparations

Name	Oral or topical forms	Dosage	Comments
Chlorhexidine gluconate (Peridex)	0.12%	Immunocompetent: 15 mL bid Immunocompromised: 10–15 mL bid–tid	

Nasal Preparations

Name	Oral or topical forms	Dosage	Comments
Budesonide (Rhinocort)	Nasal aerosol or spray: 32 µg/actuation	>6 yo: Initial: 2 sprays each nostril qam and qhs then reduce gradually to lowest effective dose	
Fluticasone (Flonase)	Nasal spray: 50 µg/actuation	>4 yo: 1 spray per nostril qd Can increase to 2 sprays per nostril qd when symptomatic	
Oxymetazoline (Afrin)	Nasal drops: 0.025%, 0.05% Nasal spray: 0.05%	2–5 yo: 2–3 drops of 0.025% solution in each nostril bid >5 yo: 2–3 sprays or 2–3 drops of 0.05% solution in each nostril bid	Do not exceed 3 days of therapy because rebound nasal congestion may occur.
Phenylephrine (Neo-Synephrine)	Nasal drops: 0.125%, 0.16%, 0.25%, 0.5% Nasal spray: 0.25%, 0.5%, 1%	>6 mo: 1–2 drops of 0.16% solution q3h prn <6 yo: 2–3 drops of 0.125% solution q4h prn 6–12 yo: 2–3 drops or 1–2 sprays of 0.25% solution q4h prn >12 yo: 2–3 drops or 1–2 sprays of 0.25% or 0.5 % solution q4h prn	Do not exceed 3 days of therapy because rebound nasal congestion may occur.

GASTROENTEROLOGY

Antidiarrheals

Name	Oral or topical forms	Dosage	Comments
Lomotil (diphenoxylate and atropine)	Sol: 2.5 mg/0.025 mg/5 mL Tab: 2.5 mg/0.025 mg	0.3–0.4 mg/kg/day div qid. Max: 20 mg.	Reduce dose once symptoms are controlled.
Loperamide (Imodium)	Cap/tab: 2 mg Liquid: 1 mg/5 mL	Initial doses: 2–6 yo: 1 mg PO tid 6–8 yo: 2 mg PO bid 8–12 yo: 2 mg PO tid >12 yo: 4 mg PO ×1 Then 0.1 mg/kg/dose PO after each loose stool with max single dose of 2 mg.	Contraindicated in acute diarrhea.

Antiemetics
See Pain Service Medication Dosing Guide, Prn Nausea/Vomiting and Pruritus.

Antacids

Name	Oral or topical forms	Dosage	Comments
Maalox (aluminum and magnesium hydroxide)	Susp: 225 mg/200 mg/5 mL Tab: 225 mg/200 mg	Infants: 1–2 mL/kg/dose PO 1–3h after meals and qhs Children: 5–15 mL/dose PO q3–6h	

		Infants: 1–2 mL/kg/dose PO 1–3h after meals and qhs
Mylanta (aluminum and magnesium hydroxide plus simethicone)	Susp: 200 mg/200 mg/20 mg/5 mL Tab: 200 mg/200 mg/20 mg	Children: 5–15 mL/dose PO q3–6h

Antiulcer—H2 blockers

Name	Oral or topical forms	Dosage	Comments
Famotidine (Pepcid)	Liquid: 40 mg/5 mL Tab: 10, 20, 40 mg Gel cap: 10 mg Disintegrating oral tab: 20, 40 mg Chewable: 10 mg	Neonates: See Neonatal Drug Recommendations. Children: IV/PO: 0.5–1 mg/kg/day bid. Max: 80 mg/day.	R.
Ranitidine (Zantac)	Tab: 75, 150, 300 mg Effervescent tab: 150 mg Syrup: 15 mg/mL Cap: 150, 300 mg Sol: 5, 10 mg/mL	Neonates: See Neonatal Drug Recommendations. Ulcer: PO, treatment: 2–4 mg/kg/day div q12h. Max: 300 mg/day. Maint: 2–4 mg/kg/day div q12hr. Max: 150 mg/day. IV: 2–4 mg/kg/day div q6–8h. Max: 150 mg/day. Gastroesophageal reflux disease/erosive esophagitis: PO: 5–10 mg/kg/day div q12hr. Max: 300 mg/day. IV: 2–4 mg/kg/day div q6–8h. Max: 150 mg/day.	R.

Antiulcer—Proton Pump Inhibitors

Name	Oral or topical forms	Dosage	Comments
Lansoprazole (Prevacid)	Cap: 15, 30 mg Susp: 3 mg/mL	<10 kg: 7.5 mg PO qd. 10–20 kg: 15 mg PO qd. >20 kg: 15–30 mg PO qd.	
Omeprazole (Prilosec)	Cap: 10, 20, 40 mg Susp: 2 mg/mL	Start with 0.6–0.7 mg/kg/dose PO qd, increase to 0.6–0.7 mg/kg/dose PO bid.	

Laxatives

Name	Oral or topical forms	Dosage	Comments
Bisacodyl (Correctol, Dulcolax)	Tab: 5 mg Supp: 5, 10 mg Enema: 10 mg/30 mL	PO: 0.3 mg/kg/day. Max: 15 mg/day. PR: <2 yo: 5 mg qd. 2–11 yo: 5–10 mg qd. >11 yo: 10 mg qd.	
Docusate sodium (Colace)	Cap: 50, 100, 240, 250 mg Tab: 100 mg Syrup: 16.7, 20 mg/5 mL Liquid: 10 mg/mL	5 mg/kg/day PO div qd-qid. Max: 400 mg/day.	

Drug	Formulations	Dosing	Comments
Glycerin	Rectal sol: 4 mL/application Supp: 10, 12, 25 mg	Neonate: See Neonatal Drug Recommendations. <6 yo: 1 infant suppository or 2.5 mL rectal solution. >6 yo: 1 adult suppository or 5–15 mL rectal solution.	
Lactulose (Cephulac)	Syrup: 10 g/15 mL	Constipation: 7.5 mL/day PO. May increase to a max of 60 mL/day. Hepatic encephalopathy: Infants: 2.5–10 mL/day PO div tid–qid. Children: 40–90 mL/day PO div tid–qid	Contraindicated in galactosemia.
Mineral oil	Rectal liquid: 133 mL Emulsion: 2.5, 2.75, 4.75 mL/5 mL Liquid: various sizes	5–11 yo: PO: 5–15 mL/day div qd–tid. >11 yo: 15–45 mL/day div qd–tid. Rectal: 5–11 yo: 30–60 mL × 1. >11 yo: 60–150 mL × 1.	Use as a laxative should not exceed 1 wk. May cause lipid pneumonitis if aspirated.
Polyethylene glycol (GoLYTELY, Miralax)	Powder for oral solution	Bowel cleansing (GoLYTELY): 25–40 mL/kg/hr PO until rectal effluent is tan. Constipation (Miralax): 8.5–17 g PO qd.	Bowel cleansing contraindicated in toxic megacolon, gastric retention, colitis, bowel perforation. Use with caution in patients with altered mental status or impaired gag.
Senna (Senokot)	Granules: 326 mg/5 mL Rectal: 652 mg Syrup: 218 mg/5 mL Tab: 187, 217, 374, 600 mg Liquid: 33.3 mg/mL	PO: 10–20 mg/kg/dose PO qhs with max by age: 1 mo–1 yr: 218 mg/day; 1–5 yr: 436 mg/day; 5–15 yr: 872 mg/day. Rectal: >27 kg: 326 mg PR qhs.	

Name	Oral or topical forms	Dosage	Comments
Sodium phosphate (Fleet enema)	Enema: 6 g Na phosphate and 16 g Na biphosphate/100 mL Pediatric size: 67.5 mL Adult: 133 mL	2–12 yr: 67.5 mL PR × 1. >12 yo: 133 mL PR × 1.	R. Contraindicated in patients with severe renal failure, megacolon, bowel obstruction, and CHF. May cause hyperphosphatemia, hypernatremia, hypocalcemia, hypotension, dehydration, and acidosis.

Other GI Agents

Name	Oral or topical forms	Dosage	Comments
Mesalamine (Asacol, Rowasa, Pentasa)	Cap. controlled release (Pentasa): 250 mg Tab, delayed release (Asacol): 400 mg Supp (Rowasa): 500 mg	Cap, controlled release: 50 mg/kg/day div q6–12h PO. Tab, delayed release: 50 mg/kg/day div q8–12h PO. Max: 4 g/day. Supp (adolescents): 500 mg bid PR × 3–6 wks.	R. Do not use in children with flulike symptoms. Contraindicated in active peptic ulcer disease, severe renal failure.
Octreotide (Sandostatin)		IV/SC: 1–10 µg/kg/day div q12–24h. Max: 1500 µg/day.	R.
Sulfasalazine (Azulfidine, Azulfidine EN-tabs, Salazopyrin EN-tabs)	Tab: 500 mg	Ulcerative colitis: >6 yo: Initial dosing: Mod/severe: 50–75 mg/kg/day div q4–6h PO. Max: 6 g/day. Mild: 40–50 mg/kg/day PO div q6h. Maint: 30–50 mg/kg/day PO div q4–8h PO. Max: 2 g/day.	R. Contraindicated in sulfa allergy, porphyria, GI obstruction. May cause orange-yellow discoloration of the skin and mucous membranes.

Ursodiol (Actigall)

Susp: 60 mg/mL
Cap: 300 mg
Tab: 250 mg

10–15 mg/kg PO qd.

Contraindicated in renal stones.

HEMATOLOGY

Anticoagulants

Name	Oral or topical forms	Dosage	Comments
Enoxaparin (Lovenox)		DVT treatment: <2 mo: 1.5 mg/kg/dose q12h SC >2 mo: 1 mg/kg/dose q12h SC. DVT prophylaxis: <2 mo: 0.75 mg/kg/dose q12h SC. >2 mo: 0.5 mg/kg/dose q12h SC.	R.
Heparin (Hepalean)		Anticoagulation: 50–100 U/kg IV bolus then maint: 10–25 U/kg/hr IV. Adjust dose q4h based on aPTT: if <50: give 50 U/kg bolus and increase rate by 10%, if 50–59: increase rate by 10%, if 60–85: keep rate the same, if 86–95: decrease rate by 10%, if 96–120: hold infusion for 30 min then resume with rate decreased by 10%, if >120: hold infusion for 60 min then resume with rate decreased by 15%. Remeasure aPTT 4 h after each change.	Check PTT q4h while adjusting dose and then qd while on steady dose.

Name	Oral or topical forms	Dosage	Comments
Warfarin (Coumadin)	Tab: 1, 2, 2.5, 3, 4, 5, 6, 7.5, 10 mg	Loading dose: baseline INR: 1–1.3: 0.1–0.2 mg/kg/dose PO qd × 2 days. Maint: 10 mg/dose. Maint: 0.05–0.34 mg/kg/day PO qd. Adjust to desired PT or INR.	R. Contraindicated in severe liver or kidney disease, uncontrolled bleeding, GI ulcers, or malignant hypertension. Many drug interactions. Monitor INR 5–7 days after new dosage before any readjustment.

Other Hematology Agents

Name	Oral or topical forms	Dosage	Comments
Erythropoietin (Epogen)		Anemia in cancer or renal failure: SC/IV: Initial dose of 50–100 U/kg/dose 3 × wk. Increase dose if hematocrit does not rise by 5–6% after 8 wks.	Iron supplementation recommended before and during therapy.
Filgrastim (G-CSF, Neupogen)		IV/SC: 5–10 µg/kg/dose qd × 14 days or until ANC >10,000/mm³. May increase dose by 5 µg/kg/day if desired effect not achieved within 7 days.	Use in caution in myeloid malignancies.
Protamine		IV: 1 mg protamine neutralizes 115 U porcine intestinal heparin or 90 U of beef lung heparin or 100 U of low-molecular-weight heparin. Max dose: 50 mg.	

NEUROLOGY

Anticonvulsants

Name	Oral or topical forms	Dosage	Comments
Carbamazepine (Tegretol, Carbatrol)	Tab: 200 mg Chewable: 100 mg Tab (ER): 100, 200, 400 mg Cap (ER): 200, 300 mg Susp: 100 mg/5 mL	<6 yo: 10–20 mg/kg/day PO div bid-tid (qid for suspension). Increase q5–7days up to 35 mg/kg/day div tid-qid PO. 6–12 yo: 100 mg PO bid. Increase 100 mg/day at 1-wk intervals. Max: 1000 mg/day. >12 yo: Initial: 200 mg PO bid, increase 200 mg/day at 1-wk intervals div bid-qid. Max: 1200 mg/day.	R. Should not be taken with clozapine due to increased risk of bone marrow suppression and agranulocytosis. Many drug interactions. Suspension should be divided qid.
Clonazepam (Klonopin)	Tab: 0.5, 1, 2 mg Susp: 100 μg/mL	<10 yo or <30 kg: Initial: 0.01–0.03 mg/kg/day PO div q8h, increase 0.25–0.5 mg/day q3days up to max of 0.1–0.2 mg/kg/day. >10 yo or >30 kg: Initial: 1.5 mg/day PO div tid, increase 0.5–1 mg/day q3days. Max: 20 mg/day.	Contraindicated in severe liver disease and acute narrow-angle glaucoma. Do not discontinue abruptly. Steady state achieved after 5–8 days of therapy with same dose.
Diazepam (Valium, Diastat)	Tab: 2, 5, 10 mg Sol: 1, 5 mg/mL Rectal gel: 2.5, 5, 10, 20 mg	Sedative: See Sedation/Analgesia. Status epilepticus: See algorithm, Chap. 19, Neurology.	May cause hypotension and respiratory depression. Do not use with protease inhibitors.
Fosphenytoin (Cerebyx)		Status epilepticus: See algorithm. Nonemergent loading dose: 10–20 mg PE/kg IV/IM. Initial maintenance dose: 4–6 mg PE/kg/day IV/IM.	R. Overdose may cause slurred speech, dizziness, ataxia, rash, nystagmus, tinnitus, diplopia. Therapeutic levels: 10–20 mg/L.

Name	Oral or topical forms	Dosage	Comments
Gabapentin (Neurontin)	Cap: 100, 300, 400 mg Tab: 600, 800 mg Sol: 250 mg/5 mL	3–12 yo: Day 1: 10–15 mg/kg/day PO div tid. Increase to the following over 3 days: 3–4 yo: 40 mg/kg/day PO div tid. >5 yo: 25–35 mg/kg/day PO div tid. Max: 50 mg/kg/day.	R. Do not withdraw abruptly.
Lorazepam (Ativan)	Tab: 0.5, 1, 2 mg Sol: 2 mg/mL	Status epilepticus: See algorithm, Chap. 19, Neurology. Sedation: See Sedation/Analgesia.	Contraindicated in narrow-angle glaucoma and severe hypotension. May cause respiratory depression.
Phenobarbital (Luminal)	Tab: 15, 30, 32, 60, 65, 100 mg Cap: 16 mg Elixir: 20 mg/5 mL	Status epilepticus: See algorithm, Chap. 19, Neurology. Maint: infants: 5–6 mg/kg/day PO/IV div qd–bid. 1–5 yo: 6–8 mg/kg/day PO/IV div qd–bid. 6–12 yo: 4–6 mg/kg/day PO/IV div qd–bid. >12 yo: 1–3 mg/kg/day PO/IV div qd–bid.	R. Contraindicated in porphyria, severe respiratory disease. May cause respiratory depression or hypotension. Therapeutic levels: 15–40 mg/L.
Phenytoin (Dilantin)	Chewable: 50 mg Prompt cap: 100 mg Cap (ER): 30, 100 mg Susp: 125 mg/5 mL	Status epilepticus: See algorithm, Chap. 19, Neurology. Sz disorder: Start with 5 mg/kg/day PO/IV div q8–12h. Usual dose range: Neonates: 5–8 mg/kg/day. 6 mo–3 yr: 8–10 mg/kg/day. 4–6 yr: 7.5–9 mg/kg/day. 7–9 yr: 7–8 mg/kg/day. > 9 yr: 6–7 mg/kg/day.	R. Contraindicated in patients with heart block or sinus bradycardia. May cause gingival hyperplasia, hirsutism, dermatitis, ataxia, lupuslike syndrome, liver damage. Many drug interactions. Therapeutic levels: 10–20 mg/L.

Valproic acid (Depakene, Depakote)	Cap: 250 mg Syrup: 250 mg/5 mL	Szs: PO: Initial: 10–15 mg/kg/day div qd–tid, increase 5–10 mg/kg/day weekly to a max of 60 mg/kg/day. Maint: 30–60 mg/kg/day div bid–tid. IV: same dose as PO but divided q6h. Migraine prophylaxis: 15–30 mg/kg/day PO div bid. Max: 1000 mg/day.	Contraindicated in hepatic disease. May cause pancreatitis, thrombocytopenia, rash, platelet dysfunction. Many drug interactions. Therapeutic levels: 50–100 mg/L.

Migraine Therapy—5HT1 Receptor Agonists

Name	Oral or topical forms	Dosage	Comments
Sumatriptan (Imitrex)	Tab: 25, 50 mg Susp: 5 mg/mL Nasal spray: 5 mg, 20 mg/ 100 μL Unit use syringe: 6 mg/0.5 mL syringe	PO: 25 mg with onset of headache. May give 25–100 mg more if no relief after 2 hrs up to a max of 200 mg/day. SC: 6 mg × 1 with onset of headache. May give additional dose if no relief up to max of 12 mg/day. Nasal: 5–20 mg/dose with onset of headache. May give up to 40 mg/day if no response in 2 hrs.	R. Contraindicated with ergotamines. Flushing and dizziness may occur.

Other Neurology Agents

Name	Oral or topical forms	Dosage	Comments
Mannitol		Cerebral edema: 0.25 g/kg/dose IV over 20–30 min. May increase to 1 g/kg/dose if needed.	R. Contraindicated in severe renal disease, active intracranial bleed, dehydration, and pulmonary edema.
Meclizine (Antivert)	Tab: 12.5, 25, 50 mg Chewable: 25 mg	>12 yo: 25–100 PO mg/day.	
Pyridostigmine (Mestinon)	Syrup: 60 mg/5 mL Tab: 60 mg Tab (SR): 180 mg	Neonates: See Neonatal Drug Recommendations. Children: PO: 7 mg/kg/day in 5–6 divided doses. Max PO dose: 500 mg. IM/IV: 0.05–0.15 mg/kg/dose q4–6h. Max IM/IV dose: 10 mg/dose.	R. Contraindicated in mechanical intestinal or urinary obstruction.

OPHTHALMOLOGY AGENTS

Antibacterials

Name	Oral or topical forms	Dosage	Comments
Erythromycin (Ilotycin)	Ophtho oint: 0.5%	Apply 0.5-in. ribbon to affected eye bid–qid.	
Neosporin Ointment (neomycin plus bacitracin plus polymyxin B)	Ophtho: Oint: 3.5 mg/400 U/10,000 U/g	Apply small amount to conjunctiva qd–qid.	

| | Ophtho oint: 0.3% | Apply a thin ribbon of ointment to affected eye bid–tid or 1–2 drops of solution to affected eye q4h. |
| Tobramycin (Tobrex) | Ophtho sol: 0.3% | |

Ocular Antiallergy Preparations

Name	Oral or topical forms	Dosage	Comments
Cromolyn sodium (Opticrom)	Ophtho sol: 4%	1–2 drops each eye 4–6×/day	
Olopatadine (Patanol)	Ophtho sol: 0.1%	1–2 drops in affected eyes bid	Do not use while wearing contact lenses.

PSYCHIATRY

Antidepressants (Selective Serotonin Reuptake Inhibitors)

Name	Oral or topical forms	Dosage	Comments
Fluoxetine (Prozac)	Liquid: 20 mg/5 mL Cap: 10, 20, 40 mg Delayed release: 90 mg Tab: 10 mg	Depression: >5 yo: 5–10 mg PO qd. Max of 20 mg/day. Adolescent max: 80 mg/day. Bulimia: 60 mg PO qam.	Divide doses >20 mg/day bid.

Name	Oral or topical forms	Dosage	Comments
Paroxetine (Paxil)	Tab: 10, 20, 30, 40 mg Susp: 10 mg/5 mL	Depression: Start with 10 mg PO qd and adjust upwards as needed q7days after 4 wks of initial therapy to max of 50 mg/day. OCD: Start with 10 mg PO qd and adjust upwards 10 mg/day q2wks to a max of 60 mg/day. Panic disorder: Start with 10 mg PO qd and adjust upwards by 10 mg/day qwk to a max of 60 mg/day. Social/generalized anxiety disorder: 20 mg PO qam.	R.
Sertraline (Zoloft)	Tab: 25, 50, 100 mg Sol: 20 mg/mL	Depression or OCD: 6–12 yo: Start with 25 mg PO qd and increase by 25 mg q3–4days up to a max of 200 mg/day. >12 yo: Start at 50 mg PO qd and increase by 50 mg qwk to max of 200 mg/day.	R.

Antidepressants—Serotonin, Norepinephrine, Reuptake Inhibitors

Name	Oral or topical forms	Dosage	Comments
Amitriptyline (Elavil)	Tab: 10, 25, 50, 75, 100, 150 mg	Depression: Children, PO: Start with 1 mg/kg/day div tid for 3 days then increase to 1.5 mg/kg/day. May increase up to a max of 5 mg/kg/day. Adolescents, PO: Start with 10 mg tid with 20 mg qhs and increase to a max of 200 mg/day. Chronic pain: Start with 0.1 mg/kg/dose PO qhs and increase over 2–3 wks to 0.5–2 mg/kg/dose qhs. Migraine prophylaxis: Adults: 25–50 mg/dose PO qhs	Contraindicated in narrow-angle glaucoma, szs, severe cardiac disorders.
Nortriptyline (Pamelor)	Cap: 10, 25, 50, 75 mg Sol: 10 mg/5 mL	Depression: 6–12 yo: 1–3 mg/kg/day PO div tid–qid. >12 yo: 1–3 mg/kg/day div tid–qid PO. Max of 150 mg/day.	Contraindicated in narrow-angle glaucoma.

Antipsychotics

Name	Oral or topical forms	Dosage	Comments
Haloperidol (Haldol)	Tab: 0.5, 1, 2, 5, 10, 20 mg Sol: 2 mg/mL	3–12 yo: Agitation: 0.01–0.03 mg/kg/day qd PO Psychosis: 0.05–0.15 mg/kg/day div bid–tid PO IM (as lactate): 1–3 mg/dose q4–8hr, max dose 0.15 mg/kg/day >12 yo: Agitation: 2–5 mg/dose IM (as lactate) or 1–15 mg/dose PO, may repeat in 1 hr. Psychosis: 2–5 mg/dose q4–8hr IM prn or 1–15 mg/day div bid–tid	Use with caution in patients with cardiac disease (risk of hypotension) or epilepsy (lowers seizure threshold). IM form comes in immediate and long acting.

Stimulants

Name	Oral or topical forms	Dosage	Comments
Adderall (dextroamphetamine and racemic amphetamine)	Tab: 5, 7.5, 10, 12.5, 15, 20, 30 mg Susp: 1 mg/mL	3–5 yr: 2.5 mg/day PO qam, increase by 2.5 mg/day qwk to a max of 40 mg/day div qd–tid. >5 yr: 5 mg/day PO, increase by 5 mg/day qwk to max of 40 mg/day div qd–tid.	Use with caution in patients with HTN or cardiovascular disease.
Dextroamphetamine (Dexedrine)	Tab: 5, 10 mg Tab (SR): 5, 10, 15 mg	3–5 yr: 2.5 mg/day PO qam, increase by 2.5 mg/day qwk to a max of 40 mg/day div qd–tid. >5 yr: 5 mg/day PO, increase by 5 mg/day qwk to max of 40 mg/day div qd–tid.	Use with caution in patients with HTN or cardiovascular disease.
Methylphenidate (Ritalin)	Tab (Ritalin): 5, 10, 20 mg Tab (ER): 8-hr (Metadate ER): 10, 20 mg, (Ritalin LA): 20, 30, 40 mg, 24-hr (Concerta): 18, 36, 54 mg Cap (ER) (Metadate CD): 20 mg Tab (SR) (Ritalin SR) : 20 mg	>5 yr: Initial 0.3 mg/kg/dose given before breakfast and lunch. Increase by 0.1 mg/kg/dose PO qwk until 0.3–1 mg/kg/day reached. Max dose: 2 mg/kg/day or 60 mg/day. Once daily dosing (Concerta): Start with 18 mg PO qam, increase qwk at 18-mg increments to max of 54 mg/day.	Contraindicated in glaucoma, anxiety disorders, motor tics, Tourette's.
Atomoxetine (Strattera)	Tab: 10, 18, 25, 40, 60 mg	<70 kg: Start with 0.5 mg/kg PO qam × 3 days, then titrate up prn to max of 1.4 mg/kg/day. >70 kg: Start with 40 mg PO qam × 3 days then titrate up prn to max of 100 mg/day.	

PULMONARY AGENTS

Beta Agonist

Name	Oral or topical forms	Dosage	Comments
Albuterol (Ventolin, Proventil, Salbutamol)	MDI: 90 µg/actuation Sol neb: 0.083%, 0.5%	Aerosol (MDI):1–2 puff q4–6h Nebulization: <1 yr: 0.05–0.15 mg/kg/dose q4–6h 1–5yr: 1.25–2.5 mg/dose q4–6h 5–12 yr: 2.5 mg/dose q4–6h >12 yr: 2.5–5 mg/dose q6h	Nebulization may be given more frequently than indicated. Always use with spacer; it enhances efficacy. Side effects: palpitations, tremor, insomnia, nervousness, nausea, and headache.
Levalbuterol (Xopenex)	Neb sol: 0.63, 1.25 mg/3 mL	<6 yr: 0.16–1.25 mg inhaled tid 6–11 yr: 0.31–0.63 mg inhaled tid pm >12 yr: 0.63–1.25 mg inhaled tid	As effective as albuterol with fewer side effects.
Salmeterol (Serevent)	MDI: 21 µg/actuation DPI: 50 µg/inhalation	>4 yo: 21–42 µg bid DPI or 50 µg bid MDI	Should not be used for acute asthma.
Terbutaline (Brethine, Bricanyl)		Continuous infusion: 2–10 µg/kg IV loading dose followed by 0.1–0.4 µcg/kg/min Titrate in increments of 0.1–0.2 µg/kg/min q30min. Max: 10 µg/kg/min	R. Tachycardia, arrhythmias may occur.

Beta Agonist Combinations

Name	Oral or topical forms	Dosage	Comments
Advair Diskus (Fluticasone + salmeterol)	DPI 100/50, 250/50, 500/50 µg/dose	100/50 µg 1 puff bid. May titrate up to effect.	May cause dysphonia, oral thrush. Less effect on suppressing linear growth compared with beclomethasone. Rinse mouth after use.

Inhaled Steroids

Name	Oral or topical forms	Dosage	Comments
Budesonide (Pulmicort Turbuhaler, Pulmicort Respules)	DPI: 200 µg/actuation Respules: 0.25 mg/2 mL, 0.5 mg/2 mL	DPI: 200 µg bid and titrate up to max of 400 µg bid Respules: 250 µg bid and titrate up to a max of 1 mg/day	Rinse mouth after use.
Fluticasone (Flovent, Flovent Rotadisk)	DPI: 50,100, 250 µg/dose MDI: 44, 110, 220 µg/actuation	MDI: 88 µg bid and titrate up to a max of 440 µg bid DPI: 50 µg bid and titrate up to max of 500 µg bid	May cause dysphonia, oral thrush. Less effect on suppressing linear growth compared with beclomethasone.

Leukotriene Inhibitor

Name	Oral or topical forms	Dosage	Comments
Montelukast (Singulair)	Chewable tab: 4, 5 mg Tab: 10 mg	2–5 yo: 4 mg PO qhs 6–14 yo: 5 mg PO qhs >15 yo: 10 mg PO qhs	Contraindicated in PKU. Adjust dose with phenobarbital and rifampin.

Others

Name	Oral or topical forms	Dosage	Comments
Dornase Alfa (Pulmozyme)	Nebulizer sol: 1 mg/mL	>5 yo: 2.5 mg qd–bid	Do not mix with other nebulized drugs.
Epinephrine (Epipen, Epipen Jr)	Epipen: 0.3 mg Epipen Jr: 0.15 mg	<30 kg: 0.15 mg/dose IM ≥30 kg: 0.3 mg/dose IM	To be used only in severe hypersensitivity reactions.
Epinephrine Racemic (Asthma-Nefrin, microNefrin)	Nebulizer sol: 2.25%	Neb: 0.5 mL/dose diluted in 3 mL NS over 15 mins	Rebound airway edema may occur.
Ipratropium Bromide (Atrovent)	Nebulizer sol: 0.02% (500 µg/2.5 mL)	250–500 µg per dose inhaled q6h	More effective in first 24 hr of reactive airway disease management. May combine with albuterol.

VITAMINS

Name	Content per	A (IU)	D (IU)	E (IU)	C (mg)	Folate (mg)	B1 (mg)	B2 (mg)	B3 (mg)	B5 (mg)	B6 (mg)	B12 (mg)	Elemental Fe (mg)	Fluoride (mg)	Others
Poly-Vi-Sol ± iron drops	1 mL	1500	400	5	35	—	0.5	0.6	8	—	0.4	2	±10	—	—
Tri-Vi-Sol drops	1 mL	1500	400	—	35	—	—	—	—	—	—	—	—	—	—
Tri-Vi-Flor drops	1 mL	1500	400	—	35	—	—	—	—	—	—	—	—	0.25	—
ADEKs drops	1 mL	1500	400	40	45	—	0.5	0.6	6	3	0.6	4	—	—	Biotin 15 µg, vitamin K 0.1 mg, zinc 5 mg, beta carotene 1 mg
Vi-Daylin liquid	5 mL	2500	400	15	60	—	1.05	1.2	13.5	—	1.05	4.5	—	—	—

	Dose														
ADEKs tab	1 tab	4000	400	150	60	0.2	1.2	1.3	10	10	1.5	12	—	—	Zinc 1.1 mg, betacarotene 3 mg, vitamin K, biotin 50 µg
Poly-Vi-Flor 1 mg tab	1 tab	2500	400	15	60	0.3	1.05	1.2	13.5	—	1.05	4.5	—	1	—
Poly-Vi-Sol tab	1 tab	2500	400	15	60	0.3	1.05	1.2	13.5	—	1.05	4.5	—	—	—
Vi-Daylin with iron tab	1 tab	2500	400	15	60	0.3	1.05	1.2	13.5	—	1.05	4.5	12	—	—

SUGGESTED READING

Briggs GG, Freeman RK, Yaffe SJ, eds. *Drugs in pregnancy and lactation*, 5th edition. Baltimore: Williams & Wilkins, 1998.

Pickering LK, ed. 2000 *Red book: report of the Committee on Infectious Diseases*, 25th ed. Elk Grove Village, IL: American Academy of Pediatrics, 2000.

Taketomo CK, Hodding JH, Kraus DM, eds. *Pediatric dosage handbook*, 9th ed. Hudson, OH: Lexi-Comp Inc., 2002.

PAIN SERVICE MEDICATION DOSING GUIDE

Patient-Controlled Analgesia

Drug	PCA dose	Lockout time	Continuous infusion rate	PCA and continuous infusion break-through pain or load-ing dose
Morphine	0.015–0.03 mg/kg/dose = 15–30 µg/kg dose	6–10 mins	0.01–0.04 mg/kg/hr = 10–40 µg/kg/hr	0.05 mg/kg
Fentanyl (Sublimaze)	0.1–0.4 µg/kg/dose	6–8 mins	0.5–1 µg/kg/hr	0.5–1 mg/kg
Hydromorphone (Dilaudid)	0.003–0.006 mg/kg/dose = 3–6 µg/kg/dose	6–10 mins	0.004–0.008 mg/kg/hr = 4–8 µg/kg/hr	0.01 mg/kg
Nalbuphine (Nubain) per anesthesia only	0.02–0.04 µg/kg	6–10 mins	10–40 µg/kg/hr	0.05 mg/kg
Meperidine[a] (Demerol)	0.2–0.3 mg/kg/dose	6–10 mins	None	0.5 mg/kg

[a]Not recommended for prolonged use.

Prn Analgesics: Oral, IV, Suppositories

Drug	Route	Dose	Frequency
Acetaminophen (Tylenol)	PO or PR	10–15 mg/kg (not >5 doses in 24 hrs)	q4–6h prn

Ibuprofen (Motrin, Advil)	PO	6–10 mg/kg (800 mg max dose)	q6–8h prn
Tylenol with codeine	PO (12 mg codeine and 120 mg acetaminophen in 5 cc)	Codeine 0.5–1 mg/kg	q4–6h prn
Oxycodone	Oral	0.05–0.15 mg/kg	q2–4h
Percocet (oxycodone with acetaminophen)	Oral (1 Tab = 5 mg oxycodone and 325 mg acetaminophen)	1–2 tabs (oxycodone 0.05–0.15 mg/kg)	q4–6h prn
Ketorolac (Toradol)	IV	IV loading dose = 0.5 mg/kg; subsequent doses 0.5 mg/kg max 30 mg for IV	q6h around the clock or prn for up to max 5 days
Morphine (MSIR)	Oral intermediate release	0.2–0.6 mg/kg	q2–4h prn
Morphine (MS Contin)	Oral SR	0.2–0.6 mg/kg	q8–12h around the clock
Morphine	Suppository	0.2–0.5 mg/kg	q4–6h prn
Morphine	IV	0.05–0.1 mg/kg	q2–4h prn
Hydromorphone (Dilaudid)	PO	0.03–0.06 mg/kg	q2–4h prn
Hydromorphone (Dilaudid)	IV	0.01–0.02 mg/kg	q2–4h prn
Meperidine (Demerol)	IV	0.5–1 mg/kg[a]	q2–4h prn
Meperidine (Demerol)	PO	1 mg/kg[a]	q2–4h prn
Oxycontin	PO	0.15–0.5 mg/kg	q12h prn
Methadone	IV	0.05–0.1 mg/kg	q6–12h
Methadone	PO	0.07–0.15 mg/kg	q8–12h

[a]Not recommended for prolonged use.

Antagonists (Always Use ABCs of Resuscitation First in Overdosed Patients)

Drug	Route	Dose	Frequency
Naloxone (Narcan): reverses opioids	IV or IM	1–2 µg/kg (for oversedation) = 0.001–0.002 mg/kg	q2–5mins.
	IV or IM	For life-threatening overdose 10–20 µg/kg = (0.01–0.02 mg/kg)	q2–3mins.
Flumazenil (Romazicon): reverses benzodiazepanes	IV	3–5 µg/kg titrate to 10–15 µg/kg total or 1 mg max dose	Avoid in patients with confirmed history of szs.

Prn Nausea/Vomiting and Pruritus

Drug	Route	Dose	Frequency
Diphenhydramine (Benadryl)	PO	0.5–1 mg/kg (max dose 50 mg) (pruritus: use with caution with opioids)	q4–6h prn
Diphenhydramine (Benadryl)	IV	0.5 mg/kg (max dose 25 mg) (pruritus: use with caution with opioids)	q4–6h prn
Hydroxyzine (Atarax/Vistaril)	PO or IM (not IV)	0.5 mg/kg (max dose 50 mg) (N/V)	q4–6h prn
Nubain	IV	25–50 µg/kg	q1–2h prn
Naloxone (Narcan)	Continuous infusion	1–5 µg/kg/hr (itching); max concentration 8 µg/mL	—

Metoclopramide (Reglan)	PO or IV	0.15–0.2 mg/kg (max dose 10 mg) (N/V)	q6h prn
Trimethobenzamide (Tigan)	Suppository	5–15 kg (50 mg), 15–40 kg (100 mg), >40 kg (200 mg) (N/V)	q8h prn
Ondansetron (Zofran)	IV	0.05–0.15 mg/kg (8 mg max)	q6h prn
Ondansetron	PO	<10 kg = 2 mg; 10–40 kg = 4 mg; >40 kg = 8 mg	q6h prn
Promethazine (Phenergan)	IM/IV	0.5 mg/kg	q6h prn
Promethazine (Phenergan)	PO/PR	0.5–1 mg/kg	q6h prn

N/V, nausea and vomiting.
From St. Louis Children's Hospital, St. Louis, Missouri, with permission.

SEDATION AGENTS

Drug	Clinical effects	Dose	Time of onset/ duration (mins)	Side effects
Sedatives				
Chloral hydrate	Sedation, motion control	20–100 mg/kg PO/PR; may repeat after 30 mins (max dose: 100 mg/kg or 2 g)	15–30/60–120	Respiratory depression, paradoxical excitement. Do not use in liver or renal failure. Best used in children <5 yrs old.
Midazolam	Sedation, motion control	PO: 0.5–0.75 mg/kg, max, 20 mg	10–30/60–90	Respiratory depression, hypotension, bradycardia.
		IN: 0.2–0.5 mg/kg, max, 7.5 mg	5–10/60–120	
		PR: 0.25–0.5 mg/kg, max, 20 mg	10/60–120	
		IM: 0.1–0.15 mg/kg, max, 10 mg	2–3/45–60	
		IV	1–3/60–120	
		<5 yrs: 0.05–0.1 mg/kg over 2–3 mins (max, 0.6 mg/kg)	—	
		6–12 yrs: 0.025–0.05 mg/kg (max, 0.4 mg/kg)	—	
Pentobarbital	Sedation, motion control	PO	15–60/60–240	Respiratory depression, hypotension.
		<4 yrs: 3–6 mg/kg (max, 100 mg)		
		>4 yrs: 1.5–3 mg/kg (max, 100 mg)		

		IV: 1–6 mg/kg, increase 1 mg/kg to desired effect, max, 6 mg/kg or 150–200 mg	3–5/60–240	Do not use in liver failure or if <6 mos old.
Analgesic				
Fentanyl (Sublimaze)	Analgesia	IV: 1 µg/kg/dose; may repeat q3mins, max, 2–3 µg/kg	2–3/30–60	Respiratory depression, stiff chest.
Ketamine	Analgesia, motion control, dissociative amnesia	IV: 1–1.5 mg/kg slowly; may repeat half dose q10mins IM: 2–3 mg/kg × 1 dose	1/dissociation 15, recovery 60	Increased ICP, nightmares, HTN, respiratory depression. Recommended for asthmatics.
Nitrous oxide	Anxiolysis, analgesia, amnesia Requires patient cooperation >4 yrs old	Preset mixture with 40% O_2	<5/<5 once off	Emesis, hypoxia.
Antagonists				
Naloxone	Opioid reversal (morphine, fentanyl)	IV/IM: 0.1 mg/kg/dose to max 2 mg/dose; may repeat q2mins	IV: 2/IM: 10–15	—
Flumazenil	Benzodiazepine reversal	IV: 0.02 mg/kg/dose, may repeat q1min to max 1 mg	1–2/30–60	Seizures.

NEONATAL DRUG RECOMMENDATIONS

Antibacterials/Antifungals/Antivirals

Drug	Dose	Interval	Mode
Acyclovir	20 mg/kg/dose	q8h	IV
Amikacin	See table below	See table below	IV/IM

Postconceptional age (wks)	Postnatal age (days)	Dose (mg/kg/dose)	Interval (h)
≤29	0–28	7.5	q24
	>28	10	q24
30–36	0–14	10	q24
	>14	7.5	q12
>36	0–7	7.5	q12
	>7	7.5	q8

Drug	Dose	Interval	Mode
Amphotericin B (no test dose required in neonates)			
Positive culture	1 mg/kg/dose	q24h	IV

Negative culture	0.5 mg/kg/dose	q24h	IV
Amphotericin B lipid complex (Abelcet) (infuse over 2 h)	5 mg/kg/dose	q24h	IV
Ampicillin	100 mg/kg/dose	q12h	IV
Aztreonam	30 mg/kg/dose	See table below	IV/IM

Weight (kg)	Age (days)	Interval (h)
<1.2	0–28	q12
1.2–2	0–7	q12
	>7	q8
>2	0–7	q8
	>7	q6

Drug	Dose	Interval	Mode
Cefazolin (Ancef)	25 mg/kg/dose	q12h	IV

Drug	Dose	Interval	Mode
Cefotaxime (reserve for suspected or confirmed CNS infection)	50 mg/kg/dose	See table below	IV

Weight (kg)	Postnatal age <7 days	Postnatal age >7 days
<2	q12h	q8h
>2	q8h	q6h

Drug	Dose	Interval	Mode
Cefuroxime	10–30 mg/kg/dose	q12h	IV/IM
Clindamycin	5–7.5 mg/kg/dose	See table below	IV

Postmenstrual age (wks)	Postnatal age (days)	Interval (h)
<29	0–28	q12
	>28	q8
30–36	0–14	q12
	>14	q8

Drug	Dose	Interval	Mode
Fluconazole	See table below	See table below	IV/PO

Postconceptional age (wks)	Postnatal age (days)	Dose (mg/kg/dose)	Interval (h)
<29	0–14	5–6	q72
	>14	5–6	q48
30–36	0–14	3–6	q48
	>14	3–6	q24
37–44	0–7	3–6	q48
	>7	3–6	q24
>44	>0	3–6	q24

Drug	Dose	Interval	Mode
Gentamicin and tobramycin	See table below	See table below	IV

Age	Dose	Interval (h)
<35 wks EGA	3 mg/kg/dose	q24
≥35 wks EGA	4 mg/kg/dose	q24
>1 mo postnatal	2.5 mg/kg/dose	q8–12

Drug	Dose	Interval	Mode
Meropenem			
Sepsis	20 mg/kg/dose	q8–12h	IV
Meningitis	40 mg/kg/dose	q8h	IV
Metronidazole	See table below	See table below	PO/IV

Age (days)	Weight (kg)	Dose (mg/kg/dose)	Interval (h)
<7	<1.2	7.5	q48
	1.2–2	7.5	q24

Age (days)	Weight (kg)	Dose	Interval
<7	≥2	7.5	q12
≥7	<1.2	7.5	q48
	1.2–2	7.5	q12
	≥2	15	q12

Drug	Dose	Interval	Mode
Nafcillin	25 mg/kg/dose	See table below	IM/IV

Age (days)	Weight (kg)	Interval (h)
≤7	<2	q12
	≥2	q8
>7	<1.2	q12
	1.2–2	q8
	≥2	q6

Drug	Dose	Interval	Mode
Penicillin			
Aqueous Pen G	50,000 U/kg/dose	q12h	IV
Procaine Pen G	50,000 U/kg/dose	q24h	IM
Piperacillin	See table below	See table below	

	Postconceptional age (wks)	Postnatal age (days)	Dose (mg/kg/dose)	Interval (h)
	≤36	≤7	75	q12
		>7	75	q8
	>36	≤7	75	q8
		>7	75	q6

Drug	Dose	Interval	Mode
Ticarcillin or ticarcillin/clavula-nate (Timentin)	See table below	See table below	IV

Age (days)	Weight (kg)	Dose (mg/kg/dose)	Interval (h)
<7	<2	75	q12
	≥2	75	q8
≥7	<1.2	75	q12
	1.2–2	75	q8
	>2 kg	100	q8

Drug	Dose	Interval	Mode
Vancomycin	15 mg/kg/dose	See table below	IV

Postmenstrual age (wks)	Interval (h)
≤29	q24
30–33	q18
34–37	q12
38–44	q8

For patients <10 days old, starting interval should not be more frequent than q12h.

Anticonvulsants

Drug	Dose	Interval	Mode
Fosphenytoin	15–20 mg PE/kg (loading)	—	IV
	4–8 mg/kg (maint)	q8–24h	IV
Lorazem (Ativan)	0.1 mg/kg	q10min × 3 prn	IV/PR
Phenobarbital	10 mg/kg (loading)	—	IV
	3–5 mg/kg (maint)	q24h	IV/PO

Blood Products

Drug	Dose	Interval	Mode
Cryoprecipitate	10–15 cc/kg	over 2–4 h	IV
Fresh frozen plasma	10–15 cc/kg	over 2–4 h	IV
Packed red blood cells	10–15 cc/kg	over 2–4 h	IV
Platelets (single donor)	10–15 cc/kg	over 2–4 h	IV

Note: All blood products should be written as CMV negative. If <1 kg, also write for irradiated and leukopoor blood products.

Cardiovascular

Drug	Dose	Interval	Mode
Dobutamine	2.5–20 µg/kg/min	gtt	IV
Dopamine	2.5–20 µg/kg/min	gtt	IV
Epinephrine	0.05–2 µg/kg/min	gtt	IV
Indomethacin	0.1 mg/kg/dose	q12–24h	IV
Propranolol (dosing for thyrotox-icosis)	0.5 mg/kg/dose	q6–12h	PO
Prostaglandin E_1	0.025–0.1 µg/kg/min	gtt	IV

Diuretics

Drug	Dose	Interval	Mode
Aldactazide	1–1.5 mg/kg/dose	q12h	PO
Furosemide (Lasix)	1 mg/kg/dose	Varies	IV
	2 mg/kg/dose	Varies	PO
Spironolactone	1–3 mg/kg/day	Divided qd–bid	PO

Gastrointestinal

Drug	Dose	Interval	Mode
Famotidine (Pepcid)	1 mg/kg/dose	q24h	IV/PO
Glycerin	0.5 ml/kg/dose	q12–24h	PR
Metoclopromide (Reglan)	0.1 mg/kg/dose	q6–8h	IV/PO
Ranitidine (Zantac)	2–4 mg/kg/day	Divided q8–12h	PO
	2 mg/kg/day	Divided q6–8h	IV

Miscellaneous

Drug	Dose	Interval	Mode
Ferrous sulfate	2–4 mg/kg (elemental iron)	qd	PO
Hydrocortisone	1 mg/kg/day (physiologic)	Divided q8h	IV
	1 mg/kg/dose (stress)	q8h	IV
Propylthiouracil	5–10 mg/kg/day	Divided q8h	PO
Pyridostigmine	0.05–0.15 mg/kg/dose	q4–6h	IM/IV
	5 mg/dose	q4–6h	PO

Ophthalmologic

Drug	Dose	Interval	Mode
Cyclopentolate 0.5%	1 gtt	q5min × 3 doses	OU
Phenylephrine 2.5%	1 gtt	q5min × 3 doses	OU

Paralytics

Drug	Dose	Interval	Mode
Cis-atracurium	0.1 mg/kg/h	gtt	IV
Pancuronium	0.1 mg/kg/h	gtt	IV
Vecuronium	0.1 mg/kg/h	gtt	IV

Note: Load or one-time dose: 0.1 mg/kg IV.

Respiratory

Drug	Dose	Interval	Mode
Albuterol	0.25–0.5 cc	q1h prn	Nebulizer

Drug	Dose	Interval	Mode
Aminophylline (IV) or theophylline (PO)			
Loading	4–6 mg/kg	—	
Maint	5–6 mg/kg/day	divided q6–8h	
Continuous[a]	0.5–1 mg/kg/h	gtt	IV
Beractant (Survanta)	4 cc/kg	q6–12h	ETT
Caffeine citrate			
Loading	20 mg/kg	—	IV/PO
Maint	6–10 mg/kg	q24h	IV/PO
Calfactant (Infrasurf)	3 cc/kg	q6–12h	ETT

[a]Therapeutic range: apnea, 7–10 µg/mL; bronchospasm, 10–15 µg/mL.

Sedation/Analgesia

Drug	Dose	Interval	Mode
Acetaminophen	10–15 mg/kg	q6–8h prn	PO
	20 mg/kg	q6–8h prn	PR

Fentanyl	1–2 µg/kg/dose	q1h prn	IV
	1 µg/kg/h	gtt	IV
Lorazepam (Ativan)	0.05–0.1 mg/kg/dose	q1h prn	IV/PO
Methadone	0.05–0.2 mg/kg/dose	q12–24h	PO
Midazolam (Versed)	50–200 µg/kg/dose	q1h prn	IV
	0.1 µg/kg/min	gtt	IV
Morphine	0.1 mg/kg/dose	q1h prn	IV/PO
	0.01 mg/kg/h	gtt	IV

CHEMOTHERAPY DRUGS

In general, most chemotherapy drugs have their onset of myelosuppression on day 4–7, nadir from day 14–21, and recovery after day 21.

Drug	Mode of action	Major adverse effects	What to do
Actinomycin D (Dactinomycin)	Inhibits RNA polymerase; intercalation/ strand breaks	MS; vesicant; N (highly emetogenic)/V/ Muc; A; malaise/fatigue, liver disease	Avoid extravasation; antiemetics; mouth care; IV integrity check

Drug	Mode of action	Major adverse effects	What to do
Bleomycin (Blenoxane)	DNA strand breaks	Lung toxicity; Muc; N (mild); hypersensitivity; Raynaud's; pruritic erythema	Pulmonary function tests; mouth care
Busulfan (Myleran)	Interferes with DNA replication/RNA transcription	Veno-occlusive disease risk; Muc; MS; A; rare pulmonary toxicity; szs	Monitor LFTs; mouth care; monitor respiratory status
Carboplatin (CBDCA)	DNA strand breaks; cross-link	Neuropathy (stocking-and-glove distribution); ototoxicity (high-frequency first); renal toxicity; MS; electrolyte disturbance (hypo Mg/Na/K/Ca); optic neuritis; death if IT	Assess renal fxn; monitor electrolytes (Ca, Mg); hearing tests prior to administration; vigorous hydration; antiemetics; electrolyte supplements (Ca, Mg); monitor vision; no Lasix
Cisplatin (Platinol; CDDP)	See Carboplatin	See Carboplatin; highly emetogenic	See Carboplatin; do **NOT** give Lasix (exacerbates ototoxicity); may require mannitol to maintain high urinary output; Mg supplements
Cyclophosphamide (Cytoxan)	Alkylating agent	Hemorrhagic cystitis; MS; N (highly emetogenic at high dose)/V/Muc; SIADH; A (at 3 wks)	Vigorous hydration; monitor for SIADH (hyponatremia, weight gain, concentrated urine; lethargy, weakness, HA, szs); antiemetics; MESNA (see pg. 359)

Drug	Mechanism	Toxicity	Monitoring
Cytarabine (Ara-C)	Inhibits DNA polymerase	Neurotoxicity (cerebellar/white matter; occurs 3–8 days after therapy; usually with high doses); szs with IT administration; pulmonary toxicity; N (highly emetogenic, including IT)/V/diarrhea/Muc; conjunctivitis/ corneal keratitis; bimodal nadir 7–9 and 15–24 days with 4–5-day courses; MS; hepatic toxicity; Ara-C syndrome (F/ N/malaise/ rigors/chest pain; usually 6–12 h after administration); life-threatening bowel necrosis; rash	Monitor neurology exam (should be withdrawn if nystagmus or ataxia occurs); steroid ophthalmologic gtt; monitor respiratory status; mouth care; Ara-C syndrome evaluation of pt; F production **may** only require cultures (no antibiotics; often responsive to corticosteroids)
Dacarbazine (DTIC)	Alkylating agent that cross-links strands (active in all phases of cell cycle); prodrug (demethylated by liver)	Vesicant; MS; N/V moderate to severe, lasting 12 hrs; flushing; rash; flulike sxs; paresthesias; anaphylactic rxn; rare liver failure from VOD/thrombosis (Budd-Chiari syndrome)	IV integrity; antiemetics (may require several days' worth of Rxs); monitor LFTs and neuro exam
Daunorubicin (Daunomycin)	Intercalates DNA, Topo II inhibitor	Vesicant; MS; cumulative cardiotoxicity; liver dysfunction; N (moderate)/V/Muc; red urine; radiation recall in post-XRT period (delay, 4–6 wks)	Monitor LFTs/bilirubin; echocardiogram/ monitor cumulative dose; antiemetics; mouth care; IV integrity check; Zinecard (see below); clearance decreases with increasing bilirubin levels
Dexamethasone	Direct cell death	Hyperglycemia; weight gain; HTN; gastritis; AVN; MS; increased fungal infections; CNS changes; osteonecrosis	Monitor VS; monitor glucose/glucosuria—may require insulin gtt; assess for gastritis (add $H_2/H+$ blockers)

357

Drug	Mode of action	Major adverse effects	What to do
Dexrazoxane (Zinecard; ICRF-187) **Nonchemotherapy Agent**	Derivative of EDTA, intracellular chelating agent that interferes with Fe-mediated free radical generation (cardioprotective)	MS; increased transaminases, amylase; N/V; diarrhea; neurotoxicity	Used primarily for pts with cumulative anthracycline (e.g., doxorubicin) dose of 300 mg/m^2 and is continuing therapy (or protocols with dose escalation); anthracycline infusion must be started before total elapsed time of 30 mins from beginning of Zinecard infusion; monitor CBCs and liver fxn
Doxorubicin (Adriamycin)	See Daunorubicin	See Daunorubicin; extreme vesicant	See Daunorubicin; extravasation: Zinecard and topical DMSO
Etoposide (VP-16)	Topo II inhibitor	Allergic rxns; hypotension with rapid infusions; MS; N (mild)/V; hemorrhagic cystitis A	Avoid rapid infusions; assess for allergic sxs (respiratory difficulty, itching, etc.); antiemetics; history of allergic sxs
Idarubicin	See Daunorubicin	See Daunorubicin	See Daunorubicin
Ifosfamide (Ifex)	Alkylating agent	Fanconi's syndrome; neurotoxicity: encephalopathy/szs (especially with renal damage and prior platinum exposure); MS; A (2–4 wks); hemorrhagic cystitis; SIADH; N (highly emetogenic with high dose); activated/inactivated by the liver	Assess renal fxn (delayed metabolism/removal increases CNS toxicity); monitor electrolytes for Fanconi's (urinary losses of amino acids, glucose, bicarbonate, uric acid, organic acids, Mg, Na, K, water; sxs include acidosis, glucosuria/polyuria with high pH >5.5, SG 1.010–1.015, mild albuminuria); vigorous hydration; use MESNA; monitor for SIADH

L-Asparaginase (Elspar; Pegaspargase)	Metabolizes L-asparaginase	Allergic reaction; pancreatitis; coagulopathy (deficiencies/imbalances in: fibrinogen, FII, FV, FVII, FVIII-X, AT III, prot. C)/thrombosis; MS	Watch for anaphylaxis (have epinephrine, benadryl, hydrocortisone, and IV fluids at bedside); check amylase/lipase; make sure adequate platelet count
6-Mercaptopurine (6-MP)	Antimetabolite	MS; hepatotoxicity; can crystallize in urine with high doses; competitive with allopurinol; hyperuricemia	Make sure pt is not receiving allopurinol; vigorous hydration; monitor LFTs
6-Thioguanine (6-TG)	Antimetabolite	See 6-Mercaptopurine; exception: administration of allopurinol is not a problem	See 6-Mercaptopurine
Methotrexate	Dihydrofolate reductase inhibitor; antimetabolite	N (moderate)/V/Muc; interaction with weak acids; renal and liver dysfunction (high dose); MS; leukoencephalopathy (months to years after IT: paralysis/szs/coma)/arachnoiditis with IT (2nd to 3rd week: CN palsy, szs, coma); rash; photosensitivity	Mouth care; ensure no signs of gastroenteritis; avoidance of weak acids (e.g., ASA, NSAIDs, Septra); monitor LFTs/renal fxn; vigorous hydration; maintain leucovorin schedule (provides folinic acid)
MESNA (Mesnex) **Nonchemotherapy Agent**	A thiol, which binds and detoxifies acrolein and other urotoxic metabolites (prevents hemorrhagic cystitis from ifosfamide and cyclophosphamide)	Allergic/anaphylactic rxns; malaise; HA; diarrhea; N/V; limb pain; rash/itching	Watch for allergic rxns; see Ifosfamide and Cyclophosphamide
Mitoxantrone (Novantrone)	See Daunorubicin	See Daunorubicin; blue-green urine	See Daunorubicin

Drug	Mode of action	Major adverse effects	What to do
Paclitaxel (Taxol)	MT stabilization	Allergic rxns; peripheral neuropathy; mental status changes; A	History of allergic rxns (**always** premedicate with Benadryl/dexamethasone); assess for neuropathy; assess CNS changes
Prednisone	Direct cell death	MS; hyperglycemia; weight gain; HTN; gastritis; AVN	Monitor VS; monitor glucose/glucosuria—may require insulin gtt; assess for gastritis (add H_2/H+ blockers)
Topotecan (Hycamtin)	Topo I inhibitor, prevents replication (S phase)	MS; paresthesia; dyspnea; HA; A; N/V (low); thrombocytopenia	Monitor CBC/platelets; transaminases; increased toxicity with cisplatin
Vinblastine (Velban)	Disrupts MTs mitotic spindle formation	Vesicant; peripheral neuropathy; A; N (mild); more MS than vincristine	Assess for neuropathy; IV integrity check; check for constipation—bowel regimens
Vincristine (Oncovin)	Disrupts MTs mitotic spindle formation	Vesicant; peripheral neuropathy; A; SIADH	Assess for neuropathy; IV integrity check; check for constipation—bowel regimens

ESTIMATED COMPARATIVE DAILY DOSAGES FOR INHALED CORTICOSTEROIDS

Drug	Low dose	Medium dose	High dose
Adults (>12 years of age)			
Beclomethasone dipropionate (Beclovent, Vanceril)	166–504 µg	504–840 µg	>840 µg
42 µg/puff	4–12 puffs—42 µg	12–20 puffs—42 µg	>20 puffs—42 µg
84 µg/puff	2–6 puffs—84 µg	6–10 puffs—84 µg	>10 puffs—84 µg
Budesonide Turbuhaler (Pulmicort) 200 µg/dose	200–400 µg (1–2 inhalations)	400–600 µg (2–3 inhalations)	>600 µg (>3 inhalations)
Flunisolide (Aerobid) 250 µg/puff	500–1000 µg (2–4 puffs)	1000–2000 µg (4–8 puffs)	>2000 µg (>8 puffs)
Fluticasone (Flovent)	88–264 µg	264–660 µg	>660 µg
MDI: 44, 110, 220 µg/puff	2–6 puffs—44 µg or 2 puffs—110 µg	2–6 puffs—110 µg	>6 puffs—110 µg—220 µg >3 puffs—220 µg
DPI: 50, 100, 250 µg/dose	2–6 inhalations—50 µg	3–6 inhalations—100 µg	>6 inhalations—100 µg >2 inhalations—250 µg
Fluticasone/salmeterol (Advair) DPI: 100/50, 250/50, 500/50	100 µg[a] (1 inhalation bid)	100–250 µg (1 inhalation bid)	500 µg (1 inhalation bid)
Triamcinolone acetonide (Azmacort) 100 µg/puff	400–1000 µg (4–10 puffs)	1000–2000 µg (10–20 puffs)	>2000 µg (>20 puffs)

361

Drug	Low dose	Medium dose	High dose
Children (<12 years of age)			
Beclomethasone dipropionate (Beclo-vent, Vanceril)	84–336 µg	336–672 µg	>672 µg
42 µg/puff	2–8 puffs—42 µg	8–16 puffs—42 µg	>16 puffs—42 µg
84 µg/puff	1–4 puffs—84 µg	4–8 puffs—84 µg	>8 puffs—84 µg
Budesonide (Pulmicort) 200 µg/dose	100–200 µg	200–400 µg	>400 µg
Turbuhaler 200 µg/dose	1 inhalation—200 µg	1–2 inhalations—200 µg	>2 inhalations—200 µg
Respules: 0.25 mg, 0.5 mg	0.25 mg per nebulizer	0.5 mg per nebulizer	1 mg per nebulizer
Flunisolide (Aerobid) 250 µg/puff	500–750 µg (2–3 puffs)	1000–1250 µg (4–5 puffs)	>1250 µg (>5 puffs)
Fluticasone (Flovent)	88–176 µg	175–440 µg	>440 µg
MDI: 44, 110, 220 µg/puff	2–4 puffs—44 µg	4–10 puffs—44 µg or 2–4 puffs—110 µg	>4 puffs—110 µg or >2 puffs—220 µg
DPI: 50, 100, 250 µg/dose	2–4 inhalations—50 µg	2–4 inhalations—100 µg	>4 inhalations—100 µg
Triamcinolone acetonide (Azamacort) 100 µg/puff	400–800 µg (4–8 puffs)	800–1200 µg (8–12 puffs)	>1200 µg (>12 puffs)

Note: The most important determinant of appropriate dosing is the clinician's judgment of the patient's response to therapy. The clinician must monitor the patient's response on several clinical parameters and adjust the dose accordingly. The stepwise approach to therapy emphasizes that once control of asthma is achieved, the dose of medication should be carefully titrated to the minimum dose required to maintain control, thus reducing the potential for adverse affect. (*continued*)

MDI dosages are expressed as the actual dose per actuation (the amount of drug leaving the canister and delivered to the patient), which is the labeling required in the United States. This is different from the dosage expressed as the valve dose (the amount of drug leaving the valve, all of which is not available to the patient), which is used in many European countries and in some of the scientific literature. Dry powder inhaler (DPI) doses (e.g., Turbuhaler) are expressed as the amount of drug in the inhaler following activation.

Some dosages may be outside package labeling.

[a]Advair not currently indicated in mild persistent asthma.

From St. Louis Children's Hospital, St. Louis, Missouri, with permission.

Reference Values

HEMATOLOGY REFERENCE VALUES

Age groups	WBC ($\times 10^3$/mm³)	HGB (g/dL)	HCT (%)	MCV (µm³)
0–1 wk	5–30	14.5–22.5	45–66	88–123
1 wk–1 mo	5–20	10–18	31–55	85–123
1 mo–6 mos	6–17.5	9–14.9	28–42	74–115
6 mos–2 yrs	6–17.5	10.5–13.5	33–39	70–86
2 yrs–6 yrs	5–15.5	11.5–13.5	34–40	75–87
6 yrs–12 yrs	4.5–13.5	11.5–15.5	35–45	77–95
12 yrs–adult				
Male	3.8–9.8	13.8–17.2	40.7–50.3	80–97.6
Female	3.8–9.8	12.1–15.1	36.1–44.3	80–97.6

Age groups	Bands (%)	Segmented neutrophils (%)	Lymphocytes (%)	Monocytes (%)	Eosinophils (%)	Basophils (%)
0–4 yrs	0–4	16–60	20–70	0–7	0–8	0–1
4–16 yrs	0–4	33–70	21–55	3–13	2–12	0–3
16 yrs–adult	0–4	44–80	8–44	2–11	0–6	0–3

- Platelet count: 140–440 $\times 10^3$/mm³
- Reticulocyte count
  - Week: 1–5%
  - 1 wk–adult: 0.5–1.5%

CHEMISTRY LAB REFERENCE VALUES

Test	Ages	Reference ranges
Albumin (g/dL)	0–30 days	2.5–5.0
	1–3 mos	3.0–4.2
	3–12 mos	2.7–5.0
	1–18 yrs	3.2–5.0
	>18 yrs	3.6–5.0
Alkaline phosphatase (IU/L)	0–3 yrs	110–320
	3–9 yrs	140–420
	9–15 yrs	130–550
	15–20 yrs	70–260
	>21 yrs	38–126
Ammonia (mmol/L)	0–6 mos	<120
	6 mos–18 yrs	<40
	>18 yrs	9–33
Amylase (IU/L)	Term–2 mos	Undetected
	2 mos–18 yrs	15–130
Bilirubin (mg/dL)	All ages >1 wk	
Unconjugated		0.3–1.1
Conjugated		0.0–0.2
BUN (mg/dL)	0–18 yrs	9–18
Calcium, total (mg/dL)	0–30 days	8.0–11.5
	>30 days	8.6–10.3
Calcium, ionized (mg/dL)	0–18 yrs	3.9–5.2
Carboxyhemoglobin (%)	All ages	0.0–0.3
Creatinine (mg/dL)	0–3 yrs	0.1–0.5
	4–19 yrs	0.2–1.2
Creatinine kinase (IU/L)	0–18 yrs	0–300
Electrolytes (mmol/L)		
Sodium	All ages	135–145
Potassium	All ages	3.3–4.9 plasma; 3.5–5.1 serum
Chloride	All ages	97–110
CO_2 total	0–30 days	17–24
	1 mo–16 yrs	20–28

APPENDIX C: REFERENCE VALUES

Test	Ages	Reference ranges
Gamma–glutamyl transferase (IU/L)	0–3 mos	71–295
	3 mos–1 yr	0–115
	>1 yr	11–50 (boys); 7–32 (girls)
Glucose (mg/dL)	0–1 mo	40–100
	>1 mo	65–115
HgbA1C (%)	0–18 yrs	4.5–5.7
Iron (µg/dL)	0–1 mo	100–250
	1 mo–12 yrs	50–120
	>12 yrs	45–160
Lactate (mmol/L)	All ages	0.5–1.5
Lactate CSF (mmol/L)	All ages	1.1–2.3
LDH (IU/L)	0–5 yrs	425–975
	5–12 yrs	350–840
	12–16 yrs	300–700
	>16 yrs	300–540
Lipase (U/L)	0–18 yrs	20–200
Magnesium (mEq/L)	All ages	1.3–2.2
Methemoglobin (%)	All ages	0.0–2.0
Osmolality (mOsm/kg)	All ages	275–300
Phosphorus (mg/dL)	0–30 days	4.2–9.0
	1 mo–18 yrs	3.0–6.0
Protein, total (g/dL)	0–1 yr	5.5–7.5
	>1 yr	6.5–8.5 plasma; 6.2–8.2 serum
Pyruvate (mmol/L)	All ages	0.03–0.08
Pyruvate CSF (mmol/L)	All ages	0.03–0.11
SGOT/ALT (IU/L)	0–5 days	0–225
	0–12 yrs	10–60
	12–18 yrs	10–40
SGPT/AST (IU/L)	0–2 yrs	6–50
	3–12 yrs	10–35
	12–16 yrs	10–55
	>16 yrs	7–53

Test	Ages	Reference ranges
Total iron-binding capacity (µg/dL)	1 mo–18 yrs	250–450
TSH (µIU/mL)	Euthyroid	0.5–6.2
	Hyperthyroid	<0.35
	Hypothyroid	>12.0
T_4 (µg/dL)	3–6 days	11.0–21.5
	1–4 wks	8.2–16.6
	1 mo–5 yrs	6.5–14.5
	6–10 yrs	6.0–13.5
	11–15 yrs	5.0–12.0
	16–20 yrs	4.2–11.8
Uric acid (mg/dL)	0–12 yrs	2.0–6.0
	>12 yrs	3.0–8.0 (boys), 2.5–7.5 (girls)

VITAL SIGNS AND FACTS

Age	Premature	Term	3 mos	6 mos	9 mos	1 yr	1.5 yrs	2 yrs	3 yrs	4 yrs	5 yrs	6 yrs	8 yrs	10 yrs	12 yrs	14 yrs
Wt. (kg)	<3	3–4	5–6	7	8–9	10	11	12	14–15	16–17	18	20	24–25	30–32	40	45
Pulse	130–160	120–150	120–140	120–140	120–140	120–140	110–135	110–130	100–120	95–115	90–110	90–110	80–100	75–95	70–90	60–90
SBP	45–60	60–70	60–100	65–120	70–120	70–120	70–125	75–125	75–125	80–125	80–125	85–120	90–120	90–125	95–130	110–130
Respiratory rate	40–60	30–60	30–50	25–35	23–33	20–30	20–30	20–28	20–28	20–28	20–25	20–25	16–24	16–24	16–24	15–20
Endotracheal tube	2.5–3.0	3.0–3.5	3.5	3.5–4.0	3.5–4.0	4.0–4.5	4.0–4.5	4.5	4.5–5.0	5.0	5.0–5.5	5.5	5.5–6.0	6.0–6.5	6.5–7.0	7.0–7.5
Blade	0	1	1	1	1	1	1	1–2	2	2	2	2	2	2–3	3	3
Nasogastric tube (Fr)	5–6	6–8	6–8	6–8	6–8	8	8–10	8–10	8–10	8–10	10–12	10–12	12–14	12–14	12–14	14–16
Foley (Fr)	6	6	6	6–8	6–8	8–10	8–10	8–10	8–10	8–10	8–10	8–10	10	10–12	10–12	12–14
CT (Fr)	10–12	10–12	10–12	12–16	12–16	12–18	12–20	16–22	16–22	16–22	18–24	20–26	20–28	24–34	24–34	24–36

Patient Data Tracking Form

Name:	
DOB	Age
Admitted	Discharged
Allergies	

HPI

PMH/PSH

Admission Meds

SH   FH

ROS

Admission

T	P	R	BP
O2		Wt	Ht

MCV=
RDW=

Ca		T bili		PTT			
Mg		D bili		PT			
Phos		AST		INR			
TP		ALT		Amylase			
Alb		Alk Ph		Lipase			

Previous Labs: Growth:

CXR   wt_____ (____%)

Admission: length/height_____ (____%)

Previous: OFC_____ (____%)

Previous Studies:

Admission	Discharge
❏ Old data	❏ Placement
❏ Old records	
❏ DDx	❏ Home care
❏ Admit orders	
❏ Interview	❏ D/C orders

Problems:

APPENDIX D: PATIENT DATA TRACKING FORM

Brief Course

☐ H&P
☐ Schedule tests
☐ Read

☐ Transport

Date							
Overnight Complaints							
	CP		SOB		CP		SOB	
	N/V		Abd		N/V		Abd	
	Urine		Ap/wt		Urine		Ap/wt	
	Fatig		BM		Fatig		BM	
	HA		Vis		HA		Vis	
	Aud				Aud			
Meds							
Relevant Tests							
T (Tmax)							
P							
R							
BP							
SaO$_2$							
I/O							
Accu							
Physical Exam							

Other Labs				
Tasks	☐ Pre-round ☐ Notes in chart ☐ Vitals ☐ Meds ☐ Labs ☐ Micro ☐ Note ☐ Order tests ☐ AM Labs	☐ Change meds ☐ Call consults ☐ Read consults ☐ Test results ☐ Chat with pt	☐ Pre-round ☐ Notes in chart ☐ Vitals ☐ Meds ☐ Labs ☐ Micro ☐ Note ☐ Order tests ☐ AM Labs	☐ Change meds ☐ Call consults ☐ Read consults ☐ Talk with other team members ☐ Test results ☐ Chat with pt and loved ones
A/P				

Index

Page numbers followed by *f* indicate figures; page numbers followed by *t* indicate tables.

Index

Nuclear medicine, 243–244
Nursemaid's elbow, 206

21-OH deficiency, 103–104
Onychomycosis, 72
Oral contraception, 29
Osgood-Schlatter disease, 207
Osteosarcoma, 139–140
Out-toeing, 209
Oxygen, in asthma therapy, 218

Pain, floor calls for, 16–17
Pain service medication, dosing guide
    for, 336–339
Pancreatitis, abdominal pain in, 114
Parenteral nutrition. *See* Total
        parenteral nutrition, cal-
        culation of
Paroxysmal disorders, 196
Patient data tracking form, 369–370
Peak flow, in asthma therapy, 218
Pediatrics
    on call in, 2–3
    note writing in, 2
    post-rounds in, 1
    preround organization in, 1
    rounds in, 1–2
    sign out in, 2
Pediculosis pubis, in adolescents, 24t
Pelvic inflammatory disease, in ado-
        lescents
    diagnostic criteria for, 25
    follow-up exam for, 26
    hospitalization criteria for, 25
    parenteral treatment for, 26
Penicillins, formulary for, 287–290
Pericardial effusion, 44–46, 131
Pericarditis, 44
Peripheral neuroectodermal tumor, 141
Pharyngitis, 162
Pityriasis alba, 70
Pleural effusion, 131
Pneumoperitoneum, evaluation of,
        236–238, 237f, 238f
Pneumothorax, evaluating for,
        232–233, 233f
Poisoning, 82–86
    elimination of ingested poison in,
        83–84, 84f
    secondary elimination in, 84,
        85t–86t
Port wine stain, 68

Potassium replacement, in diabetic
        ketoacidosis treatment, 97
Prader-Willi syndrome, 195
Prescriptions, writing, 6
Protein, in total parenteral nutrition, 12
Proteinuria
    differential diagnosis, 181–182
    epidemiology of, 178
    management of, 182
    measurement of, 178–179
    mechanisms of, 178
    workup of, 179–181
Pulseless arrest, algorithm for, 269f
Pyelography, intravenous, 241

Quinolones, formulary for, 290–291

Radial head luxation, 206
Radiology exam, 229–230
Rashes, neonatal, 67–68
Reflexes, primitive, 122
Renal function
    evaluation of, 174–177
        evaluating urine and, 174
        three essential attributes to, 174
    history of, 174–175
    lab evaluation of, 175–176, 177t
    physical exam of, 175
Renal scan, 243
Renal tumor, 139
Respiratory distress syndrome, 170
Retinoblastoma, 141–142
Retinopathy, of prematurity, 173
Retropharyngeal abscess, 160, 162
Rhabdomyosarcoma, 140–141
Rheumatic fever, 251–253
Rickets, prevention of, 13
RSV immunoglobulin, 282

Scabies, in adolescents, 24t
Scoliosis, 212
Sedation
    equipment for, 88
    formulary for, 340–341
    IV, 87–88
    monitoring, 88, 89t
Seizure, 133, 196–197
    febrile, 197–201
        etiology of, 198
        risk factors for, 198–199
        treatment of, 199–201
    partial, 197